Essentials of
Immediate
Medical Care

Essentials of
Immediate
Medical Care

Dr C John Eaton MB BS Dip IMC RCS(Ed)

General Practitioner
Member of the British Association for Immediate Care
Saffron Walden
Essex, UK

CHURCHILL LIVINGSTONE
EDINBURGH LONDON MADRID MELBOURNE NEW YORK AND TOKYO 1992

First published 1992
Reprinted 1993 with revisions

ISBN 0-443-04575-5

British Library Catologuing in Publication Data
A catalogue record for this book is available from the British Library.

Library of Congress Cataloguing in Publication Data
A catalogue record for this book is available from the Library of Congress.

Accurate indications, adverse reactions, and dosage schedules for
drugs are provided in this book, but it is possible that they may change.
The reader is urged to review the data information sheet of the
manufacturers for the medications mentioned.

The author has made every effort to trace the copyright holders for
borrowed material. If he has inadvertently overlooked any, he will be
pleased to make the necessary arrangements at the earliest opportunity.

Produced by Longman Singapore publishers Pte Ltd
Printed in Singapore

The
publisher's
policy is to use
paper manufactured
from sustainable forests

Preface

These notes have been produced primarily for the doctor who is either practising, or considering practising Immediate Care, and in particular for the doctor preparing for the Diploma in Immediate Medical Care of the Royal College of Surgeons of Edinburgh (Dip IMC RCS Ed). It should also be of interest to doctors involved in hospital medical and surgical teams, doctors staffing minor casualty departments, which may have a triaging role in very rural areas, doctors in the armed forces on detatched duty, doctors practising in remote areas and both extended trained and non-extended trained ambulancepersonnel.

Immediate Care is a relatively new sub-speciality, and at present there are very few texts devoted to the subject. Most American texts are designed primarily for the paramedic, and with few exceptions most British texts are either multiauthor, or have been written by experts who are primarily hospital orientated.

This book has been written in the form of a series of notes, each using the same format and style, so as to facilitate their use as revision material, and as a ready reference. The use of one author, albeit with input from many experts and sources, hopefully has avoided the duplication and differing styles so often found in multiauthor books.

Although intended to be reasonably comprehensive, no attempt has been made to cover anything other than the Immediate Care aspects of most problems, and references are given at the end of the book for further reading should the reader wish to research any particular subject in greater depth. Anatomy and physiology have not been covered as there are already many excellent textbooks which cover these subjects admirably.

Guidelines where shown are those most universally agreed, and not necessarily the latest (but controversial) state of the art. Drug information is based on that in the current edition of the British National Formulary.

This book began life as a set of personal revision notes for the Diploma in Immediate Medical Care, but having produced them I realised that there was a need for a book specifically on Immediate Medical Care and that my notes would hopefully, after criticism and resulting amendments, become that definitive book. The initial Coures Notes on Immediate Care were produced in rather a hurry for the Cambridge Immediate Care Courses, organised by Dr John Scott, a member of the BASICS Education Committee. They were corrected and revised after a lot of help and constructive comments from a large number of experts, and became the second edition. Following this a third edition was produced and became the final proof for this book.

This book has now been substantially revised and this reprint incorporates the revised guidelines recently developed by the British Thoracic Association for the management of acute asthma; the new guidelines produced by Medical Commission on Accident Prevention for the out of hospital management of hypothermia; the guidelines of the joint working party of the British Paediatric Association, the College of Anaesthetists, the Royal College of Midwives and the Royal College of Obstetricians and Gynaecologists for basic and advanced resuscitation of the newborn; the revised Paediatric Resuscitation Chart produced by Dr Peter Oakley, and the revised guidelines issued by the Meningitis Trust for the diagnosis and management of bacterial meningitis, and the new guidelines for resuscitation published by the European Resuscitation Council in November 1992. This book was the first attempt, as far as I am aware, to develop universal guidelines for all aspects of pre-hospital emergency medicine (or Immediate Medical Care) which encompasses the pre-hospital aspects of emergency surgery, medicine, anaesthetics, obstetrics and gynaecology, toxicology and therapeutics.

C.J.E., 1993

Dedication

This book is dedicated to all of those involved in Immediate Care, past, present, potential and future, and in particular to the father of Immediate Care, Dr Kenneth Easton, and my personal mentor in Immediate Care, Dr Robin Winch, without either of whom this book would not exist, in the hope that it will enable the victims of trauma or sudden serious illness to receive the best possible pre-hospital treatment.

Foreword

Immediate Care has become a recognised and rewarding speciality within General Practice, Community and Hospital Practice. In the past, I believe some of the resistance to establishing new Immediate Care Schemes, was due to lack of experience and suitable reading material, rather than a lack of willingness on the part of the physician. Medical schools are now teaching more basic and advanced resuscitation skills, and they are being introduced into both qualifying and postgraduate examinations, providing further impetus and encouragement to doctors to carry appropriate resuscitation equipment at all times and to form BASICS schemes.

With the introduction of "The Diploma in Immediate Medical Care" by the Royal College of Surgeons of Edinburgh, we finally have a higher professional qualification, by which we can both evaluate and recognise a competent Immediate Care doctor. Appropriate literature to prepare for this examination has previously been scattered throughout many textbooks. Now that the practical skills can be refreshed at several Immediate Care courses throughout the United Kingdom, this timely volume provides an excellent, comprehensive and appropriate text, not only for use during the course, but for many years to come.

Judith M Fisher MB BS FRCGP

Immediate Past Chairman, the British Association for Immediate Care

Technical Note

The manuscript for this book was produced by the author on Acorn Archimedes computers, using Computer Concepts' Impression II document processing software. The diagrams were scanned in using a Computer Concepts' Scanlight Professional image scanner, and the entire book was then down-loaded onto two Syquest 44 Mbyte removable hard disc drive cartridges supplied by Atomwide. These were then processed, using a Linotronic Imagesetter to produce the film, which was then supplied to the printer.

Acknowledgements

I am very grateful to all those doctors and other experts (see list of contributors), who have very kindly and so freely given me much constructive criticism and helpful advice, and I hope they will see that I have listened to them! It came as a very pleasant surprise to me, that without exception, they have all been so tremendously helpful. I hope that all those that use this book will also give me their comments, good and bad, so that future editions will be as comprehensive as possible.

I would like to acknowledge the help of the Resuscitation Council and Laerdal (UK) for their generous permission to use material and diagrams from *Resuscitation for the Citizen, Guidelines in Cardiopulmonary Resuscitation* and the *ABC of Resuscitation*. I am also grateful to Dr Brian Robertson, the editor of the *Basics Journal* for his permission to use line drawings from that journal; to the Officer Commanding HQ Search and Rescue Wing, RAF Finningley for his assistance in obtaining line drawings of the Wessex and Sea King helicopters; to Little Brown & Company of Boston USA, for permission to use diagrams from *Emergency Care in the Streets* by Nancy Caroline; to HMSO and the Home Office (Fire Department) for permission to use various diagrams from the *Manual of Firemanship;* to Richard D Meyer M D to incorporate the diagrams on helmet removal; to Dr Peter Oakley and the *British Medical Journal* for permission to use his Paediatric Resuscitation Chart; to Hoechst UK Ltd for permission to use ECG tracings from their *ECG Atlas* and to Emma Williams who has produced a large number of the line drawings for me, including those on airway devices.

I am most grateful to Dr John Scott for using the precursors of this book as the core material for the BASICS Education courses on Immediate Care and Advanced Cardiac Life Support, held in Cambridge, and for his constructive advice and enthusiasm, to Drs Kenneth Easton and John Scott for proof reading the manuscript, and to Claire Clenshaw, my secretary, and my wife and partner Dr Catherine Brown who have provided me with much needed support and advice. I am also very grateful to Tim Hodgetts for his all his considerable help with the corrections, additions and ammendments incorporated into this revised reprint.

Finally I would like to thank Richard O'Hanlon, Mike Capaldi and Dee Drinkwater and her staff, of SmithKline Beecham for all their assistance in the production of the precursors of this book, and Peter Richardson, Ian Dick and Lucy Gardner of Churchill Livingstone for all their invaluable help and advice over the prolonged gestation period of this book, without which it would never have seen the light of day.

C John Eaton
Saffron Walden, 1993

Contributors: list of those who have given valuable advice and criticism

Dr C M C Allen MA MRCP MD,
Consultant Neurologist,
Addenbrooke's Hospital,
Hills Road,
CAMBRIDGE CB2 2QQ

Mr David H. Austwick MB BS FRCS,
The Old Orchard,
Village Street, Hexton,
HITCHIN,
Herts SG5 3JG

Dr J H Baker BSc MB MRCP,
Welsh Spinal Injury Centre,
Rookwood Hospital,
Fairwater Road,
CARDIFF CF5 2YN

Dr N D Barnes MA MB FRCP,
Consultant Paediatrician,
Addenbrooke's Hospital,
Hills Road,
CAMBRIDGE CB2 2QQ

Dr P J F Baskett BA MB BChir FRCAnaes,
Consultant Anaesthetist,
Frenchay Hospital,
BRISTOL
BS16 1LE

Mr J Belstead MB FRCS Ed FRCS Ed Orth,
Consultant in A & E Medicine,
6 Stanwell Road,
ASHFORD
Middx. TW15 3ER

Mr M. V. Bright FRCOG FRCS,
Consultant Obstetrician and Gynaecologist,
4 Brookside,
Exning,
NEWMARKET, Suffolk

Surgeon Captain S A Bussell Royal Navy,
Assistant Director, Naval Dental Services,
Ministry of Defence,
First House, High Holborn,
LONDON WC1V 6HE

Dr C J Carney MB BS,
Magnolia House,
SUNNINGDALE,
Berkshire
SL5 0QS

D Carrington Esq.,
Chief Ambulance Officer
Area Headquarters, Scottish Ambulance Service,
55 Greenbank Drive,
EDINBURGH EH10 5SA

Dr D A Chamberlain MD FRCP,
Consultant Cardiologist,
Royal Sussex County Hospital,
Eastern Road, BRIGHTON,
Sussex BN2 5BE

Dr J Chappel MB BS,
1 Cheriton High Street,
FOLKESTONE,
Kent
CT19 4PW

Dr M Colquhoun BSc MB BS MRCP MRCGP DRCOG
The Surgery,
Court Road,
MALVERN
Worcs WR14 3BL

Mr P T Doyle FRCS,
Consultant Urologist,
Addenbrook's Hospital,
Hills Road,
CAMBRIDGE CB2 2QQ

Dr K C Easton MB BS DObs RCOG FRCGP OStJ OBE,
The Orchard, 10 High Green,
Catterick Village,
RICHMOND,
North Yorkshire DL10 7NL

Dr O M Edwards MD FRCP MA,
Consultant Physician,
Addenbrooke's Hospital,
CAMBRIDGE
CB2 2QQ

Mr P D M Ellis MA MB BChir FRCS,
Consultant ENT Surgeon,
Addenbrooks Hospital,
Hills Road,
CAMBRIDGE CB2 2QQ

Dr P Ernst LRCP MRCS,
Consultant in A & E Medicine,
Orsett Hospital,
GRAYS,
Essex RM16 3EU

Dr R Fairhurst MB BS MRCS LRCP DObs RCOG,
The Travellers Medical Service,
Golden Square,
PETWORTH,
West Sussex GU28 0AP

Dr J M Fisher MB BS FRCGP,
Baileys Cottage,
2 The Terrace,
WOODFORD GREEN,
Essex IG8 1TB

Mr D G Hardy FRCS,
Consultant Neurosurgeon,
Addenbrooke's Hospital
Hills Road,
CAMBRIDGE CB2 2QQ

Dr B D W Harrison FRCP
Consultant Physician in Respiratory Disease,
West Norwich Hospital,
Bowesthorpe Road,
NORWICH NR2 3TU

Brig. I R Haywood FRCS FRCS(Ed), L/RAMC,
Comanding officer,
Queen Elizabeth Military Hospital,
Stadium Road, WOOLWICH
London SE18 4QH

Dr J A Henry MB FRCP,
Consultant Physician,
National Poisons Centre,
New Cross Hospital
LONDON   SE14 5ER

Major T J Hodgetts MB BS MRCP DipIMC RAMC,
Senior Registrar in Accident and Emergency Medicine,
Royal Army Military College,
Millbank0,
LONDON SW1 4RJ

Mr A E Holmes MB MA BChir FRCS(Ed) FRCS(Eng),
Consultant Neurosurgeon,
Addenbrooke's Hospital
Hills Road,
CAMBRIDGE CB2 2QQ

Dr I James MB BS PhD FRCP,
Reader in Therapeutics, Dept. of Medicine,
Royal Free Hospital,
Pond Street, HAMPSTEAD,
London   NW3 2QG

Mr J Keast-Butler FRCS FCOphth,
Consultant Ophthalmic Surgeon,
Saffron Walden Hospital,
Radwinter Road,
SAFFRON WALDEN, Essex

Mr W T Lamb MA MB BS BDS FRCS
Consultant Facio-Maxillary Surgeon
Addenbrooke's Hospital
Hills Road
CAMBRIDGE CB2 2QQ

Wing Commander S D Milnes MB BS DipIMC RAF,
Headquarters Royal Air Force Support Command,
Royal Air Force Brampton,
HUNTINGDON
Cambs PE18 8QL

Mr A Marsden MB ChB FRCS(Ed),
Consultant in Accident and Emergency Medicine,
Pinderfields General Hospital, Aberford Road,
WAKEFIELD,
Yorkshire   WF1 4DG

Dr Virginia Murray MSc MFOM,
Hon Consultant Occupational Toxicologist,
National Poisons Centre,
New Cross Hospital
LONDON   SE14 5ER

Dr P J Nicholson MB BS MRCGP AFOM DAvMed,
Late Senior Medical Officer,
RAF Sealand,
DEESIDE,
Clwyd

T J Nuttall SRN REMT
A&E Department,
Duchess of Kent's Military Hospital,
Catterick Garrison,
N. Yorks DL9 4DF

Surgeon Commander H Oakley Royal Navy,
Head of Survival and Thermal Medicine,
Institute of Naval Medicine,
Alverstoke, GOSPORT,
Hants. PO12 2DL

Dr David Rubenstein MD BS FRCP
Consultant Physician
48 Lensfield Road
CAMBRIDGE
CB2 1EG

Dr J A D Settle OBE M Phil FRCS (Ed),
Director, Yorkshire Regional Burns Centre,
Pinderfields General Hospital, Aberford Road,
WAKEFIELD,
Yorkshire   WF1 4DG

Mr P Sherry FRCS
Norfolk and Norwich Hospital,
St Stephens Road,
NORWICH,
NR1 3SR

Dr P Silverston
Mill Road Farm,
Lt. Wilbraham,
CAMBRIDGE,
CB1 5LG

Mr D Skinner FRCS,
Consultant in Accident & Emergency Medicine,
 John Radcliffe Hospital,
Headington
OXFORD OX3 9DU

Surgeon Commander J J W Sykes FFOM Royal Navy
Head of Undersea Medicine,
Institute of Naval Medicine,
Alverstoke, GOSPORT,
Hants. PO12 2DL

Mr R N Villar BSc MS FRCS,
Consultant Orthopaedic Surgeon,
Saffron Walden Community Hospital,
SAFFRON WALDEN,
Essex

Mr F C Wells MS BSc (Hons) FRCS MB BS,
Consultant Cardiothoracic Surgeon,
Papworth Hospital,
PAPWORTH EVERARD,
Cambridge CB3 8RE

Mr R H Whitaker FRCS,
Consultant Urologist,
21 High Street,
GT. SHELFORD,
Cambridge

M Willis Esq,
Regional Chief Ambulance Officer,
Norfolk Ambulance Service HQ,
Hospital Lane,   Helesdon,
NORWICH   NR6 5NA

Dr D A Zideman BSc MB BS FRCAnaes,
Department of Anaesthetics,
Royal Postgraduate Medical School,
Hammersmith Hospital, Du Cane Road,
LONDON W12 0HS

Contents

Glossary of abbreviations

A&E	Accident and Emergency
ACCOLC	Access overload control
ACLS	Advanced Cardiac Life Support
AF	Atrial fibrillation
ALS	Advanced Life Support
AM	Amplitude modulation
AMI	Acute myocardial infarction
amp	ampoule
ARDS	Adult respiratory distress syndrome
ATLS	Advanced Trauma Life Support
AV	Atrio-ventricular
BA	Breathing apparatus
BP	Blood pressure
BP	British Pharmacopoeia
BLS	Basic Life Support
CNS	Central nervous system
CO	Carbon monoxide
CO_2	Carbon dioxide
COAD	Chronic obstructive airways disease
CSF	Cerebral spinal fluid
CVA	Cerebral vascular accident
CT	Computed tomography
DC	Direct current
DGH	District General Hospital
DTs	Delirium tremens
ECG	Electrocardiogram
EMD	Electromechanical dissociation
ENT	Ear, nose and throat
ERC	Emergency reserve channel
FG	French gauge
FM	Frequency modulation
HACO	High altitude cerebral oedema
HANE	Hereditary angio-oedema
HAPO	High altitude pulmonary oedema
HAZCHEM	Hazardous chemical
HBIG	Hepatitis B immunoglobulin
HCO_3	Bicarbonate
Hg	Mercury
HIV	Human immunodeficiency virus
HPPF	Human plasma protein fraction
Hrs	Hours
GI	Gastrointestinal
ID	Identity
iv	intravenous
im	intramuscular
ITU	Intensive therapy unit
LED	Light emitting diode
LMA	Laryngeal mask airway
LTB	Laryngotracheobronchitis
LSCS	Lower segment caesarian section
MAOI	Monoamine oxidase inhibitor
mmHg	millimetres of mercury (pressure)
MIO	Medical Incident Officer
NAI	Non accidental injury
NATO	North Atlantic Treaty Organisation
N_2O	Nitrous oxide
NSAID	Non steroidal anti-inflammatory drug
O_2	Oxygen
PAC	Premature atrial contraction
PASG	Pneumatic anti-shock garment
PAT	Paroxysmal atrial tachycardia
PEEP	Positive end expiratory pressure
PEFR	Peak expiratory flow rate
pCO_2	Partial pressure of carbon dioxide
pO_2	Partial pressure of oxygen
PTLA	Pharyngeal tracheal lumen airway
PTSD	Post-traumatic stress disorder
PVC	Poly-vinyl chloride
PVCs	Premature ventricular contractions
RTA	Road traffic accident
RTS	Revised trauma score
SA	Sino-atrial
SaO_2	Arterial oxygen saturation
SCUBA	Self-contained underwater breathing apparatus
Sec	Seconds
SIDS	Sudden infant death syndrome
SOCO	Scenes of crimes officer
s/r	sustained release
SWG	Standard wire gauge
SVT	Supraventricular tachycardia
TIG	Tetanus human immunoglobulin
TT	Tetanus toxoid
TREM	Transport emergency
UHF	Ultra high frequency
UKHIS	UK hazard information system
VF	Ventricular fibrillation
VHF	Very high frequency
VSD	Ventricular septal defect
VT	Ventricular tachycardia

The concept and history of Immediate Care

Definition of Immediate Care

"Immediate (Medical) Care is the provision of skilled medical help at the scene of an accident, medical emergency, or during transport to hospital".

It consists of the recognition, resuscitation and stabilisation of the seriously injured and it extends beyond the preservation of life to the prevention of complications and the relief of suffering.

As such it may only be rendered by doctors and ambulance personnel who have received special training, using equipment specifically designed or adapted for use in the pre-hospital environment.

The chain of survival begins with self help and progresses to bystander First Aid, then with the arrival of an ambulance progresses to Ambulance Aid of varying sophistication depending on the training of those rendering it, and can vary from basic ambulance aid to that rendered by those with paramedic skills. Finally if an appropriately trained doctor arrives, he or she will practice Immediate Medical care.

Rationale

It has been realised increasingly over the last five decades, that if the seriously ill or injured patient receives effective immediate medical treatment, "Immediate Care", then the morbidity and the mortality are significantly reduced. In fact, it has recently been shown that in the critically injured, for every 20 minutes delay in instituting treatment, there is a threefold increase in mortality. This reduction in mortality and morbidity is due to a combination of the early performance of life saving procedures, and the prevention and treatment of life threatening pathophysiological events.

If the application of Immediate Care is to be effective, it must be rendered in a thoroughly disciplined, intelligent and rational manner, because time is of the essence; and once a procedure has been forgotten or not performed, there is seldom the opportunity for it to be done later, and for its full benefit to be experienced by the patient.

The history of BASICS

During the Second World War doctors became fully conversant with the requirements of emergency care, and were involved professionally with the rescue services and the public in the devastating effects of warfare waged upon the civilian population and armed forces alike. This expertise was a bonus to their patients during the post-war years of resettlement into general practice, the momentous commitment to a National Health Service in 1948, and the gradual evolution of the professional ambulance service. At the same time road traffic was increasing, although the roads were inadequate, and road traffic accidents accounted for more deaths and disabilities than had resulted from the previous armed conflict. Dr Kenneth Easton first became involved in this programme in 1949, when as Senior Medical Officer to the RAF Regiment Depot, Catterick, North Yorkshire, he was allowed to organise on-site medical care for the victims of road traffic accidents on the 15 mile stretch of the A1, a long way from the nearest hospital and where accidents occurred with monotonous regularity. He entered general practice at Catterick in 1950, retaining links with the RAF. After meeting several farseeing colleagues including Dr William Pickles, Dr Ekke Kuenssberg, Dr John Hunt, and Dr Ken Pickworth, who were later instrumental in forming the College of General Practitioners, he was invited to give lectures on "Immediate Care at road accidents" to groups of enthusiasts.

Deaths and injuries from road traffic accidents reached a peak in 1965, when it was obvious that these *ad hoc* rescue units needed improved co-ordination and co-operation between the statutory emergency services and general practitioners and hospital doctors, if unnecessary deaths and disabilities were to be prevented. Contact was made with Professor Eberhard Goegler of Heidelberg who had just published the results of a highly organised and funded scheme based on his University Surgical Clinic. By filling the "therapeutic vacuum" between the occurrrence of the accident and hospital admission, Goegler had reduced the mortality and morbidity following serious injury by 20%, within a radius of 20 miles of his hospital. There seemed to be no reason why this "therapeutic vacuum" should not be filled in the United Kingdom by forming "Immediate Care Schemes", utilising the nearest general practitioners to provide this specialised medical care.

An approach made to Parliament asking both for the integration of the rescue services, and for better rescue equipment for the fire services, met with a surprising reply. Not only were fire services not obliged to attend persons trapped in road accidents, but any improvements in rescue procedures would necessarily depend upon local voluntary action. Thus the ground was prepared for the starting of the pilot Immediate Care scheme: "The Road Accident After Care Scheme (RAAC)" of the North Riding of Yorkshire, which covered 1,000 square miles and utilised the voluntary services of 34 doctors. The RAAC (Registered Charity No. 256843) went into operation in December 1967, and although its main concern was to be with road traffic accidents, all types of sudden illness and accidents were to be attended. Dr K.C. Easton and the late Dr E.L.R. McCallum addressed the BMA Annual Scientific Conference in July 1967, calling upon the profession to study the needs for establishing similar schemes in their own localities.

The Chairman of the BMA Scientific Conference of 1967, the late Mr Norman Capener, CBE, FRCS, was also Chairman of the Medical Commission on Accident Prevention, and he invited representation from the RAAC on that commission, their aims being mutual.

This avuncular relationship gave rise to the far ranging associations of the parent body, including the Royal Colleges, many eminent members of which joined in the First International Conference on Immediate Care held at Scotch Corner in May 1969. As new schemes came into existence, often as a result of lecture tours and enquiries, it was important to have national cohesion, a centre for information, and a source of help and encouragement to others. This role was fulfilled by the Immediate Care Subcommittee of the Medical Commission on Accident Prevention's Rescue and Resuscitation Committee. An evaluation of the efficiency of the schemes extant in 1977 was commissioned by the Department of Health and Social Security. This indicated a 20% improvement in the care expected and achieved.

The Medical Commission on Accident Prevention understood that the schemes would eventually become autonomous, and this came about in June 1977 with the formation of the British Association of Immediate Care Schemes (Registered Charity No. 276054). This title was later changed to the British Association for Immediate Care and the constitution altered so that individual doctors could become members as well. A room for a central office was made available to BASICS by The Royal College of General Practitioners in Princes Gate, until the needs of the College and BASICS occasioned a move out of London to Ipswich.

The aims of BASICS are to foster co-operation between existing Immediate Care Schemes, to encourage and aid the formation and extension of schemes in the United Kingdom and its surrounding waters; to strengthen and develop co-operation between all services in dealing with emergencies resulting in injury or risk to life; to encourage and assist research into all aspects of Immediate Care and accident prevention; and to raise the standards of Immediate Care and the training of all who undertake to practise the discipline.

Trauma and sudden illness have emerged as the pandemic of modern society. By the end of the 1980s, the annual accident toll in the United Kingdom had risen to 15,000 killed, 300,000 seriously injured, and some 5,000,000 hurt. One third of these arose from road traffic accidents. In 1990 the cost to society of one road traffic accident fatal casualty was nearly £740,000 and £23,270 for each seriously injured casualty. If these figures were related to some other disease they would shock both the medical profession and the general public into demanding urgent action.

By 1991 BASICS had a membership of nearly 2500 doctors in about 100 Immediate Care schemes. Schemes vary in size from one individual doctor working in close co-operation with the emergency services, to some with over 200 doctors. They cover between one third and one half of Scotland, England, Wales and Northern Ireland. The doctors involved give their time and expertise entirely without financial reward. BASICS has formed a valuable liaison with the statutory emergency services, especially the ambulance service, and with the Honorary Medical Advisers of the Royal National Lifeboat Institution; the latter forming one of BASICS schemes. Other organisations which have recently joined BASICS include the British Association of Aeromedical Practitioners (BAMPA), the British Association of Rally Doctors (BARD), the British Medical Equestrian Association, and the Mountain Rescue Committee.

Despite the recommendations of the House of Commons Expenditure and Social Services Committee in January 1974 that Immediate Care Schemes should have financial support and that "One Minister should have overall responsibility for the organisation of rescue services and for procedures for dealing with all types of accidents"; it was not until 1978, and then only through the good offices of the Parliamentary All Party Disablement Group under the chairmanship of Mr Jack Ashley, CH, MP, that Parliament asked the Department of Health and Social Security to provide financial assistance. A "pump priming" grant was made to BASICS for central administrative expenses only, for a limited period under Section 64. After several years this grant was reduced and eventually ceased altogether in 1988. Mr Ashley's group considered that moral and financial help should also be forthcoming from the Ministry of Transport and the Department of the Environment, thus reflecting the team effort required to provide effective Immediate Care on-site.

Although BASICS started as a national organisation, it has now become internationally recognised. In 1980 in association with the Association of Emergency Medical Technicians (AEMT, now Paramedic UK) and the Centre for Emergency Medicine, Pittsburgh, USA, it organised the First Brighton International Congress on Immediate Care. There is great value in the extension of these international links, which have continued to grow through BASICS representation on international bodies including the World Association of Emergency and Disaster Medicine.

It is the aim of BASICS to strengthen still further its ties with the Ambulance Service, and with the Casualty Surgeons' Association (now the British Association for Accident and Emergency Medicine). Through its various committees, working parties and publications, it is constantly seeking to extend its work in the fields of research and data collection and dissemination, radio-communications and emergency equipment, and in the education and training of the general public and medical profession in emergency medical procedures. It is hoped that there will be a concerted effort on the part of the Deans of Medical Schools and Postgraduate Deans of Universities to establish tuition in Immediate Care as a basic professional requirement. This aim was partially achieved in 1988, when after considerable input from leading members of BASICS, the Royal College of Surgeons of Edinburgh introduced a diploma examination in Immediate Medical Care.

BASICS members have played a full and active part in the recent series of major incidents including the King's Cross fire, the Lockerbie and Kegworth air crashes, the sinking of the Marchioness in the river Thames, and the train crashes at Purley and Clapham, following which an independent investigation under the chairmanship of Anthony Hidden QC into the Clapham Junction Railway Accident acknowledged the valuable part that BASICS members had played and in his recommendations advised the Department of Health to consider the role of BASICS in emergency planning and to review BASICS' funding arrangements. Similarly the recent Department of Health circular on major incidents, HC 90/25, recognised the value of Immediate Medical Care teams at major incidents and the role of the Medical Incident Officer.

Thus after several decades, the value of Immediate Medical Care rendered by BASICS doctors and specially trained ambulance service personnel has eventually been recognised and given credence both by the medical profession and the Government. There is however a long way to go before this dawning recognition is translated into active support, and this will only come about after all those practising Immediate Medical Care show themselves to be thoroughly professional in every aspect of their practice, even though most of them may be working in a voluntary capacity.

1

Guidelines for Immediate Medical Care

Guidelines for Immediate Medical Care

Introduction

- The principle of working to a set of guidelines, which with time and practice becomes automatic, will reduce thinking time and save lives, whatever the circumstances of the emergency.
- These guidelines are based on recognised ACLS, PHTLS and ATLS guidelines and should be used as the basis for all your actions. The Immediate Care situation may introduce many variables, and these guidelines should not be adhered to mindlessly, but used as a basis for action by the thinking person.
- Assessment/examination of any patient follows the simple protocol: look, listen and feel.
- The aim of all treatment is to produce a neurologically intact survivor, with a reasonable quality of life.
- Remember that the patient may be suffering from more than one type of problem at the same time.

Safety

- Protect yourself:
    - Wear appropriate protective identifying clothing
- Do not expose yourself unnecessarily to any hazards (present or potential), e.g. adverse weather, overexertion, infection.
- Protect the scene, if necessary.

Scene assessment

- Look for, identify and then neutralise or remove any life threatening hazards if possible, so as avoid any avoidable injury to the rescuers and any further injury to the sick or injured. If necessary, remove the casualty to a place of relative safety.
- Ascertain:
    - What has happened and how and why did it happen?
    - What injuries or problems might you expect?
- Assess the number and severity of casualties/patients with medical problems, and the resources needed for their management and evacuation.

Triage (if there is more than one casualty)

- Rapidly sort (triage) the patients according to their priority for treatment and transportation.

Primary survey and resuscitation

- This is the simultaneous assessment, identification and management of any immediate life threatening problems, followed by an assessment of the potential for developing other serious life threatening problems or complications.
- In the time critical patient, the identification and management of life threatening conditions is the first priority, and Immediate Care may not progress beyond the primary survey.

Guidelines for the primary survey

- **A**ssessment: rapid assessment of the patient whilst approaching them and preparing for the examination.
- **A**irway (with in line cervical spine stabilisation, if trauma is involved).
- **B**reathing and the maintenance of adequate ventilation.
- **C**irculation (with control of haemorrhage, if trauma is involved).
- **D**isability of the central nervous system (brief neurological examination).
- **E**xposure of the whole patient to allow identification of any significant conditions not otherwise obvious.

Note: - If a life threatening problem is identified during the primary survey, it should be managed immediately, rather than waiting until the end of the survey.

Airway assessment and management

- Initial assessment should be done without moving the neck (if possible):
    - It *must* be assumed that the casualty (especially if they are unconscious or has any significant injury above the clavicles) has a cervical spine injury, until this possibility can be reasonably excluded (*think spinal, do airway*).
- Is the airway clear or obstructed?
- Is there any risk of obstruction developing? e.g.:
    - In the unconscious/sedated patient (especially if he is lying on his back, trapped, sitting up, etc.)
    - In faciomaxillary injuries
    - In laryngotracheal injuries
    - From fractured dentures/teeth, bony fragments, foreign bodies (remove if present).
- Insert an airway if necessary:
    - Oropharyngeal airway (Guedel):
        - May provoke vomiting/retching and result in neck movement and a rise in intracranial pressure.
    - Nasopharyngeal airway:
        - May cause nasal haemorrhage, and should *not* be used if a basal skull fracture is suspected.
- If the patient has persistent obstruction of the airway:
    - Consider cricothyrotomy.
- If the patient has no gag reflex; protect the airway from pulmonary aspiration of gastric contents:
    - Intubate with an endotracheal tube, maintaining in-line cervical stabilisation (intubation may be deferred until the secondary survey, if there is no immediate risk).
- Rapidly examine the neck for:
    - Tracheal deviation
    - Engorged neck veins
    - Swelling/deformity
    - Lacerations.
- Apply a rigid cervical collar, and only remove it to examine the neck further.

Breathing (ventilation)

- Assess:
    - Whether there is spontaneous respiration.
    - Whether respiration is effective.
    - Whether there is any evidence of respiratory depression or distress.
- Count the respiratory rate:
    - Is it normal? (12-20 respirations per minute)
    - If it is:
        - Under 12 or greater than 20 respirations per minute:
            - Consider oxygen administration.
        - Under 10 or greater than 30 respirations per minute:
            - Consider ventilation.
- If respiration is absent, impaired or inadequate:
    - Ventilate the patient.
- If you suspect a chest problem, or if the patient has required ventilation:
    - Expose and examine the chest:
        - Look for chest movement:
            - Is it present and equal?
        - Auscultate for breath sounds
            - Are they normal and present on both sides?
- Monitor the patient's arterial oxygen saturation (SaO_2) with a pulse oximeter.
- If the patient is hypoxic or there is a risk of hypoxia:
    - Administer oxygen at 15 l/min through a tight fitting face mask with reservoir.

Circulation care with control of haemorrhage

- Is there any obvious major haemorrhage?:
    - If so, elevate and control with firm direct pressure (tourniquets should *only* be used when major haemorrhage can be controlled no other way or the limb is deemed to be non-viable).
- Check the patient's:
    - Skin: colour, temperature (a warm pink patient is rarely suffering from hypotension)
    - Pulse: presence or absence, rate, regularity (or irregularity), character
    - Blood pressure.

PRACTICAL POINT: Estimating blood pressure:
- *If the carotid pulse is palpable: the systolic BP >60 mmHg.*
- *If the femoral pulse is palpable: systolic BP >70 mmHg.*
- *If the radial pulse is palpable: systolic BP >80 mmHg.*

- If necessary, perform basic and advanced cardiac life support, including defibrillation.
- Is there any evidence of hypovolaemic shock *or* of hypovolaemic shock developing? e.g. from:
    - Internal injuries
    - Pelvic or long bone fractures, etc.
- If so:
    - Put up two intravenous infusions, using:
        - Peripheral veins (antecubital fossae)
        - Large bore cannulae (14 or 16 swg)
        - Colloid initially, followed by crystalloid.
    - Splint any long bone fractures.
    - Consider using a pneumatic anti-shock garment (PASG).

Disability (neurological state)

- Rapidly assess the patient's central (brain) and peripheral (spinal cord) neurological status.
    - Central nervous system:
        - AVPU scale:
            - **A** - Alert
              V - Responds to verbal stimuli
              P - Responds to pain
              U - Unresponsive/unconscious.
        - Assess the pupils: size, equality and reactivity.
        - Ask the patient to put their tongue out.
    - Peripheral nervous system:
        - Ask the patient if they can feel:
            - Their fingers
            - Their toes.
        - Ask the patient to:
            - Squeeze your hand with their fingers
            - Wriggle their toes.

Exposure of the patient

- Expose the whole patient if appropriate/necessary for the management of immediate life threatening problems (it is usually best to wait until the patient is in a place of relative safety, e.g. in the ambulance, if the incident has occurred outside, before removing all the clothing for a full examination).
- Only remove as much clothing as is necessary to determine the presence or absence of a suspected condition or injury.
- Be aware of hypothermia, which can precipitate and aggravate shock, and is a major problem in the injured patient. Cover any exposed area as soon as the examination (and treatment) is complete.

Secondary survey and management

Subjective interview

- This is most useful in medical emergencies.
- If possible try to obtain information from bystanders as well as the patient.
- Try to ascertain:
    - What has happened?
    - What is the patient complaining of?
    - The patient's significant past medical history (see below).

Objective examination

- The casualty should be completely undressed to enable a complete, comprehensive, head to toe examination, allowing identification and appropriate early management of the patient's injuries/illness.
- This should not result in any undue delay in the evacuation of the time critical trauma patient.

Guidelines for the secondary survey

- Systematic examination of the whole body in the following order:
    - **H**ead (including neurological status) and **N**eck
    - **C**hest
    - **A**bdomen and **P**elvis
    - **E**xtremities
    - **S**pine and **B**ack.
- Obtain the **M**edical history (this should be considered first in the absence of a history of trauma).
- **R**eassessment and evaluation of patient's response to treatment:
    - If there is any unexplained deterioration in the patient's condition, go back to the beginning of the primary survey and start again.

General appearace

- Pale and/or sweating
- Cyanosed
- Pink.

Examination of the head

Neurological state
- Monitor the patient's level of consciousness
- Note and record the patient's Glasgow coma scale score.

Scalp
- Perform a rapid visual inspection to reveal any obvious injuries.
- Palpate the scalp from posterior to anterior checking for:
    - Lacerations
    - Swellings
    - Depression
    - Fractures at the base of lacerations.
- Haemorrhage from the scalp should be stopped with :
    - Pressure dressing.

Base of skull
- Look for mastoid staining/bruising.
- Look for CSF:
    - Rhinorrhoea
    - Otorrhoea.

Eyes
- If the patient is unconscious, test the:
    - Pupillary and corneal reflexes.
- Look for:
    - Evidence of a penetrating injury
    - Foreign bodies under the eye lids
    - Haemorrhages.

Face
- Palpate the face on both sides feeling for deformities and tenderness.
- If there is a facial injury:
    - Check for loose or lost teeth.
    - Grasp the upper incisors and check for instability of the maxilla (suggesting a middle third fracture).
    - Identify any fractures or injuries which may compromise the airway, and if necessary:
        - Pull the relevent fractured facial segment forward
        - Pull the tongue forward.
- Does their breath smell: alcohol, ketones?
- Is there evidence of haemoptysis or haematemtesis?
- Look inside the mouth: lacerations, burns.

Examination of the neck

- If trauma is involved and a cervical spine injury is suspected:
    - Leave the neck undisturbed in a hard cervical collar until the patient reaches hospital.
    - Repeat the neurological examination to assess the patient's peripheral:
        - Sensation
        - Motor power
        - Reflexes.

Examination of the chest

- Identify and treat any immediate or potential life threatening conditions, e.g. tension pneumothorax.
- Inspect the anterior and posterior chest wall for:
    - Tracheal deviation
    - Signs of respiratory obstruction: stridor, intercostal recession, tracheal tug.
    - Asymmetrical chest movement
    - Wounds
    - Bruising.

Chest wall and lungs
- Examine the chest wall for:
    - Parodoxical chest movement (indicates flail chest):
        - If the patient shows signs of respiratory distress, consider:
            - Intubation and ventilation.
    - Open chest wound:
        - Cover with occlusive dressing on three sides (will then act as a flutter valve)
        - Consider insertion of a chest drain.
    - Tenderness and crepitus over the ribs and sternum:
        - If this is so painful that respiration is impaired, consider:
            - Analgesia.
    - Surgical emphysema.
    - Hyperresonance ⎫
- Auscultate for: ⎬ Indicates a pneumothorax: if tension, perform a needle decompression
    - Reduced air entry ⎭   and insert a chest drain.
- Monitor:
    - SaO_2.

Heart
- Suspect myocardial contusion/injury if the patient has suffered:
    - Massive deceleration
    - Penetrating thoracic injury.
- Examine the neck for engorged neck veins.
- Auscultate for:
    - Muffled heart sounds: if so perform:
        - Needle pericardiocentesis (pericardial aspiration).
- Perform an ECG if an acute myocardial infarction (AMI), cardiac dysrrhythmia or cardiac contusion is suspected.

Examination of the abdomen/pelvis

- Look for:
    - Bruising
    - Movement
    - Open wounds; if present cover with saline soaked pads.
- Palpate for localised tenderness:
    - If there is bruising and tenderness over the lower ribs; suspect injury to the liver or spleen:
        - Monitor the haemodynamic state carefully, put up two intravenous infusions using wide bore cannulae and be prepared to infuse large volumes of fluid rapidly if there is any deterioration.
    - Abdominal palpation may be unreliable, especially if the patient is head injured or intoxicated.
- If there appears to be gastric distension:
    - Insert a naso-gastric tube.
- Pelvic springing to elicit pain/movement/crepitus (may be unreliable as an indication of a pelvic fracture).

Examination of the extremeties

- Inspect for:
    - Bruising
    - Wounds
    - Deformities
    - Burns.
- If any injuries are found; check:
    - Distal pulses
    - Sensation.
- Reduce and splint any fractures/subluxations:
    - Re-check the distal pulses and sensation after reduction
    - Record the position before and after reduction with polaroid photography.
- Cover and seal (after first taking a polaroid photograph):
    - Compound fractures
    - Degloving injuries.
- Collect any extruded fracture fragments and place in clean container for conveyance with the patient.

Examination of the spine

- If spinal injury is suspected:
    - Do *not* move the patient unnecessarily:
        - If movement *is* necessary, move the patient with great care, in the horizontal axis only.
    - Look for:
        - Sensory deficit
        - Motor defecit
        - Abnormal reflexes
        - Priapism.

Examination of the back

- Log roll the patient, but with great care, if a spinal injury is suspected; and:
    - Examine the back for:
        - Bruising
        - Lacerations/open wounds.
    - Auscultate the back of the chest.
    - Examine the spine for:
        - Tenderness or muscular spasm
        - Boggyness
        - Irregularity (step deformity) of the contour of the spinous processes.

Assessment and management of pain

- Assess whether the patient:
    - Is in pain
    - Is likely to develop pain during the extrication process.
- If so administer adequate and appropriate analgesia:
    - Nitrous oxide/oxygen (Entonox) (but not for chest injuries where pneumothorax is a possibility)
    - Opiates
    - Non steroidal anti-inflammatory drugs.
- Consider sedation if the patient is distressed, or violent and hypoxic:
    - Hypnovel
    - Diazepam.

Medical history

- **A**llergies
- **M**edicines
- **P**ast medical history
- **L**ast meal
- **E**vents leading to the injury.

Unexplained deterioration

- If there is any sudden, severe or unexplained deterioration in the patient's condition:
    - Go back to the primary survey.

Monitoring/reassessment of the patient

- This should be continuous, so as to detect any changes in the patient's condition and will allow modification of their management accordingly.
- Is their condition:
    - Improving?
    - Deteriorating?: if so why? what can you do about it?
    - The same.

Monitor

- Airway patency.
- Breathing:
    - Appearance/colour
    - Respiratory rate
    - Chest expansion
    - SaO_2 .
- Circulation:
    - Pulse rate
    - Blood pressure
    - Capillary refill
    - Peripheral pulses.
- Disability/neurological status:
    - Glasgow coma scale.
- Pain severity.
- Drug and fluid administration.

Trending

- This allows early assessment of changes in the patients condition, i.e. any improvement or deterioration, and gives a guide as to the efficacy of their management.

Monitoring equipment/devices

- Sphygmomanometer: electronic/automatic
- Pulse oximeter
- ECG monitor
- End tidal CO_2 monitor
- Trauma scoring.

Recording information

- Patient report form
- Photography
- Print out from monitor.

2

Basic life support

Basic life support

Introduction

- Basic Life Support, which is life support using no aids (other than a simple airway device or protective shield), to maintain the airway and support breathing and the circulation, is something in which every health care professional should be proficient.
- Many lives that are lost would be saved if a significant proportion of the population were trained in Basic Life Support, because no matter how good the emergency services are, it has to be the bystander who starts treatment.
- Survival from cardiac arrest is greatest if the event is witnessed; if a bystander starts resuscitation; if the heart arrests in ventricular fibrillation; and when defibrillation is carried out soon after the arrest-- "the Chain of Survival".
- Regular practice using training aids will help maintain skills, if there is not enough real life experience.

Guidelines

- Even for the experienced, it is advisable to stick to a set of guidelines when dealing with life threatening problems, so that initial actions become automatic and rapid, rather than action interspersed with thought, which takes longer!
- The first objective of the Basic Life Support is to assess the patient rapidly, and obtain help early during the resuscitation attempt, especially for the casualty with an absent pulse. The rationale behind this is that the commonest treatable cause of sudden cardiac arrest is ventricular fibrillation and the only effective management of this is early defibrillation. The rest of the guidelines are designed to maintain the patient's ventilation and circulation, preserving the cerebral blood supply, until the arrival of medical/ambulance Advanced Life Support with a defibrillator.

Approach

- Do not rush headlong into the situation, but try to assess what has happened.
- Look out for dangers to yourself, e.g. electricity, gas, road traffic, dangerous chemicals and falling masonry.

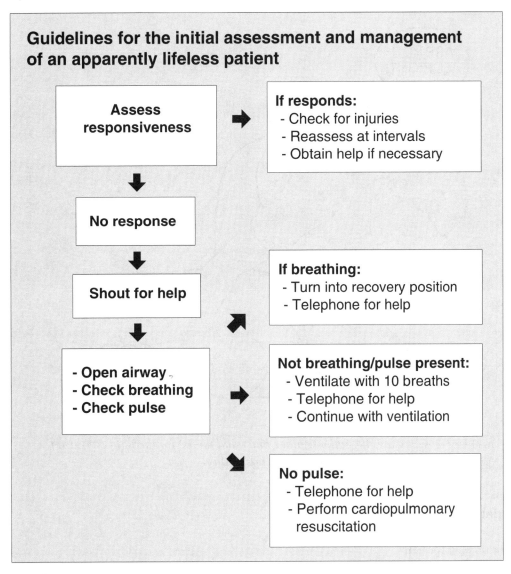

Guidelines for the initial assessment and management of an apparently lifeless patient

Assess responsiveness

➡️ **If responds:**
- Check for injuries
- Reassess at intervals
- Obtain help if necessary

⬇️

No response

⬇️

Shout for help

If breathing:
- Turn into recovery position
- Telephone for help

⬇️

- **Open airway**
- **Check breathing**
- **Check pulse**

➡️ **Not breathing/pulse present:**
- Ventilate with 10 breaths
- Telephone for help
- Continue with ventilation

No pulse:
- Telephone for help
- Perform cardiopulmonary resuscitation

Assessment

General appearance

- Is the patient unconscious, pale or cyanosed?

Responsiveness

- Shake the patient gently (be careful not to exacerbate any injuries especially of the neck, chest or spine).
- Ask loudly: "Are you all right?", "What's happened?", or give a command such as "Open your eyes".

Management

- If the patient responds by answering or moving:

- Leave the patient in the position in which you found them (provided they are not in further danger).
- Check for any injuries.
- Reassess their responsiveness at regular intervals and obtain further help if necessary.

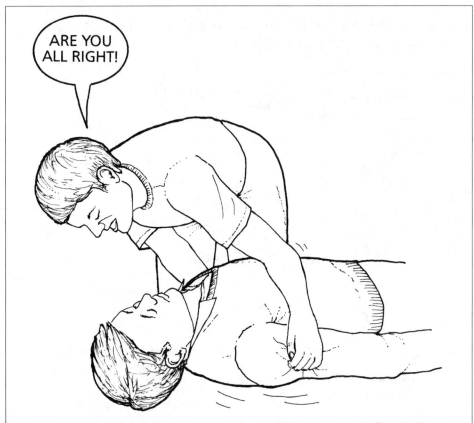

Figure 2-2 Assessing the patient (place one hand on the forehead to stabilise the head/neck if a cervical spine injury is a possibility).

- **If the patient is unresponsive:**

    - Shout or send for help.

Airway

- If the patient is not breathing, they may have an obstructed airway:
    - Airway obstruction may be caused by:
        - The tongue falling back onto the posterior pharyngeal wall, e.g. in unconsciousness
        - Vomit or blood.
        - Foreign bodies, e.g. false teeth or food impacted in the oropharynx (sometimes both conditions may be present).

Management

- Loosen any tight clothing around the patient's neck.
- Remove any obvious obstruction from the mouth including loose dentures, but leave well fitting dentures in place (don't waste time trying to find hidden obstructions.)
- If possible, leave the patient in the position in which you found them, and open the airway.
- If there is any possibility of a neck injuriy, only tilt the head enough to obtain a clear airway (see method 2, jaw thrust, which is preferable).

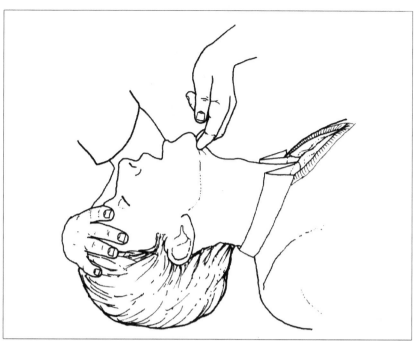

Figure 2-3 Head tilt, chin lift

Method 1
- Head tilt:
    - Place one hand along the hairline, keeping the thumb and index finger free to close the nose, in case ventilation is necessary, and exert gentle pressure to tilt the head.
- Chin lift:
    - Lift the chin with the tips of the index and middle fingers of other hand under the point of the chin (this will often allow breathing to restart).

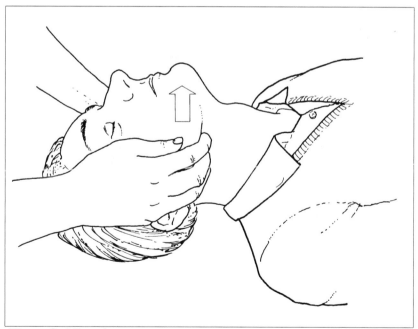

Figure 2-4 Jaw thrust

Method 2 (this is the method of choice when cervical spine injury is a possibility)
- Jaw thrust:
    - Put one hand under each angle of the jaw, and lift it forwards and upwards.

Breathing

- Once the patient has a clear airway, the rescuer should check that they can breathe spontaneously.

Method
- Put your cheek close to the patient's mouth looking along his chest and:
    - *LOOK* for chest movement
    - *LISTEN* at the mouth for breath sounds } for 5 seconds before deciding that breathing is absent.
    - *FEEL* expired air on your cheek.

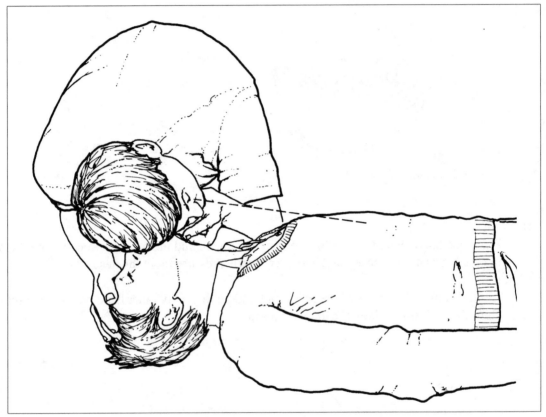

Figure 2-5 Look, listen and feel for signs of spontaneous respiration

- Causes of respiratory arrest include:
    - Airway obstruction by the tongue due to unconsciousness and an unprotected airway
    - Airway obstructed by vomit, or foreign body
    - Head injury
    - Chest injury
    - Poisoning from toxic gases or drug overdose
    - Near drowning.

Circulation

Assessment

- Check for a pulse (the best pulse to feel in any emergency is the carotid).
- Palpate for the pulse for at least 5 seconds before deciding that it is absent (indicating a cardiac arrest).

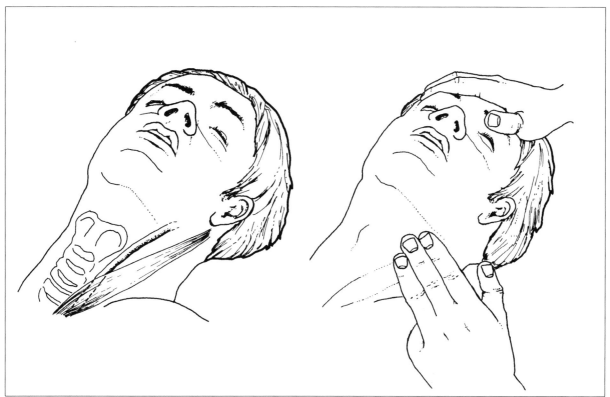

Figure 2-6 Palpation of the carotid pulse

Management

- If the patient is breathing spontaneously, but unconscious:

- Put them into the recovery position, unless this would exacerbate any injuries (see below).
- Go or telephone for help.
- Return and keep them under close observation, checking that they are breathing freely.

- If the patient is not breathing, but a pulse is present:
- Turn them onto their back, if necessary.
- Give 10 breaths of expired air ventilation:

Expired air ventilation

- Expired air contains 16-17% oxygen (atmospheric air 21% oxygen), which is more than sufficient to sustain life.
- Expired air ventilation is most easily performed with the patient lying on his back, but can be done in almost any situation, e.g. swimming pool, when trapped, etc.

Mouth to mouth ventilation

-   This is the most widely used method of expired air ventilation.

Method
-   Ensure that the patient's head is tilted and the chin is lifted.
-   Pinch the nose with the index finger and thumb of one hand (which is already pressing on the forehead).
-   Allow the patient's mouth to open a little, while still maintaining chin lift.
-   Take a deep breath and seal your lips firmly around those of the patient.

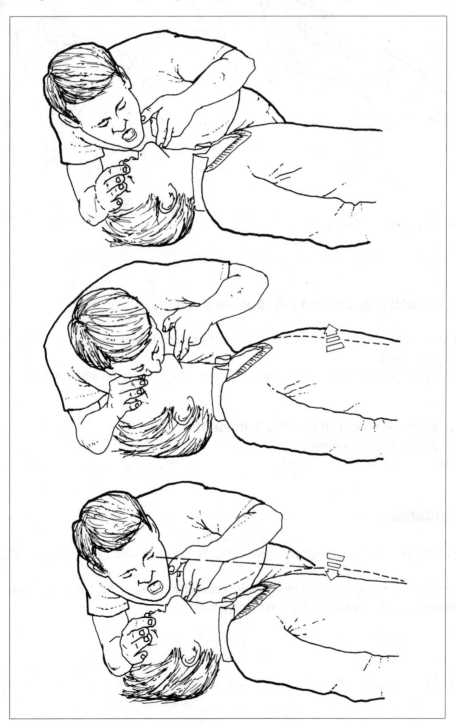

Figure 2-7 Mouth to mouth ventilation

- Blow out slowly and gently into the patient's mouth, until you can see the chest rise (about two seconds for full inflation).
- Lift your head away, maintaining head tilt and chin lift and allow the expired air to come out of the patient's mouth, while you take another breath in.
- Allow the patient's chest to deflate fully (usually 2-4 seconds), before inflating again.
- Continue to do ventilations until you have given a total of 10 ventilations (taking about one minute).

Note:- Only a small amount of resistance should be felt during mouth to mouth ventilation.
- The desired tidal volume in an adult is about 800-1200 ml in an adult, which is the volume required to produce visible lifting of the chest.

CAUTION
- If you try to inflate too rapidly, the resistance will be greater, less air will enter the lungs and gastric and oesophageal distension may occur, resulting in gastric regurgitation and pulmonary aspiration.

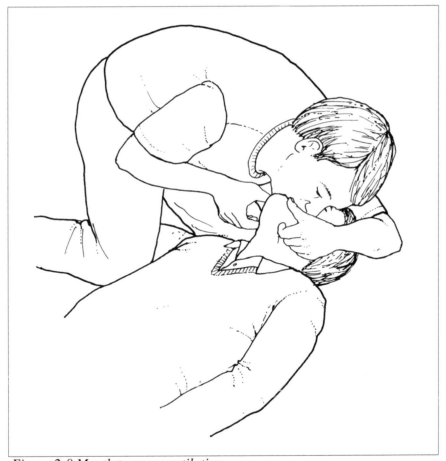

Figure 2-8 Mouth to nose ventilation

Mouth to nose ventilation

- This may be aesthetically more acceptable than mouth to mouth ventilation especially if the patient has vomited.
- May be indicated: if the patient has a clenched jaw (trismus), a mandibular injury or during water rescue.
- May not be possible: if the patient has nasal obstruction or a nasal or maxillary injury.

Method
- Open the airway with head tilt and chin lift.
- Seal the patient's lips with the hand supporting the chin, but remember to open the mouth during the expiratory phase to allow expiration.
- Take a deep breath, form a tight seal with your lips around the patient's nose and blow out.
- Otherwise the method is similar to mouth to mouth ventilation.

- **After 10 ventilations:**
  - Go for help/telephone for an ambulance.
  - Return to the patient and reassess consciousness, breathing and pulse as above.
  - If a pulse is still present, continue doing ventilations alone, but recheck the pulse after every 10 breaths, starting full CPR if the pulse disappears.
  - If the patient starts to breathe spontaneously, put them onto their side in the recovery position.

Airway obstruction

- If the chest does not rise with each ventilation, the airway is obstructed. Causes include:
  - Failure to extend the neck enough (extend the neck a bit further).
  - Failure to make an efficient seal around the mouth or nose (maker a better seal).
  - Obstruction by vomit, blood or a foreigh body (see under Choking).

Cross infection and expired air ventilation

- Hepatitis B and herpes viruses have been known to be transmitted by saliva and nasal discharge, and so it is advisable to avoid direct contact with these if possible, by using a simple and effective barrier device, e.g. a pocket mask (see chapter on Airway Management).
- For HIV virus disease, contact with infected blood is the only risk, and even then the incidence of transmission is extremely low. Recent studies have shown that the HIV virus does not survive in human saliva.
- About 70% of cardiac arrests occur in the home where the patient is known to the rescuer.

Circulation: cardiac arrest

- **If the patient has no pulse:**

- **Go or telephone for help**

- **Give two expired air ventilations**

- **Start external chest compressions**
  - Return and position the patient on their back on a firm flat stable surface (if possible), preferably with the legs elevated (to aid the venous return).
  - Open the airway by tilting the head and lifting the chin.
  - Ventilate the patient by giving two breaths of expired air ventilation.
  - Locate the xiphisternal notch by running the index and middle fingers of one hand up the lower margins of the rib cage and find the point where the ribs join.

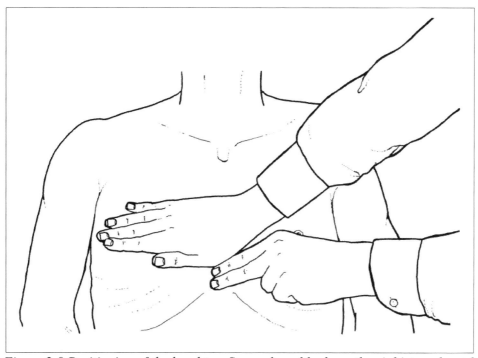

Figure 2-9 Positioning of the hand two fingers breadth above the xiphisternal notch

- With your middle finger over the xiphisternum, place the tip of your index finger on the sternum above.
- Place the heel of your other hand on the upper sternum, and slide it down towards the first hand until it touches the index finger. This should be the middle of the lower half of the sternum.
- The heel of the first hand should then be placed on top of the other hand and the fingers interlocked, so that pressure is not applied over the ribs.
- Lean well over the patient, so that your shoulders are positioned directly above the hands, with the arms held straight at the elbows.

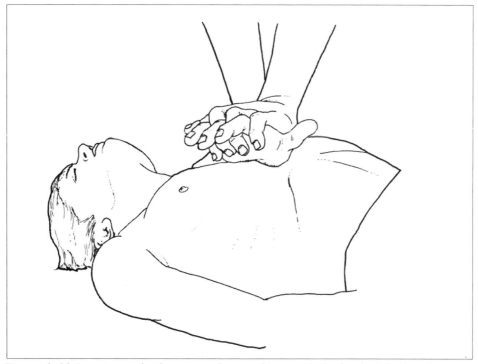

Figure 2-10 Intertwine the fingers and press down with the heel of the hand

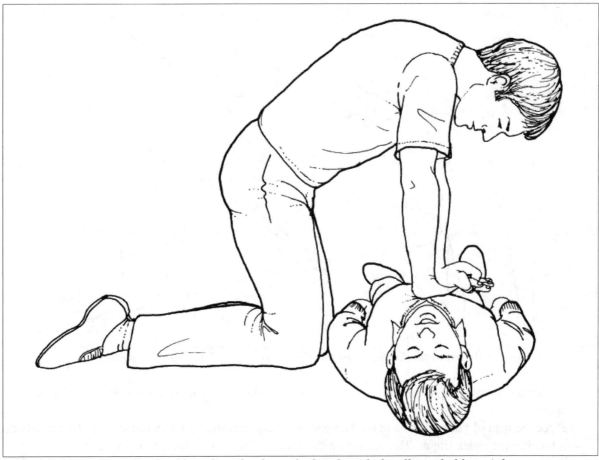

Figure 2-11 Position the shoulders directly above the hands with the elbows held straight

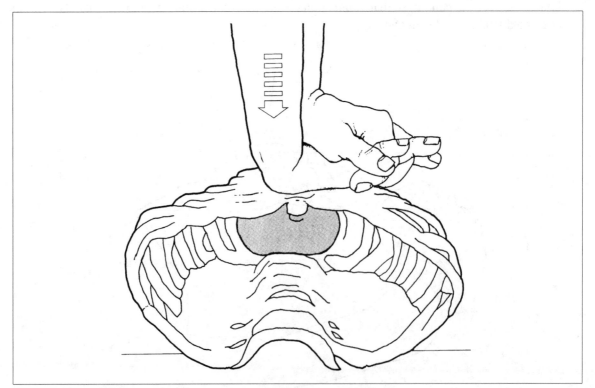

Figure 2-12 Showing direction of pressure on the sternum (although it may not in fact directly compress the heart against the spine as shown here)

- Press down firmly and vertically on the sternum using just enough force to depress it 1.5-2 inches (4-5 centimetres) without allowing your elbows to flex. The movement should be well controlled. Erratic or violent action is dangerous and may cause unnecessary injury to the patient.
- Release the pressure, still keeping your hand on the patient, and repeat the procedure at a rate of approximately 80 compressions per minute.
- The compression phase should last at least 50% of the cycle.
- Do not waste time checking for a pulse as it is unlikely that effective spontaneous cardiac function will return, without using advanced life support techniques including defibrillation.
- If the patient makes a movement or takes a spontaneous breath, check the carotid pulse, to see if the patient has any productive cardiac output, taking no more than 5 seconds to do so. Otherwise *Do NOT interrrupt* resuscitation.
- Combine ventilations and chest compressions.

Note: - A new device, the Ambu Cardiac Pump has recently been introduced, which enables the chest to be actively decompressed as well as compressed. This has theoretical advantages, but has not yet been fully assessed.

Organisation

Single rescuer BLS

- The single rescuer should do two initial expired air ventilations, followed by 15 chest compressions, two expired air ventilations and then 15 chest compressions and so on.
- Do not stop to check for a pulse.
- If the patient moves or takes a spontaneous breath, check the carotid pulse to see if the patient has any effective cardiac output.

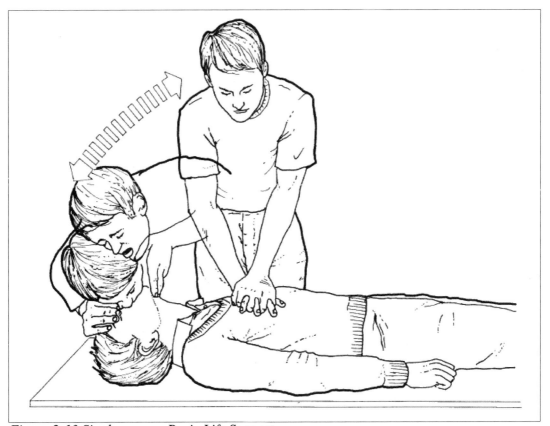

Figure 2-13 Single rescuer Basic Life Support

Two rescuer BLS

- The first rescuer (lung ventilator) should look after the airway, beginning with two inflations, following which the second rescuer (chest compressor) should do five chest compressions, counting out loud between compressions, as they do so.
- At the end of every five compressions, the second rescuer should pause just long enough for the first rescuer to do one lung inflation, but no longer. They should not remove their hands from the patient's chest.
- Sellick's manoeuvre (cricoid pressure to compress the oesophagus) helps to reduce the risk of gastric regurgitation and if indicated is usually performed by the lung ventilator.
- When the second rescuer becomes tired, the rescuers should exchange positions.
- If the pulse returns and spontaneous respiration begins, the patient should be put into the recovery position (see below), and their condition carefully monitored.
- The usual convention is for the first rescuer to be in charge, and to give instructions to the second.

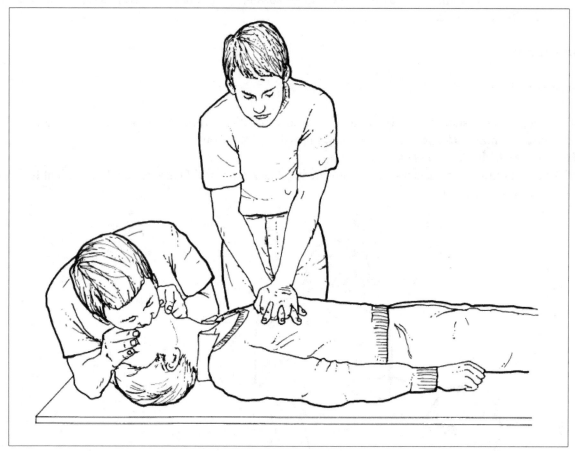

Figure 2-14 Two rescuer BLS

Recovery position

- If the patient is breathing, but unconscious, put them into the recovery position.
- The procedure should minimise the movement of the patient, especially the cervical spine.
- The patient's head, neck and trunk should be kept in a straight line.
- The position should:
    - Allow the tongue to fall forward away from the posterior pharyngeal wall.
    - Allow drainage of liquid from patient's mouth by gravity.
    - Be stable, i.e. not allow the patient to roll over.
    - Allow the patient to be nursed or carried on a stretcher.

Method
- Remove the patient's spectacles and any bulky objects from their pockets.
- Turn round (rotate) any rings, so that the stones are on the palmar aspect of the finger.
- Kneel beside the patient and make certain that both their legs are straight.
- Open the airway by tilting the head and lifting the chin.

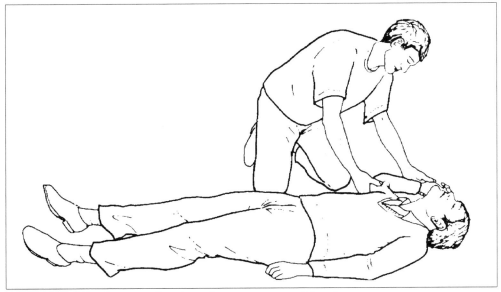

Figure 2-15 Putting a patient into the recovery position 1

- Take the arm nearest you, and place it at right angles to the body with the elbow bent and the palm of the hand uppermost.

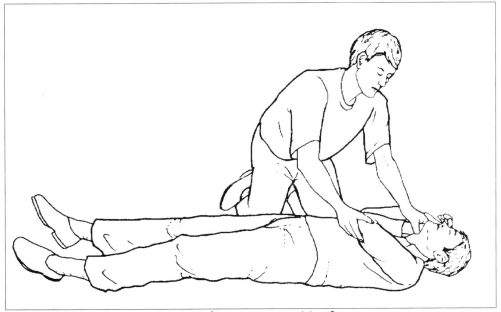

Figure 2-16 Putting a patient into the recovery position 2

- Bring the furthest arm across the chest, and place the back of the hand against the patient's nearest cheek.

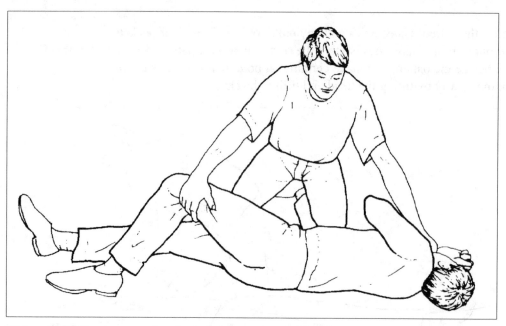

Figure 2-17 Putting a patient into the recovery position 3

- With your other hand grasp the far leg, just above the knee, and pull it up, bending the knee, but keeping the foot on the ground.
- Pull on the leg to roll the patient towards you on their side.
- Adjust the upper leg so that both the hip and the knee are bent at right angles.
- Tilt the head back so that the airway remains open.

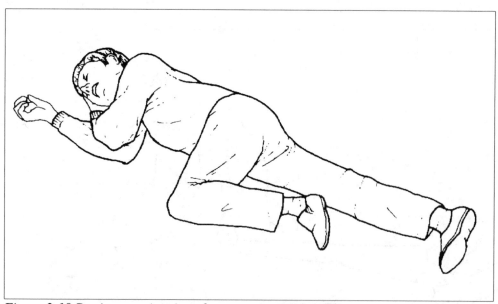

Figure 2-18 Putting a patient into the recovery position 4

- Adjust the hand under the cheek, as necessary, so that the head stays tilted.
- Check the breathing and pulse regularly.

Turning a patient onto their back

Method
- Kneel down beside the patient and place the arm nearest to you above their head.
- Turn their face away from you.

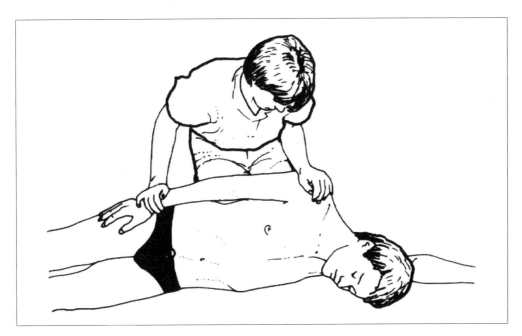

Figure 2-19 Turning a patient onto their back

- Hold the far shoulder with one hand and the hip with the other, at the same time clamping the wrist to his hip.
- With a steady pull, roll the patient over against your thighs.
- Lower them gently to the ground on their back, supporting the head and shoulders as you do so, and place the extended arm by their side.

Cervical spine injury

- Particular care should be exercised if there is any suspicion that the patient may have sustained a cervical spine injury with possible damage of the spinal cord, for example in:
    - Road traffic accidents
    - Falls from heights
    - Falls down stairs
    - Riding accidents
    - Rugby football accidents: scrum collapse
    - Diving accidents into shallow water
    - The unconscious head injured patient.

- If cervical spine injury is suspected:
    - The neck should be immobilised with gentle in-line cervical stabilisation
    - Avoid moving the neck any more than necessary
    - Avoid over extending the neck to maintain the airway
    - If turning is necessary, log roll the patient (see chapter on Spinal Injury).

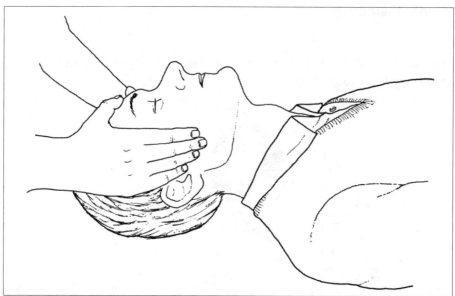

Figure 2-20 Immobilisation of the neck with gentle in-line cervical stabilisation

Choking/airway obstruction

- Choking occurs when a foreign body, e.g. a bit of food gets stuck in the back of the throat, obstructing the airway.
- The patient will have difficulty with breathing, and may appeared cyanosed.
- If conscious they may indicate that they are choking by grasping their neck with their hands or point to their throat.

Management

- If the airway is only partially obstructed, the casualty may often able to dislodge the foreign body by coughing.
- If airway obstruction is complete, urgent intervention is indicated to prevent asphyxia.

- **If the patient is conscious and breathing, despite evidence of obstruction:**
    - Obtain their confidence and encourage them to cough; this allows them to use their own muscles and so exert as much pressure as possible to expel the foreign body (this is successful in the majority of patients).

- **If obstruction appears to be complete, and the casualty shows signs of exhaustion or cyanosis, consider:**

- **Back slaps**

Method
    - Stand behind and to the side of the patient.
    - Lean the patient forwards, with the head down, (preferably over the back of a chair or alternatively support the front of their chest with one hand). This allows gravity to assist you.
    - Give up to five firm blows smartly with the heel of the other hand to the middle of the back, between the scapulae.

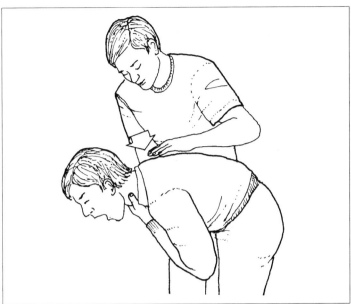

Figure 2-21 Back blows: patient bending over

- **If back slaps are unsuccessful, consider:**

- **Abdominal thrusts**

  - The sudden inward and upward movement of the upper abdomen against the diaphragm forces air up the oesophagus, and helps expel the foreign body.

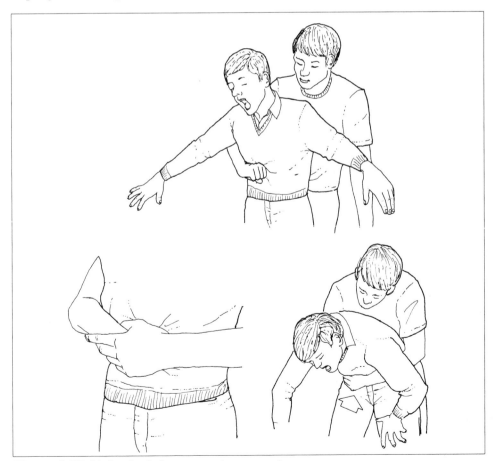

Figure 2-22 Abdominal thrusts: patient conscious

Method
- Stand or kneel behind the patient, and put both your arms round the patient's upper abdomen.
- Clench one fist and place it with the thumb inwards, immediately below the patient's xiphisternum.
- Grasp the fist with your other hand, and pull both hands inwards and upwards towards you, with a quick thrust from the elbows.

CAUTION
- Excessive force may result in injury to the stomach, liver, diaphragm, spleen and aorta.
- Not recommended in pregnancy, gross obesity, or in infants and children.

- If neither method is successful, consider giving back blows alternating with finger sweeps followed by abdominal thrusts.

- **If the casualty is unconscious, administer:**

- **Finger sweeps**

Method
- Use an index finger to sweep inside the mouth and try to remove the foreign body digitally (well fitting dentures, however, may help to maintain a mouth seal during ventilation, so do not remove).

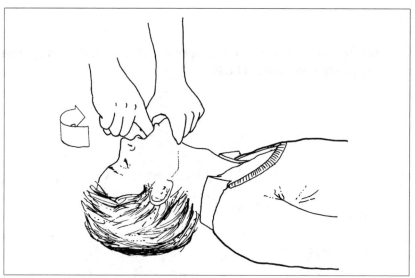

Figure 2-23 Finger sweeps

Abdominal thrusts *(may also be used if the patient is obese or pregnant)*

Method
- Kneel astride, or if this is not possible, beside the patient.
- Place the heel of one hand in the patient's epigastrium and cover it with the other hand, keeping the wrist dorsiflexed.
- With both arms straight, give a quick inwards and upwards thrust towards the patient's upper thoracic spine.
- Repeat this up to four times as necessary.

Chest thrusts

Method
- Use the same technique as for chest compressions during cardiac arrest.

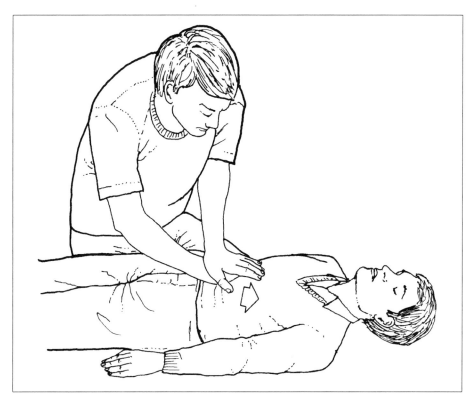

Figure 2-24 Abdominal thrusts: patient unconscious

Resuscitation: when to stop

- When resuscitation attempts are obviously unsuccessful.
- When the rescuers are exhausted.
- In the elderly.
- Where there is evidence of irreversible brain damage:
    - The presence of *dilated pupils* is an unreliable sign of cardiac arrest, circulatory failure or established/ irreversible brain damage and should *not* be used to influence the management of a patient during or after cardiopulmonary resuscitation.
- Exceptions:
    - Hypothermia
    - Drug overdosage
    - Drowning
    - Electrocution
    - In children.

Notes

3

Airway care

Airway care

Introduction

- Basic airway care is covered in the previous chapter on Basic Life Support.
- Rapid assessment, and if appropriate, management of the airway must be the first potential problem to be addressed in every patient. The treatment is simple and may be lifesaving.
- Bystander failure to recognise and treat airway obstruction is a common but preventable cause of death on all too many occasions: it is estimated that one in five of all preventable deaths following road traffic accidents is from an obstructed airway.

Respiratory failure

- Occurs when there is a failure of normal gas exchange in the lungs.

Aetiology

Unsuitable respirable atmosphere
- Carbon monoxide, smoke or other toxic constituents.
- Hypoxic environment.
- High altitude hypoxia.
- Drowning.

Airway obstruction
- Above the larynx:
    - Excess mucus
    - Enlarged tonsils: severe quinsy
    - Enlarged/hypertrophied adenoids
    - Foreign body: food, false teeth
    - Faciomaxillary injury
    - Angioneurotic oedema.
- Laryngeal:
    - Tumours, acute epiglottitis, laryngeal trauma, burns.
- Below the larynx:
    - Trauma, inhaled foreign body, tracheitis, burns.
- In the lungs:
    - Asthma, bronchitis, bronchiolitis, pneumonia, lung contusion.

Bellows failure
- Central depression:
    - Drugs: narcotics, hypnotics, tranquillizers, alcohol
    - Accidents: severe head injury, cerebral vascular accident.
- Neuromuscular paralysis:
    - Cervical spine injury
    - Tetanus, polyneuritis, poliomyelitis
    - Myasthenia gravis
    - "Nerve" gases (organophosphates).
- Breach in the integrity of the thoracic cage:
    - Flail chest, pneumothorax, ruptured diaphragm, stab wound.

Failure of oxygen transfer and utilisation
- Poisoning: carbon monoxide, cyanide.

Pathophysiology

- Normal gas exchange fails, resulting in:
    - A reduction in the level of oxygenation of the blood (hypoxaemia)
    - An increase in the levels of deoxygenated haemoglobin in the blood (cyanosis)
    - A build up of carbon dioxide levels in the blood (hypercapnia)
    - A resultant metabolic acidosis.

Symptoms/signs

- Depend on the underlying pathophysiology.

Respiratory distress
- Hypoxia:
    - Disturbance of cerebral function, restlessness
    - Pallor, sweating
    - Dyspnoea, tachypnoea, irregular respiratory effort, inability to cough, tracheal tug
    - Use of accessory muscles, intercostal recession
    - Increase in heart rate, unless severe hypoxia, when heart rate starts to decrease
    - Oliguria: this is a relatively late development and therefore not usually relevant in Immediate Care.
- Hypercapnia:
    - Vasodilation: warm extremities
    - Tachycardia with a high volume pulse.
    - Flapping tremor and drowsiness.

Impending death
- Cyanosis:
    - Discolouration of tongue and lips: not usually seen until the pO_2 is less than 60 mmHg.
    - Does not occur if the patient is very anaemic.
- Drowsiness.
- Irregular respiration, absence of rhonchi (silent chest).
- Tachycardia >150 bpm, hypertension or hypotension.

Measurement

Pulse oximetry

- This is a most valuable development in Immediate Care, in which a non-invasive device is used for determining the percentage oxygen saturation of arterial haemoglobin (SaO_2) and the pulse rate.

How it works
- Photoplethysmography as used in pulse oximetry depends on the principle that oxy- and deoxy-haemoglobin absorb different wavelengths of infra-red light (so do carboxy- and met-haemoglobin, but they are not usually present in the circulation in any significant quantity, except in burns).
- Infra-red light generated by a light emitting diode in a probe passes through the tissues, where the two different wavelengths of the infra-red light are absorbed to a greater or lesser extent by oxy- and deoxy-haemoglobin depending on the the amount of these substances present, which in turn depends on the oxygen saturation of the arterial haemoglobin. The remaining infra-red light is then picked up by a photo-detector and converted into an electronic signal, which is then processed and displayed to give analogue digital readouts for the arterial waveform, oxygen saturation (SaO_2) and pulse rate, with high and low alarm settings for both.
- The light source and detector are housed in a clip probe, which is usually attached to a digit, the nasal septum or an ear lobe.

Normal values
- Normal range: 97-100% (at sea level)
- Mild hypoxia: 90-96%
- Moderate hypoxia: 85-90%
- Severe hypoxia: <85%

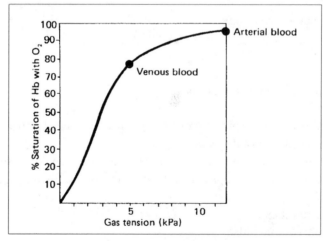

Figure 3-1 Oxygen dissociation curve for haemoglobin

Uses
- For detecting reduced arterial oxygen saturation (which will result in tissue hypoxia) and monitoring the pulse rate.

Note:- There must be an effective arterial circulation in the part being monitored.
- The site to which the probe is clipped, must permit the transmission of light.
- An initially satisfactory pulse oximetry reading does *not* indicate satisfactory positioning of the endotracheal tube following intubation, if the patient has been preoxygenated. This is because the lungs act as an oxygen reservoir, and it may take up to 8 minutes for the arterial oxygen saturation levels to fall.

Applications
- Determining/monitoring:
  - Efficacy of ventilation:
    - Patency of the airway
    - Adequacy of ventilatory effort
    - When to stop suctioning
    - Confirming the correct position of an endotracheal tube or other ventilation device (but see above)
    - Adequacy of oxygen therapy
    - Efficacy of analgesia in fractured ribs.
- Effectiveness of the circulation, e.g. checking the distal circulation in limb fractures.
- Estimating the degree of hypovolaemic shock:
  - The contour of the plethysmograph waveform loses the sharpness of its upward point and dicrotic notch and becomes rounded as the arterial pressure falls.
- As an aid to diagnosis:
  - Assessing whether a patient's confusion is due to hypoxia, e.g. in silent pulmonary embolism.
- Pulse oximetry has an important role in the following situations:
  - Trauma:
    - Head injury: obstructed airway
    - Chest injury: flail chest, haemothorax or pneumothorax
    - Multiple injuries: hypovolaemic shock
    - Limb injuries: assessing the adequacy of the distal circulation.
  - Medical emergencies:
    - Unconsciousness: upper airway obstruction
    - Asthma: degree of hypoxia
    - Respiratory depression: overdose, alcohol
    - Cardiogenic shock and arrest
    - Hypovolaemic and bacterial shock.

Disadvantages
- Pulse oximetry may not be accurate when there is poor peripheral perfusion, e.g. when the ambient temperature is very low, and there is peripheral vasoconstriction.
- It will give a false high result in carbon monoxide poisoning (common when there has been smoke inhalation), as the photo-detector is unable to distinguish oxyhaemoglobin from carboxyhaemoglobin.

PRACTICAL POINTS
- *Pulse oximetry may produce artefacts and inaccurate results if:*
  - *The patient has painted her finger and toe nails, as some nail varnish pigments (notably black, purple and blue) do not allow the light to pass through them.*
  - *The probe is attached to skin which is covered in dirt, oil, grease (low) or dried blood (high)*
  - *The probe is uncovered in bright sunlight.*
  - *The patient is shivering or is in a moving vehicle (movement artefact).*
  - *The probe is taped too tightly to the patient.*
  - *The patient is peripherally shutdown: hypovolaemia, cold environment.*
  - *The patient is a heavy smoker (over estimation).*

Management

- Treatment of the cause.
- Improvement in tissue oxygenation: oxygen therapy.

Oxygen therapy

- This is the treatment of choice for respiratory failure and hypoxia, independant of the cause.

Mode of action

- Increases the haemoglobin oxygen saturation.
- Increases the amount of oxygen carried in solution in the blood.
- Should be administered with caution in some patients, i.e. those with chronic obstructive airways disease (COAD) who depend on their hypoxic drive to maintain respiration (provided that there is no other cause for their hypoxia). This is not a problem if they are being ventilated.

Administration

Oxygen mask

- Oxygen is usually given at inadequate flow rates, (e.g. 4-6 litres per minute); but ideally it should be given at 8-12 litres per minute.
- Concentration varies with the type of mask used:

Ventimask
   - Designed to provide some oxygen enrichment of inspired air.
   - Only allows minimal rebreathing of expired air.
   - Delivers 24/28/35/40/60% oxygen (the Edinburgh mask has an adjustable flow rate of 24-35%).

Polymask, MC Mask
   - Designed to provide a moderate concentration of oxygen in inspired air.
   - Delivers about 60% oxygen at a flow rate of 8 litres per minute.

Oxygen mask with rebreathing reservoir
   - Allows rebreathing of expired air.
   - Delivers 98-100% oxygen at a flow rate of 8 litres per minute.

Nasal cannulae (double nasal cannulae inserted into the nostrils)

Advantages
   - Do not permit the rebreathing of carbon dioxide.
   - Are well tolerated and do not interfere with speech, etc.

Disadvantages
   - Produces unpredictable oxygen levels, but at a flow rate of 2 litres per minute gives about 30% oxygen.
   - May be irritant at high flow rates, and there is a risk of gastric distension.
   - Can be difficult to keep attached to the patient in field conditions.

CONCLUSION
   - Not often used in Immediate Care.

PRACTICAL POINT: Oxygen supports combustion, and so should be kept away from naked flames, cigarettes, and cutting equipment in use.

Advanced airway care (use of an artificial aid/appliance to maintain the airway)

Introduction

- Effective airway care is the first priority in the care of the seriously ill or injured patient, for without a patent airway the patient will die in minutes.
- In addition to the airway itself, the possibility of a cervical spine injury should *always* be borne in mind especially if the patient is unconscious following an injury above the chest, and the neck handled with appropriate care.

Simple airways

Oropharyngeal airway (Guedel)

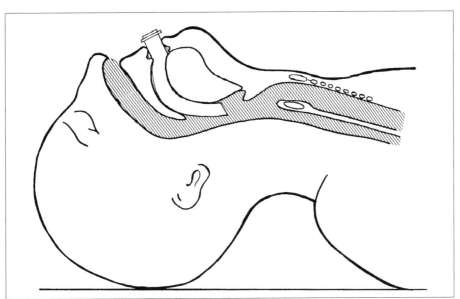

Figure 3-2 Oropharyngeal airway (the head and neck should NOT be hyperextended if injury to the cervical spine is a possibility, but stabilised with in-line immobilisation)

Indications
- It improves airway patency in the unconscious patient by preventing the tongue falling backwards and obstructing the airway.

Disadvantages
- May cause oropharyngeal stimulation and vomiting unless the patient is deeply unconscious.
- If too long, may impunge on the epiglottis and bend it over the laryngeal opening.
- If too short, may not support the tongue.

Sizes
- 00 - infant   0 - small child   1 - child   2 - small adult   3 - medium adult   4 - large adult

PRACTICAL POINT: The correct length for an airway is the same distance as that from the corner of the mouth to the ear lobe.

Method of insertion
- Invert the device and insert it into the mouth turning it through 180° as the end of it passes under the palate and into the oropharynx (except in infants/small children, when it should be inserted the right way up under direct vision).
- May require supplementary jaw support.

Nasopharyngeal airway

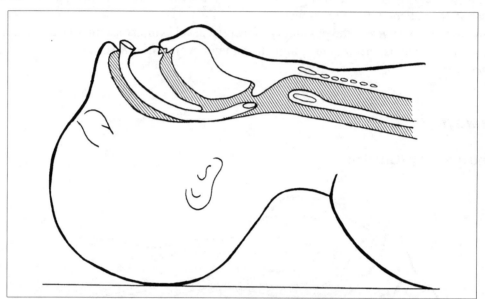

Figure 3-3 Nasal airway (the head and neck should NOT be hyperextended if injury to the cervical spine is a possibility, but stabilised with in-line cervical immobilisation)

Indications
- Patients who do not tolerate an oropharyngeal airway.
- Severe faciomaxillary injury.
- Trismus (clenched jaw).

Disadvantages
- May cause haemorrhage from the nasopharynx.
- Should not be used in patients with a known or suspected anterior fractured base of skull.

Sizes
- Female: 6.0 mm.   Male: 7.0 mm.

Method of insertion
- Prepare the device by putting a safety pin through the proximal end to prevent it being lost inside the nose and lubricate it well.
- Carefully insert the device into the right nostril, parallel to the palate.
- If resistance is experienced, withdraw the device and try the left nostril.

PRACTICAL POINT: If no nasopharyngeal airway is available: a size 6 or 7 endotracheal tube may be used instead. It should be cut to length and a safety pin inserted through the proximal end.

Linder balloon

- This is a development of the nasopharyngeal airway, but uses a soft deflatable introducer, which is less likely to cause nasopharyngeal trauma and resultant haemorrhage.

Ventilation airways

- Combine airway support and ventilation ability.

Requirements
- It should:
    - Provide adequate tongue support
    - Provide a mouth seal
    - Have provision for rescuer protection/isolation with a valve for expired gas
    - Have a facility for ventilation, with a minimum lumen diameter of 6 mm
    - Be very portable: small, lightweight and easily pocketed
    - Be inexpensive
    - Be easy to assemble and use.

SALAD/Safar airway

- Two Guedel airways connected back to back.
- Provides adequate tongue support.
- Does not provide rescuer protection in the form of either a mouth seal or airway isolation.

Brook airway

- Simple model: has no tongue support.
- Professional model: has a tongue support.

Advantage
- Provides expired air protection.

Disadvantage
- Rather bulky, has no mouth seal, low tidal volume.

CONCLUSION: used to be the device of choice for the professional rescuer.

Vent Easy airway

- A mask with valves, but it has no tongue support, and is rather bulky.

Lifeway airway

- Basically a modified Brook airway.

Sussex airway

- An oral tube with valves.

Advantage
- It provides tongue support, and the rescuer does not have to remove his mouth from the device to inhale.

Disadvantage
- It is rather bulky.

Modified pharyngeal and laryngeal airways

Pharyngeal tracheal lumen airway (PTLA)

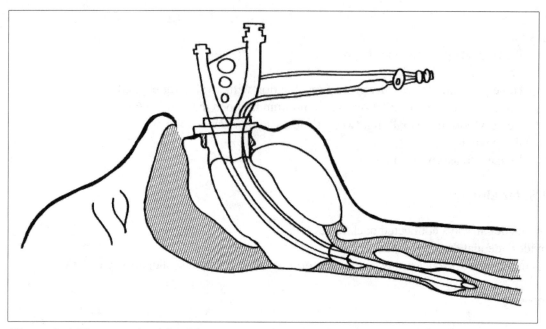

Figure 3-4 Pharyngeal tracheal lumen airway (the head and neck should NOT be hyperextended if injury to the cervical spine is a possibility, but stabilised with in-line immobilisation)

Description
-   The PTLA consists of two parallel tubes of differing length, held together by a length of moulded semi rigid plastic, which conforms to the shape of the oropharynx.
-   The shorter tube has a large inflatable cuff proximal to its distal end, while the longer tube has a smaller inflatable cuff at its distal end. These cuffs are high volume, low pressure and are inflated via a single air entry port, with a one way valve and a universal connector. Air can be directed selectively to either cuff with the aid of a slide clamp on the air inlet to the longer tube.

Indications
-   Requirement for ventilation/ airway protection in the presence of a cervical spine injury.
-   Difficult access to an unconscious patient with an obstructed/unprotected airway, e.g. trapped, sitting up in a vehicle.
-   When the operator is not trained/experienced in endotracheal intubation.

Method of insertion
-   Lift the jaw: there is no need to move the neck.
-   Insert the device with its curvature following the natural curve of the oropharynx, until the tooth guard is reached.
-   If resistance is met: The device should be withdrawn and reinserted.
-   Inflate the cuffs by first blowing air into the cuff air entry port, and then into the short tube, following which check for breath sounds and chest expansion.
-   If ventilation is satisfactory:
     - Attach a bag or ventilator to the short tube.
-   If air does not enter the lungs:
     - Remove the stylet from the long tube, blow air down the long tube, and check for breath sounds/ chest expansion.

- If ventilation is satisfactory:
    - Attach a bag or ventilator to the long tube.
- If air still does not enter the lungs:
    - Look for airway obstruction.
- Secure the device with the neck strap.
- Once the device is in position:
    - Check for air leaks continually especially if the long tube is in the oesophagus.
- If a leak does occur:
    - Clamp the long tube, and reinflate the oral cuff until the leak is controlled.

Advantages
- Easy to use.
- Rapid insertion is possible, without the need for instrumentation.
- Neck movement is unnecessary.
- Controlled ventilation is possible.

Disadvantages
- The tube is of fixed length, and care has to taken using the device in very small or very large adults.
- Airway obstruction may occur with the longer tube in the oesophagus.

CONCLUSION
- Gaining increasing acceptance for use in Immediate Care, but is a bit complicated to use initially.

Laryngeal mask airway (LMA): Brain airway

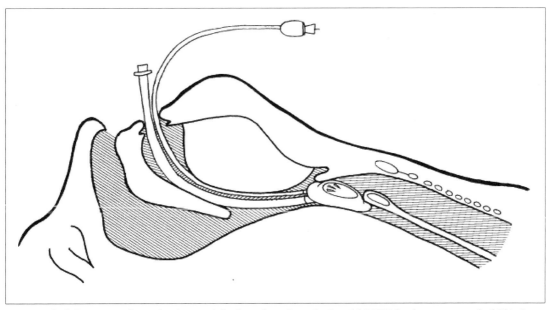

Figure 3-5 Laryngeal mask airway (the head and neck should NOT be hyperextended if injury to the cervical spine is a possibility, but stabilised with in-line immobilisation)

Description
- The LMA consists of an oropharyngeal tube inserted into the upper end of a spoon shaped mask through a perforated window.
- The mask is surrounded by an inflatable cuff, which forms a seal around the larynx when it is adequately inflated.

Indications
- Requirement for ventilation in the presence of a cervical spine injury.
- Facial injuries and supraglottic trauma, where use of a face mask is difficult.
- When endotracheal intubation is not possible due to the shape of the patient's neck/larynx.
- When the operator is not trained/experienced in endotracheal intubation.

Sizes
- Children: 1, 2
- Average adult female: 3
- Average adult male: 4

Method of application
- Prior to insertion, prepare the mask by actively deflating it (by sucking it flat with a syringe).
- Insert the mask over the teeth, and carefully push it down over the middle of the back of the tongue.
- Then push it further down the oropharynx, until the tip comes to rest in the triangular shaped hypopharynx (further insertion is not possible unless excessive force is used). This signifies a definite end point which indicates correct placement of the mask around the laryngeal outlet.
- Inflate the cuff with 20-30 mls of air through the pilot tube, which isolates the larynx from the rest of the pharyngeal space.
- Correct placement may be accompanied by slight bulging of the soft tissues at the front of the neck.

Advantages
- Easy to insert: the technique is simple and is much less traumatic than endotracheal intubation, and does not require laryngoscopy.
- It allows controlled ventilation, provided inflation pressures below 20 cm of water are sufficient.
- It requires minimum cervical movement for insertion.
- It can be inserted with the operator sitting in front of the patient.
- The mouth needs to be opened less than for endotracheal intubation.
- It is particularly useful in patients with "bull necks".

Disadvantages
- Leaking may occur around the cuff when using ventilatory pressures greater than 20 cm of water.
- There is a risk of gastric aspiration, especially in those patients in whom the mask does not seal the hypopharynx precisely.
- Easily dislodged.

CONCLUSION
- Potentially useful; the risk of aspiration makes its use inadvisable at present, except possibly in the sitting trapped patient in whom access does not allow intubation.

Endotracheal tube

- A tube with an inflatable cuff near its distal end is inserted through the vocal cords and into the trachea.

Advantages
- Provides a patent and secure airway, through which effective positive pressure ventilation can be applied.
- Protects the airway from aspiration of foreign material.
- Allows access for tracheal suction.
- Allows release of skilled medical staff for other tasks.

Disadvantages
- It is difficult for the inexperienced to perform.
- It requires anaesthesia in the conscious patient, e.g. in severe facial burns.
- There is a danger of:
    - Local trauma during insertion
    - Aspiration during insertion
    - Intubating the right main bronchus
    - Oesophageal intubation.

Indications
- Apnoea
- Upper airway obstruction
- Respiratory insufficiency
- Risk of gastric regurgitation or blood entering the lungs
- Raised intracranial pressure requiring hyperventilation
- Risk of airway compromise, e.g. after facial burns, continuous fitting inspite of administration of intravenous diazepam.

Tube sizes (external diameter)
- Approximately the size of the little finger.
- Adults: Male 9.00 mm
       Female 8.00 mm.

Tube length:
- Twice the length from the corner of the mouth to the tip of the ear lobe.
- Adults: Males: approximately 23 cm.
       Females: approximately 21 cm.

Endotracheal intubation: essential equipment

Laryngoscopes
- Usually have detachable blades:
    - Straight blade: probably better for the intubation of infants and small children.
    - Curved blade: better for adults.
- Illumination may be:
    - Bulb in the blade.
    - Fibre optic lighting system (better as the light source is brighter and less bulky).

Syringe
- For inflating the cuff (5-10 ml).

Lubricant
-   For lubricating the tube.

Magill's forceps (not often used in Immediate Care).
-   For manipulating the endotracheal tube through the cords or removing objects obstructing the airway.

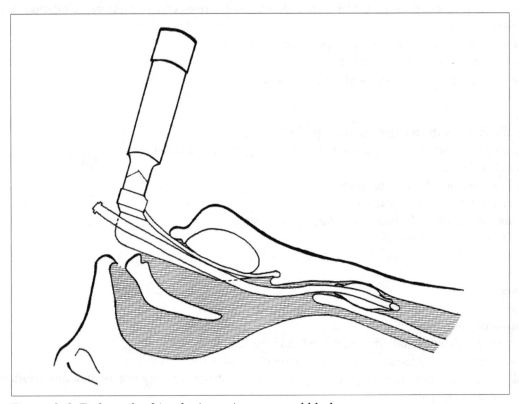

Figure 3-6 Endotracheal intubation using a curved blade

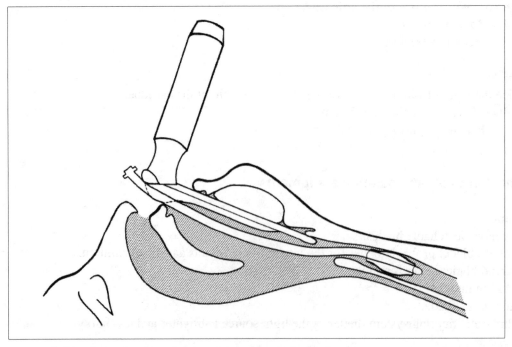

Figure 3-7 Endotracheal intubation using a straight blade

Endotracheal intubation: method of insertion

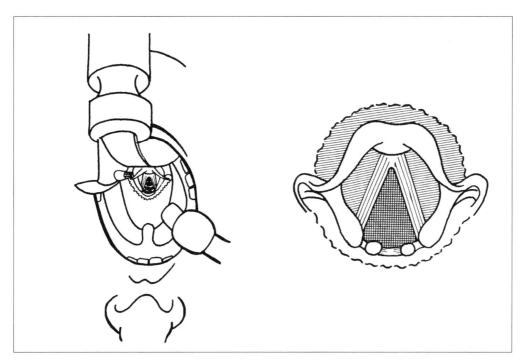

Figure 3-8 Endotracheal intubation 1: Visualise the larynx

- Assemble the equipment and make certain there is an appropriately sized tube cut to the correct length.

PRACTICAL POINT: Always pre-cut and pre-assemble tubes ready for immediate use.

- Always pre-oxygenate the patient.
- Position the patient correctly: with cervical flexion and head extension (sniffing the morning air), unless the patient has a possible cervical spine injury, when all neck movement should be avoided.
- Holding the laryngoscope in the left hand, insert the blade into the right side of the mouth, making sure that the lower lip is not trapped between the blade and lower teeth.
- Advance the tip of the blade, aiming it towards the larynx in the midline, displacing the right side of the tongue to the left as you do so.
- Lift the laryngoscope handle upwards and forwards, slide the tip of the curved blade laryngoscope into the space between the base of the tongue and the root of the epiglottis, maintaining the position of the patient's head with your right hand as you do so. (If you are using a straight bladed laryngoscope, the tip of the blade should be placed below the epiglottis.)
- Be careful not to press the laryngoscope blade against the patient's teeth, as this can result in damage to them.
- Visualise the larynx, adjusting the position of the blade, so as to obtain the best view. Thyroid pressure may make the larynx easier to see, especially if neck movement is contraindicated.
- Insert a lubricated endotracheal tube into the right hand corner of the patient's mouth, and pass it through the vocal cords under direct vision.
- Continue inserting the tube until the cuff has completely passed through the vocal cords.
- Inflate the cuff with air using a syringe attached to the cuff port, and apply positive pressure ventilation, checking for air leaks as you do so. Cease inflating the cuff when the sound of leaking air disappears. If this does not happen after fully inflating the cuff, check that the tube has not been misplaced in the oesophagus, under direct vision.
- Ventilate the patient using the tube, making certain that it is correctly placed by checking for chest expansion and air entry into both sides of the lungs.
- Secure the tube with tape.

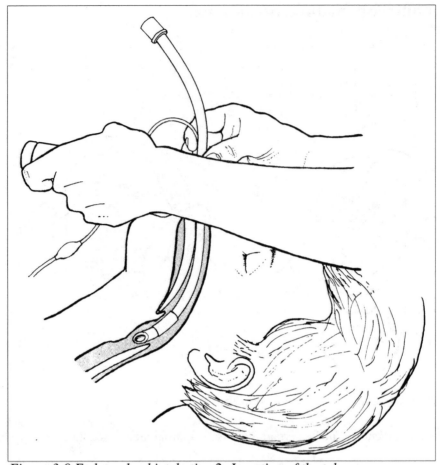

Figure 3-9 Endotracheal intubation 2: Insertion of the tube

Note: - This procedure should take no longer than 30 seconds in the apnoeic patient. If you have not been successful within this time, ventilate the patient for a few minutes with oxygen, before trying again.

PRACTICAL POINT: If endotracheal intubation is difficult: pass a laryngeal mask airway. Ensure that there is lung inflation and then pass a bougie, following which remove the LMA, and pass the endotracheal tube down over the bougie. Check satisfactory placement (see above).

Endotracheal intubation: useful equipment

Gum elastic bougie
- This is passed down through the cords before passing the endotracheal tube, which is then passed down over it.
- Useful for inexperienced intubators and if laryngeal oedema is present.

Light wand
- A stylet with a light source at its tip used as an aid to endotracheal intubation.

End tidal CO_2 monitor

- This is a device which detects and measures the amount of carbon dioxide in the patient's expired gases (end tidal CO_2). The sampling part of the device is attached between the connector of the endotracheal tube and the catheter mount.
- It gives an indication as to whether the tube is in the oesophagus or trachea.

- There are two types of device:
    - Disposable monitor:
        - This uses a chemical pH indicator to detect the presence of carbon dioxide.
        - The colour varies from mauve, indicating a CO_2 level of <0.5% (inspiration), to yellow, indicating a CO_2 level of 2-5% (expiration).
    - Electronic device.

Problems
- Little or no CO_2 may be produced during cardiac arrest.
- Disposable monitor:
    - Gastric acid contamination causes a permanent orange colour.
    - Endotracheal lignocaine or adrenaline will cause a permanent yellow colour.
    - May not work when it is very cold.
- Electronic device:
    - Expensive
    - Relatively heavy and bulky.

CONCLUSION
- Useful devices when conditions make assessment of the correct placement of the tube difficult.
- Provides a simple and non invasive method of measuring blood flow during resuscitation, and can indicate the return of spontaneous circulation.

Sellick's manoeuvre
- Cricoid pressure to protect the airway from gastric regurgitation.

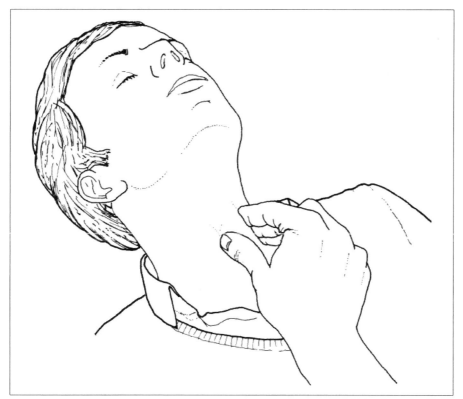

Figure 3-10 Sellick's manoeuvre

Method
- Apply continual downward pressure to the cricoid cartilage with the thumb and index finger of one hand, whilst exerting counter pressure to the back of the neck.

Endotracheal intubation: alternative methods

Blind digital intubation

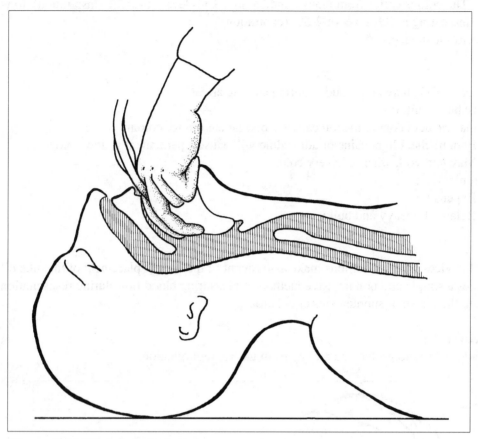

Figure 3-11 Blind digital intubation

Indications
- When intubation using a laryngoscope is not possible, because of the patient's position, e.g. trapped, sitting upright in a vehicle.

Method of insertion from the front
- May only be used in the deeply unconscious patient.
- The endotracheal tube should be lubricated with gel, a gum elastic bougie inserted into it, and made into a "J" shape.
- Place yourself on the patient's right side, facing towards their head. Put the right index and middle fingers into the right corner of the patient's mouth, holding back the tongue.
- Move your fingers along the lower border of the teeth until they reach the back of the tongue.
- Insert the tube, guiding it down between your fingers, and manoeuvre it just behind the epiglottis before slipping it into the larynx.
- Once the tube is in place, withdraw the bougie, and inflate the cuff to confirm correct placement of the tube.

CONCLUSION: Requires practice (and long fingers) and is *rarely used* in Immediate Care.

Nasotracheal intubation

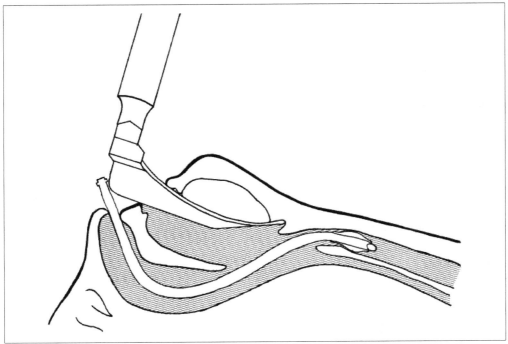

Figure 3-12 Nasotracheal intubation

Indications
- When intubation is indicated but the patient has a potential cervical spine injury and orotracheal intubation is not possible, e.g. in certain maxillo-facial injuries, or there is an abnormal anatomical configuration, e.g. in ankylosing spondylitis. (should *not* be used if there is a basal skull fracture).

Disadvantages
- Relatively difficult to perform.
- Risk of causing nasal haemorrhage.
- Possibility of introducing infection from the upper (nasal) to the lower respiratory tract.

Tube size
- 1 mm smaller than that used for normal intubation.

Method of application
- Spontaneous respiration is necessary if the tube is to be passed successfully without a laryngoscope.
- Lubricate the tube with gel.
- If possible try to position the head and neck in the clear airway position, by applying gentle pressure to the occiput.
- Insert the tube through the right nostril and gently push it backwards in a straight line. If resistance is met, try the left nostril.
- Continue inserting the tube, until it enters the nasopharynx, and try to manipulate it through the glottis into the trachea, if necessary using a laryngoscope to obtain direct vision.
- If difficulty is experienced with insertion of the tube into the larynx, tracheal displacement and direct manipulation using Magill's forceps may help.
- Once the tube is in place, inflate the cuff to confirm the correct placement of the tube.
- If the patient is breathing spontaneously, correct placement is indicated by the presence of breath sounds.

CONCLUSION: Not often used in Immediate Care.

Airway obstruction: surgical management

Aetiology

- Trauma:
    - Severe faciomaxillary injury resulting in:
        - Tongue displacement
        - Gross retroposition of the middle third of the maxilla
        - Actual or potential oedema of the pharynx or glottis
        - Uncontrollable oronasopharyngeal haemorrhage, e.g. from the lingual artery.
    - Laryngeal injury.
    - Blast, burn or missile injury to the face.

- Infection:
    - Larynx or epiglottis (epiglottitis).

- Physical obstruction:
    - Foreign body: Incompletely chewed food, children's toy, soft tissue swelling of neck, etc.

- Allergy:
    - Acute laryngeal oedema, e.g. insect stings, drug anaphylaxis.

Management

Cricothyrotomy

- Minimum lumen for prolonged effective spontaneous ventilation: 6.0 mm.
- Assisted ventilation by a bag or ventilator may be effective with a smaller lumen.

Advantages
- It is a rapid and safe procedure in trained hands.
- The anatomical landmarks in the adult are usually easy to identify.
- There is little danger of causing oesophageal damage.
- There are rarely any overlying veins, thyroid isthmus, muscles, or calcification to cause problems.

Disadvantages
- It may cause haemorrhage within the airway.
- It may result in trauma to the posterior laryngeal wall.
- There is a risk of faulty placement of the tube in the subcutaneous tissues.
- The procedure should not be performed in infants unless the situation is desperate, because the larynx/trachea is soft.

Complications
- Asphyxia
- Aspiration
- Cellulitis
- Oesophageal perforation
- Haemorrhage
- Perforation of the posterior tracheal wall.

Cricothyrotomy devices

Needle cricothyrotomy (using a 12 or 14 gauge intravenous cannula).

- Can give temporary oxygenation and ventilation, if placed through the cricothyroid membrane, using a flow rate of 15 litres of oxygen per minute.

Method
- With the patient in the supine position (if possible), extend the neck, palpate the larynx and identify the cricothyroid membrane.
- Attach the cannula to a 5-10 ml syringe, and pierce the skin directly over the membrane in the midline.
- Direct the needle towards the feet at an angle of 45°.
- Carefully insert the needle through the lower part of the cricothyroid membrane, withdrawing the plunger on the syringe as you do so.
- Aspiration of air indicates entry into the trachea.
- Continue to insert the needle, being careful not to perforate the posterior wall, withdrawing the stylet as you do so.
- Attach the tube to an adaptor and "Y" piece, and oxygen tubing.
- Ventilate the patient to ensure its correct placement.
- Secure the needle with tape and adjust the oxygen flow rate to 15 l/min.

Ventilation
- The patient may be ventilated by placing a thumb over the open end of the "Y" piece, using a rhythm of 1 second on to 4 seconds off.

Note: - Using this method, a patient can be adequately oxygenated for only 10-15 minutes.
- It is essential that the larynx is patent, so exhalation can occur through the mouth or nose.

CONCLUSION: Method of choice for children.

Mini Trach II

- Originally developed for the treatment of post-operative sputum retention.

Method
- Position yourself at the head of the patient, with the patient in the supine position (if possible) and extend the neck.
- Palpate the larynx and identify the cricothyroid membrane.
- Stretch the skin over the cricothyroid membrane with the thumb and index finger of the left hand and, holding the guarded scalpel in the right hand with the blade pointing towards the patient's feet, incise the skin and cricothyroid membrane vertically in the midline up to the guard.
- Withdraw and discard the scalpel, and without moving the fingers of the left hand, take the introducer and insert it through the stab incision and into the trachea.
- With the end of the introducer well inserted into the trachea, pass the cannula over the introducer and into the trachea.
- Hold the flange in place against the skin and withdraw the introducer.
- Ventilate the patient using the device, to check that it is correctly positioned.
- Secure the device with the neck tapes.

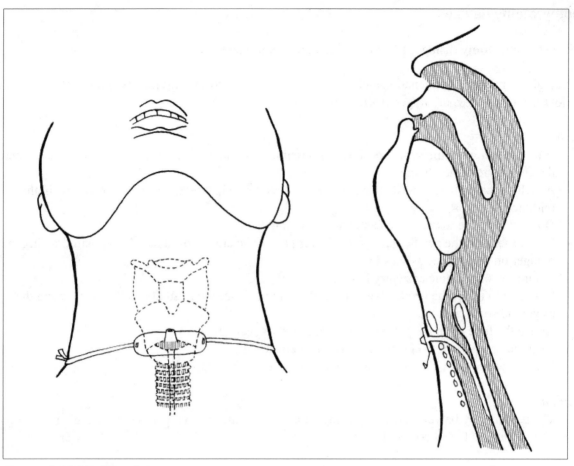

Figure 3-13 Mini Trach II

Complications
- As for needle cricothyrotomy, but there is less risk of damaging the posterior pharyngeal wall, as the scalpel has a guard which prevents the blade being inserted too far.
- Malpositioning in the tissues of the neck, especially if the left hand is released and the tissue alignment is lost.

CONCLUSION: Possibly the *device of choice* in Immediate Care, but the 4 mm tube usually suffices to give *only temporary relief.*
Not for use in children.

Quicktrach

- A new curved cricothyrotomy device, incorporating a syringe.
- Available in two sizes:
    - Adult: 4 mm.
    - Paediatric: 2 mm.

Method
- Assemble the device by attaching the syringe to the Quicktrach, making certain that the depth gauge and the red markers are adjacent to each other.
- Position the patient in the supine position (if possible) and extend the neck slightly.
- Palpate the larynx and identify the cricothyroid membrane.

- Hold the device vertically by the syringe.
- Puncture the skin overlying the cricothyroid membrane in the midline with the Quicktrach, gently withdrawing the plunger as you do so.
- Move the syringe so that it makes an angle of 45° to the horizontal and continue insertion. The device is in the trachea when air enters the syringe freely.
- Continue inserting the device until the depth gauge is reached.
- Remove the depth gauge, holding the the needle firmly by the syringe, and slide the cannula down over the needle until the hub of the cannula is reached.
- Withdraw the syringe and attached needle, and ventilate the patient via the device to confirm that it is correctly positioned.
- Secure the device with the neck tape provided.

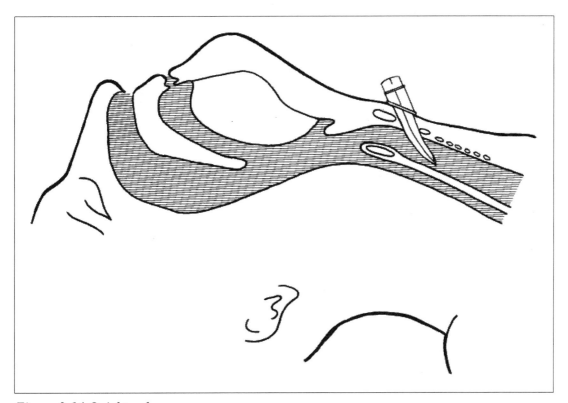

Figure 3-14 Quicktrach

Complications
- As needle cricothyrotomy.

CONCLUSION
- A new device, whose use in Immediate Care has not yet been evaluated.
- Not suitable for long term ventilation as the lumen is only 4 mm.

Nutrach

- A new device similar to the Quicktrach, but it also incorporates a set of trochar dilators, of increasing diameter. These are used to dilate the opening in the cricothyroid membrane, until finally a tube of 6.0-6.5 mm diameter can be placed in the trachea.

CONCLUSION:
- Possibly the device of choice in Immediate Care, as it allows satisfactory long term ventilation.

Small tracheotomy tube (surgical cricothyrotomy).

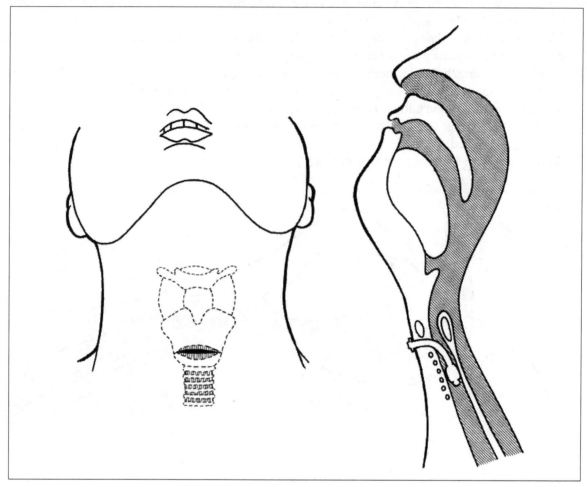

Figure 3-15 Surgical cricothyrotomy

Method
- With the patient in the supine position (if possible), palpate the larynx and identify the cricothyroid membrane.
- Stabilise the thyroid cartilage with the left hand, and with a scalpel in the right hand, incise the skin and underlying membrane horizontally, over the lower half of the membrane.
- Insert the scalpel handle (or ideally tracheal dilators if available) through the incision and rotate it through 90° to enlarge the opening.
- Insert a small tracheotomy tube through the opening, inflate the cuff and ventilate the patient.
- Auscultate the chest to confirm correct placement of the tube.
- Secure the device in place with neck tapes.

Complications
- As needle cricothyrotomy, with the addition of:
    - Creation of a false passage in the tissues
    - Subglottic/laryngeal stenosis
    - Mediastinal emphysema
    - Vocal cord damage: hoarseness, paralysis.

CONCLUSION
- Can give adequate ventilation and oxygenation, and should be seriously considered in Immediate Care.

Tracheotomy

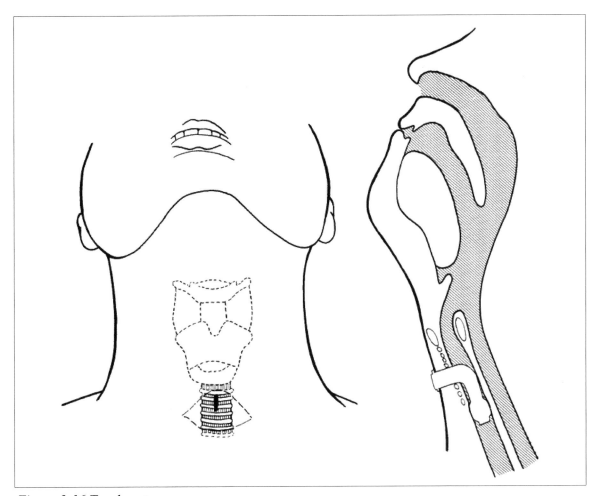

Figure 3-16 Tracheostomy

- Should not really be considered as an emergency procedure; cricothyrotomy is preferable.

Indications
- As cricothyrotomy.

Method
- Make a vertical incision from the cricoid cartilage to just below the thyroid isthmus.
- Divide the second to fourth tracheal rings.
- Insert tracheal dilators.
- Insert the tube.

Airway management devices

Suction equipment

- This is a vital piece of equipment for resuscitation which is used to clear the oropharynx of: blood, saliva, vomit and other secretions.

Requirements

- They should have:
  - The ability to exert an adequate vacuum and flow rate to enable the effective and rapid removal of both liquid and semisolid material
  - A container of adequate size or an overflow for aspirated matter
  - The facility for the easy attachment of a suction catheter or Yankauer sucker
  - An integral power source.
- They should be:
  - Lightweight, portable and easy to use
  - Easy to dismantle for cleaning and maintenance and reassemble without error
  - Reliable and robust.
- In the prehospital situation, they may be:
  - Hand powered:
    - *Advantage*
      - Lightweight.
    - *Disadvantages*
      - Requires the operator both to power the device and manipulate the suction tip with the same hand, and may therefore be difficult to control accurately.
      - When full, may overflow over the operator's hands.
  - Foot powered:
    - *Advantage*
      - Allows hands free operation.
    - *Disadvantages*
      - May be difficult to operate on uneven ground or in a moving vehicle.
      - Fairly heavy.
  - Electrically (battery) powered:
    - *Advantage*
      - Allows hands free operation.
    - *Disadvantages*
      - Relatively heavy and bulky.
      - The battery has a limited useful life.
  - Gas powered: Usually powered by the oxygen cylinder connected to a ventilator.
    - *Advantage*
      - Very effective.
    - *Disadvantage*
      - Uses up a considerable amount of oxygen.

Suction tips

- There are two basic types:
  - Yankauer:
    - Rigid, only used for sucking out the upper airway.
  - Soft:
    - Flexible (not recommended for use in Immediate Care).

Breathing (ventilation)

Introduction

- Once the airway has been secured, attention should be paid to the patient's breathing, and the chest examined.
- The maintenance of adequate ventilatory support is essential for the successful resuscitation of the severely ill and injured.

Symptoms/signs

- Expose the chest completely and evaluate the patient's breathing by:
    - Observing their respiratory movement and quality of respiration
    - Palpating the chest wall
    - Auscultation.
- In particular look for:
    - Intercostal and supraclavicular muscle retraction
    - The signs of chest injury
    - Evidence of impending hypoxia (often subtle and difficult to detect):
        - An increase in respiratory rate
        - A change in the breathing pattern, with respiration usually becoming more shallow.

Management

Severe spontaneous pneumothorax
- Needle decompression

See chapter on
Chest Injuries

Tension pnemothorax
Open pneumothorax
Massive Haemothorax

Flail chest
- Assisted ventilation.

Assisted ventilation

Indications

- Hypoxia
- Apnoea
- Excessive respiratory work
- Ventilatory insufficiency
- In severely head injured patients to prevent hypoxia.

Expired air ventilation

- May be:
    - Mouth to mouth } described under Basic Life Support.
    - Mouth to nose
    - Mouth to mask, e.g. pocket mask
    - Mouth to tube.
- In small children: mouth to mouth and nose.

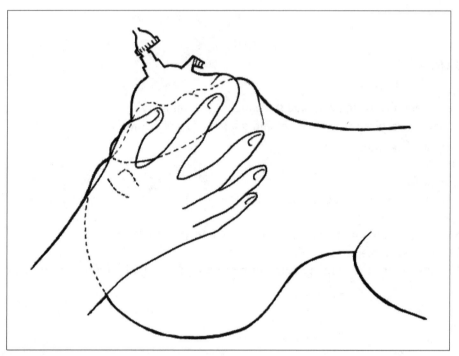

Figure 3-17 Pocket mask

Air ventilation

- Resuscitation bag/mask: bag, valve and mask (a Guedel airway may or may not be inserted first).
- Resuscitation bag/tube: bag, valve and cricothyrotomy device or endotracheal tube.

Resuscitation bag

- A self inflating bag with two one-way valves, which can be connected at one end to a mask or airway, and at the other an oxygen reservoir with inlet.

Advantage
- Provides a higher inspired oxygen concentration than expired air ventilation.

Disadvantage
- Can be a difficult technique to perform and is is usually less effective if performed unassisted.

Supplemental oxygen

Pocket mask (Laerdal) with oxygen inlet:
- Probably the best device available at present to supplement the inspired oxygen concentration with expired air ventilation.
- Delivers up to 55% Oxygen with flow rates of 8-10 litres per minute.

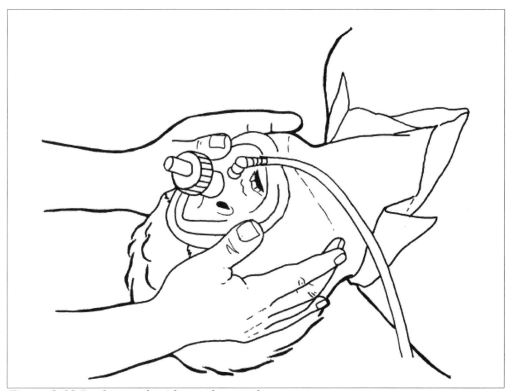

Figure 3-18 Pocket mask with supplemental oxygen

Bag/valve/mask (Laerdal/Ambu):
- Use of an oxygen mask with rebreathing reservoir can increase the concentration of inspired oxygen up to 90%, with oxygen flow rates of 8-10 litres per minute.

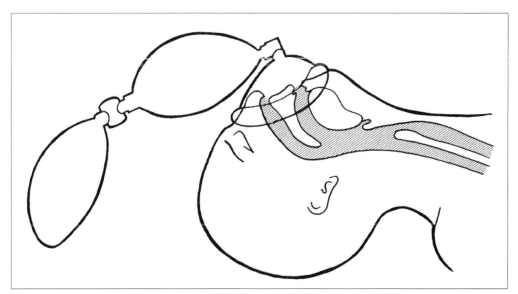

Figure 3-19 Bag and mask with oxygen reservoir

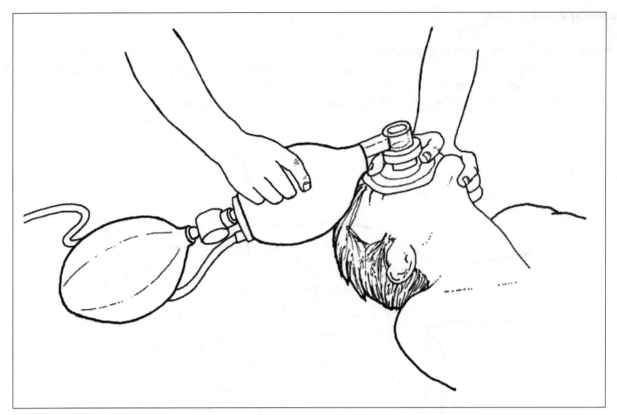

Figure 3-20 Bag and mask, showing hand positions

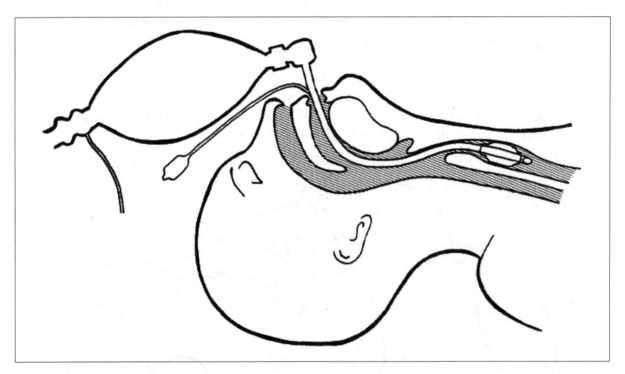

Figure 3-21 Bag and endotracheal tube

Mechanical ventilation

Manually triggered oxygen powered ventilators

- These devices have a high pressure oxygen supply attached to a manually triggered valve which when open inflates the lungs via a face mask or ventilation tube.
- Most devices incorporate a demand valve which allows the patient to breathe spontaneously when able to do so.

Advantage
- Both hands can be used to provide jaw support and apply the mask to the face, whilst lung inflation is triggered by a thumb.

Disadvantage
- They lack the "feel" that allows the trained operator to judge when lung inflation is complete or gastric inflation is occurring.

Automatic oxygen powered ventilators

- Most modern automatic ventilators used in Immediate Care can be used in either the manually triggered or the automatic mode, and may have a straight oxygen therapy facility.
- They are similar to the manual models, but have a mechanism which allows automatic ventilation.
- Usually function best when connected to a ventilation tube, i.e. endotracheal tube, PTLA, laryngeal mask airway, etc.

Requirements
- They should be:
    - Robust, reliable and require little or no maintenance
    - Lightweight, portable and easy to use
    - Self powered: usually by oxygen, ideally with air entrainment.
- They should:
    - Enable the patient who is being ventilated to trigger their own respirations, and recommence ventilation, if spontaneous breathing ceases
    - Give an audible warning of high inflation pressures (airway obstruction)
    - Provide differing tidal volumes, and rates of ventilation depending on patient size
    - Have controls situated near the patient's airway.
- An oxygen powered suction facility is also useful, but may significantly reduce the time the ventilator can be used.

Advantage
- As the manually triggered models, and if connected to a ventilation tube, it also allows hands free operation.

Disadvantages
- As the manually triggered models:
    - They are inclined to cause gastric distension if not carefully adjusted and controlled.
- Limited life of oxygen cylinders.

Oxygen cylinders

Identification

- Black cylinder with a white collar and neck.

Sizes and capacity of oxygen cylinders

Size	Capacity (litres)	Duration at 8 l/min
C	170	20 (minutes)
D	340	40
E	680	80
F	1360	160
G	3400	400

- Size C is the most portable and may fit into a carrying case for use at the scene of an incident.
- Size D is used in portable ventilators.
- Sizes C and D have an integral contents guage and can be recharged from larger cylinders using a charging valve.
- Sizes E, F and G are not readily transportable, due to their weight and size.
- Other sizes may be available, e.g.; 125, 230, and 370 litres.
- Modern cylinders are made of aluminium and are lighter than older metal cylinders.

Flow rates

- Fixed at 6, 8, 10 or 15 litres per minute.
- Variable: 2, 4, 6, 8, and 10 litres per minute.

Duration
- Cylinder capacity in litres divided by flow setting.

Maintenance
- All cylinders need to be retested ever 5 years after the date stamped on the neck of the cylinder.

CAUTION: Do not use oil to lubricate any part of the oxygen regulator valve as an oil/oxygen mixture is explosive.

4

Circulation care: shock

Circulation care: shock

Introduction

- The prevention and active management of the various types of shock, especially hypovolaemic shock, is one of those procedures, which should be performed as early as possible by those involved with the Immediate Care of the patient. It is therefore one of the most useful procedures that can be performed in the pre-hospital situation.

Definition

- Shock may be defined as "a reduction in the effective circulating blood volume, resulting in an inadequate supply of oxygen and nutrients to cells, tissues and organs, and inadequate removal of waste products". It can arise from a variety of causes:

Hypovolaemic shock
- Occurs as a result of a reduction in the circulating blood volume, e.g. as a result of haemorrhage, dehydration (prolonged vomiting, diarrhoea or heatstroke) and burns.

Cardiogenic shock
- This is caused by pump (cardiac) failure, e.g. as a result of acute myocardial infarction (only rarely associated with injury), electrocution, tension pneumothorax, myocardial contusion, cardiac tamponade, or air embolism.

Neurogenic shock
- This is caused by stimulation of the autonomic nervous system, resulting in sudden enlargement of the vascular bed, e.g. as a result of head injury, fainting or spinal cord injury.

Bacteriological shock
- This is due to cellular poisoning followed by circulatory failure, e.g. septicaemia, peritonitis.

    - **Septic shock:** Caused by Gram negative or other organisms.

    - **Toxic shock:** Caused by toxins from *Staph. aureus* or rarely by endotoxins from *Haemolytic strep.*

Anaphylactic shock
- This is caused by an acute allergic response resulting in respiratory failure, pump failure and tissue damage.

Pathophysiology

- Tissue hypoxia results in anaerobic metabolism causing an initial metabolic acidosis, which together with continuing hypoxia results in a reduction in cardiac output, and so a vicious cycle develops.
- The secondary effects of shock, which can take up to an hour to develop, include the release of various substances as a result of cellular damage-- including enzymes, kinins, hormones and complement.

Assessment

- Patient's appearance (peripheral perfusion)
    - Colour
    - Temperature.
- Measurement of the patient's:
    - Pulse rate
    - Blood pressure: systolic and diastolic (to estimate pulse pressure)
    - Capillary refill time
    - Respiratory rate
    - Pulse oximetry plethysmography: see chapter on Airway Care
    - Temperature.

Hypovolaemic shock

Incidence

- This is the commonest avoidable cause of death and morbidity following major trauma.

Aetiology

- Hypovolaemic shock may be caused by:
    - Haemorrhage
    - Oedema due to severe soft tissue injury
    - Fluid loss due to severe vomiting and/or diarrhoea.

Pathophysiology

- In haemorrhage:
    - The initial fluid loss is from the intravascular compartments.
- In oedema:
    - The initial fluid loss is from the interstitial compartment.

Physiological compensation/response

Fluid compartments
- The intravascular and interstitial compartments are normally in equilibrium with each other.
- Loss of fluid from one compartment will normally result in donation to that compartment of fluid from the other compartment.
- Intravascular fluid loss will result in depletion of the interstitial compartment by approximately 25% of the overt blood loss.

Vascular changes
  - Initially:
    - There is a reduction in the blood volume, which causes a fall in the systolic blood pressure. This in turn results in:
    - A sympathetic response resulting in release of catecholamines which cause:
        - Peripheral vasoconstriction which results in:
          - A contribution from the vascular pool of up to 1 litre
          - An increase in heart and pulse rate
          - An increase in cardiac contractility.
        - The increase in pulse rate and cardiac contractility result in an increase in myocardial oxygen demand.
    - A reduction in the venous return, which in turn results in a drop in the arterial pressure causing hypotension.
    - This arterial hypotension together with the peripheral vasoconstriction results in a reduction in tissue perfusion which with the increase in myocardial oxygen demand results in myocardial failure.
    - The reduction in tissue perfusion also results in anaerobic metabolism and a metabolic acidosis.
  - Later:
    - There is multisystem failure as sympathetic vasoconstriction ceases and the heart rate, peripheral resistance and arterial pressure fall.

Symptoms/signs

Mental state
  - This changes progressively from anxious, restless, and talkative, to aggressive, confused, drowsy and eventually unconscious (cerebral hypoxia).

Symptoms
  - Thirst (hypovolaemia).
  - Feeling cold (vasoconstriction).
  - Blurring of vision, weakness, faintness and giddiness (hypoxia and acidosis).

Skin appearance
  - Pale, cold and clammy (vasoconstriction secondary to catecholamine release).

Respiration
  - Shallow rapid respirations (hypoxia and acidosis).

Circulation
  - Tachycardia (catecholamine release).
    - Tachycardia is present when the heart (pulse) rate is more than:
      - 160 beats per minute in an infant
      - 140 beats per minute in a pre-school child
      - 120 beats per minute from school age to puberty
      - 100 beats per minute in an adult.
  - Reduced pulse pressure.
  - Reduced systolic and diastolic pressures.
  - Reduced central venous pressure (hypovolaemia and possibly myocardial insufficiency).
  - Pulse oximetry plethysmograph will show flattening of the waveform.

Urine output (not usually measured in Immediate Care): reduced (reduced renal perfusion).

Classification of hypovolaemic shock in adults

Class I haemorrhage: up to 15% (up to 750 ml)

Pathophysiology
- Blood loss of up to 750 ml is usually well tolerated and results in minimal symptoms or signs.

Symptoms/signs
- A slight tachycardia.

Fluid replacement
- Oral fluids are usually sufficient.

Class II haemorrhage: 15-30% (800-1500 ml)

Pathophysiology
- The body responds with catecholamine release.

Symptoms/signs
- Anxiety or aggression.
- A narrow pulse pressure due to a rise in the diastolic pressure (systolic pressure does not consistently fall until >30% blood volume is lost) with absent or reduced jugular venous pulses when the patient is lying flat.
- A tachycardia with a slow capillary refill (>2 sec.).

Fluid replacement
- Intravenous fluid replacement: usually a combination of crystalloid and colloid.

Capillary refill test
- Press on the skin for a few seconds. As you remove the pressure say "capillary refill" to yourself.
- If the skin is still pale at the end of this time, then the capillary refill time is prolonged (>2 sec.).

Class III haemorrhage: 30-40% (1500-2000 ml)

Pathophysiology
- The patient's compensatory mechanisms begin to fail.

Symptoms/signs
- Pallor of the face and extremities.
- Anxiousness, aggression or drowsiness.
- Shallow respiration with a marked tachypnoea.
- A marked tachycardia, with a reduction in both systolic and diastolic pressures and a weak pulse.

Fluid replacement
- Rapid fluid replacement with colloid and crystalloid followed by blood.

Class IV haemorrhage: >40% (>2000 ml)

Pathophysiology
  - This is life threatening fluid loss.

Symptoms/signs
  - Ashen complexion with cold clammy sweaty skin, especially the extremities.
  - Confusion, impaired consciousness and eventually unconsciousness, coma and death.
  - A marked tachycardia, with a profound fall in systolic and diastolic blood pressures.
  - A reduced SaO_2.

Fluid replacement
  - Rapid aggressive fluid replacement with colloid, crystalloid and blood.
  - Arrest of haemorrhage and possibly application of a pneumatic anti-shock garment (PASG).

Modifying factors

  - The patient's symptoms and signs may be modified by various factors:

Patient age
  - Relatively more severe in the very young (small blood volume) and the old (myocardial insufficiency).
  - Less severe in the young and fit who compensate for hypovolaemia very well initially (efficient catecholamine response), but may later suddenly deteriorate.

Injury severity
  - Increases if there is extensive tissue damage.

Previous medication
  - e.g. β-blockers may prevent tachycardia.

Hypothermia
  - This will exacerbate the severity of shock, and will make the patient's hypovolaemia more difficult to manage.

Pre-existing medical conditions
  - May modify the patient's response to hypovolaemia, e.g. patients with coronary artery disease may become hypotensive due to myocardial insufficiency after only modest blood loss.

Blood loss estimation

  - In acute trauma the cause of blood loss is usually obvious, but one must be aware of the potential for blood loss from internal injuries, and also from pelvic and long bone fractures.
  - Relatively minor injuries, e.g. scalp lacerations, may cause significant blood loss.

Blood loss from fractures in the first 4 hours

Pelvis: 2000 ml
Shaft of femur:1000 ml   This should be *doubled* if the fracture is compound.
Tibia: 650 ml
Ribs: 150 ml

Classification of hypovolaemic shock according to blood loss

Class of shock		I	II	III	IV
Blood loss	*(%)*	<15	15-30	30-40	>40
	Volume (ml)	<750	800-1500	1500-2000	>2000
Pulse rate (per minute)		slight tachycardia	100-120	>120 thready	>140 very thready
Blood pressure	*Systolic*	unchanged	normal	reduced	very low
	Diastolic	unchanged	raised	reduced	very low or unrecordable
Pulse pressure		normal or increased	decreased	decreased	decreased
Capillary refill		normal	>2 sec	>2 sec	undetectable
Respiratory rate (per min)		normal (14-20)	normal (20-30)	tachypnoea (30-40)	tachypnoea (>35)
Urine output (ml/hr)		>30	20-30	5-15	0-10
Extremities		normal colour	pale	pale	pale & cold
Complexion		normal	pale	pale	ashen
Mental state		alert	anxious or aggressive	anxious, aggressive or drowsy	drowsy, confused lethargic or unconscious

Management

- The aim of effective management is to maintain tissue oxygenation and restore it to normal.
- The maintenance of an adequate oxygen carrying capacity requires:
    - Normal electrolyte levels
    - Normal clotting factors
    - A normal colloid osmotic pressure
    - A packed cell volume of more than 30%.

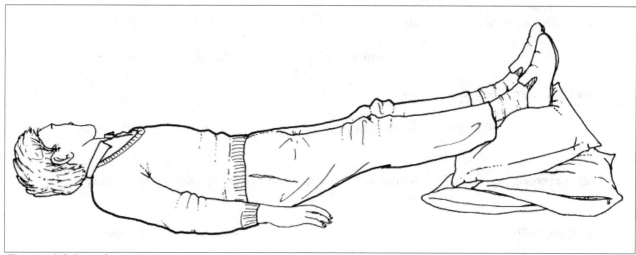

Figure 4-1 Leg elevation

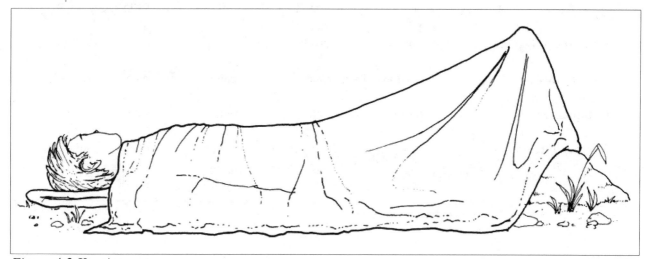

Figure 4-2 Keeping warm

Principles of management

Position
- Elevate the legs to aid the venous return.
- Make comfortable and reduce heat loss.

Airway
- Maintain an adequate airway with cervical spine control if indicated.
- Administer oxygen.

Breathing
- Maintain adequate ventilation.

Circulation
- Assess the amount of blood lost, the cause of the blood loss and the potential blood loss.
- Control the blood loss, where this is possible:
    - Limb elevation
    - Application of direct pressure with a dressing
    - Application of pressure on appropriate pressure points, e.g. femoral, popliteal.
    - Application of a tourniquet to prevent life threatening exsanguination.
- Establish intravenous access with large bore cannulae and provide adequate fluid replacement.
- Consider application of a pneumatic anti-shock garment (PASG).
- Treat the cause of the blood loss, e.g. reduction of the fracture with appropriate splinting.

Note: - The use of artery forceps/haemostats is *not* recommended, unless the bleeding point can be visualised easily.

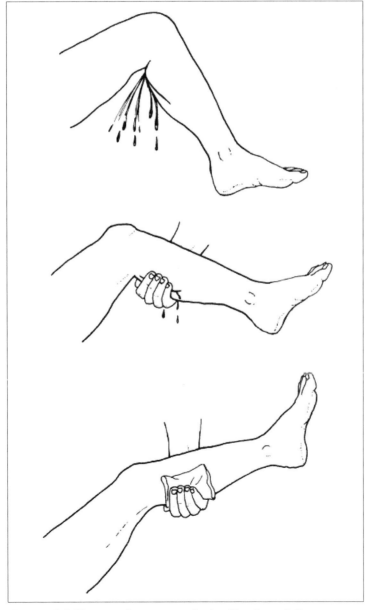

Figure 4-3 Haemorrhage control: Application of direct pressure and limb elevation

Monitoring
- Careful monitoring of the patient's:
    - Airway
    - Breathing
    - Circulation:
        - Monitor the patient's haemodynamic state: further blood loss and response to treatment.

Relief of pain (see chapter on Pain Relief)

Airway

Oxygen

- All shocked patients, especially the elderly and those with ischaemic heart disease, tolerate hypoxia badly and should be given oxygen, at as high a percentage as possible.
- In severe shock: use 100% oxygen.

Breathing

- Intubate and ventilate unconscious patients. This avoids gastric distension, which impairs effective ventilation and exacerbates shock.

Circulation

Control of blood loss

Pneumatic anti-shock garment (PASG)

- Although PASGs are widely used in the USA and several other countries, their use has not yet been generally accepted in the UK or Europe, and they are not widely available.
- They are therefore *not recommended as first line treatment* in this country at the present time.

Description
A PASG is:
- An inflatable pair of trousers, separated into different compartments:
    - One for the patient's abdomen and one for each leg.
- Usually made from radiolucent double layered polyurethane coated fabrics.
- Inflated up to 100 mmHg by a foot pump, the pressure in each compartment is indicated by a pressure gauge.

In addition:
- There is an opening in the groin to allow catheterisation, and rectal and vaginal examination without deflation.
- Each compartment is colour coded, as are the securing Velcro strips.
- Each leg can be shortened if necessary.

Mode of action
- An inflated PASG effectively transfers one and a half to two units of blood (or up to 25% of the patient's available blood volume) from the lower extremities to the upper, protecting the vital organs from the initial effects of shock.

- The exact mode of action is not fully understood but may include:
    - Reduction in the peripheral vascular capacitance/increase in the peripheral vascular resistance
    - Tamponade of bleeding vessels
    - An increase in the tone of the vascular bed
    - Autotransfusion.
- In addition it may splint lower limb and pelvic fractures reducing further blood loss and pain.

Advantages
- Reduces the initial amount of blood/fluid required to replace blood loss. This may be of particular benefit when there has been major blood loss associated with a head or chest injury, when there will be less risk of developing cerebral or pulmonary oedema secondary to large volumes of fluid infused.
- Other advantages: splinting of fractures.
- Facilitates venepuncture in the hypovolaemic patient by making the upper limb peripheral veins more prominent.

Disadvantages
- Dyspnoea may be caused by use of a PASG, which should therefore be used with caution in the patient with a chest injury or cardiac failure:
    - Management: oxygen.
- Defecation, urination and vomiting may rarely occur as a result of the raised intra-abdominal pressure
- Metabolic acidosis and compartmental syndromes have been recorded.
- There is a potential risk of puncture of the PASG from sharp objects, e.g. compound fractures, glass.

Application
- Inflate the leg compartments first and then the abdominal compartment noting the time.
- Use inflation pressures of 40-50 mmHg initially, increasing to 80 mmHg, if the systolic pressue fails to improve.

Deflation
- The garment must be deflated slowly; compartment by compartment starting with the abdominal compartment.
- This should only be performed where there are facilities for rapid blood transfusion, e.g. in an operating theatre, with two intravenous lines in place and with careful monitoring of the patient's haemodynamic state.

Indications
- Hypovolaemic shock with a systolic BP <90 mmHg, especially where the cause is haemorrhage involving the abdomen, pelvic region or lower limbs, including ruptured aortic aneurism and ruptured ectopic pregnancy.
- Neurogenic shock, e.g. spinal cord injury.
- Infective or anaphylactic shock.

Contraindications
- Absolute: None.
- Relative:
    - Head injury with a risk of raised intracranial pressure.
    - Severe chest injury, respiratory distress, cardiac failure, pulmonary oedema
    - Suspected or actual diaphragmatic rupture.

CAUTION: - Inflation of the leg compartments *only*, is advised for:
    - Pregnancy: more than 26 weeks (do *NOT* inflate abdominal compartment)
    - Abdominal evisceration or impalement.

Tourniquets

- Should only be used in: acute life threatening emergencies, e.g. sudden traumatic amputation.
- In severe crush injury application may protect the rest of the body from the toxins, i.e. potassium, myoglobin and lactic acid produced by the non-viable tissue.
- If a tourniquet is applied, the time and date of application and the name of the person applying it should be recorded.
- It is most important that the pressure exerted is sufficient to prevent arterial flow, not only when it is applied, but also when the patient's blood pressure rises to normal after resuscitation (*if too low a pressure is applied, it will act as a venous tourniquet and will make bleeding worse*).
- Should be broad (narrow tourniquets may cause permanent damage to the underlying tissues, e.g. nerves, just distal to the site of application). If only a narrow touniquet is available, apply it over padding.
- May be removed after an effective pressure bandage has been applied.

Intravenous fluid replacement

Introduction

- It is far better to infuse vigorously and prevent the onset of shock, with all its associated problems, than to wait for it to occur and then treat it.
- Two large bore cannulae, i.e. 13 to 16 gauge, should always be used, so as to provide an adequate rate of flow.
- The patient's symptoms and clinical signs can act as an aid to estimating the amount of fluid loss.

Normal blood volumes

- The blood volume of an individual is approximately 8% of their total body weight, i.e. 80 ml/kg.

Children	12 months	10 kg	800 ml
	10 years	30 kg	2400 ml
Adults	Male	70 kg	5600 ml
	Female	55 kg	4400 ml

Intravenous fluid flow rates

- These are dependent on the diameter and length of cannula, the viscosity of the fluid, and the pressure at which it is infused (pressure differential).
  - 14 gauge: 1 litre in 3 minutes.
  - 16 gauge: 1 litre in 6 minutes.
  - 18 gauge: 1 litre in 20 minutes.

- Elevation of the fluid container may increase the pressure differential and hence increase the rate of flow.

Intravenous cannulation sites

- The usual route for fluid replacement in Immediate Care is intravenous, although the intraosseous and rectal routes may be used in special circumstances, e.g. in children when intravenous cannulation is difficult.

Peripheral venous cannulation

- Peripheral veins are usually better than some central veins, e.g. subclavian, for fluid replacement in hypovolaemic shock:
    - Fewer risks
    - Easy access for the non-anaesthetist
    - Faster flow rates.
- The usual sites are:
    - The lateral cephalic vein in the wrist
    - The cephalic, median cubital, and basilic veins in the antecubital fossa
    - The long saphenous vein at the ankle.

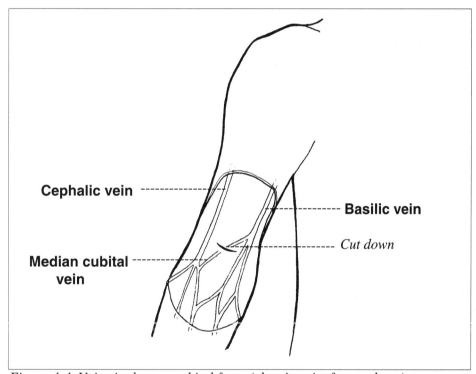

Figure 4-4 Veins in the antecubital fossa (showing site for cut down)

Venous cut down

- A cut down is rarely if ever necessary in Immediate Care, unless there is very considerable delay in initiating fluid replacement.
- The best sites are:
    - The long saphenous vein in the ankle
    - The median cephalic vein in the antecubital fossa
    - The sapheno-femoral vein in the groin.

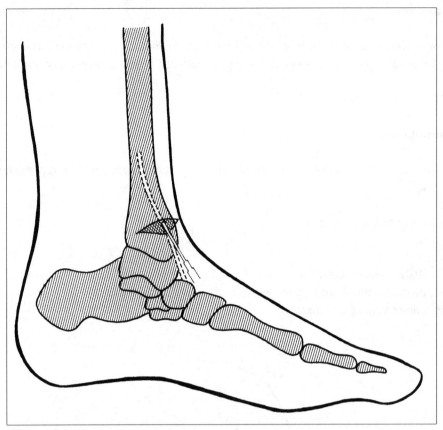

Figure 4-5 Site for long saphenous cut down

Long saphenous vein cut down

Method
- Identify the long saphenous vein, which lies just anterior to the medial malleolus at the ankle (it is not always visible).
- Cleanse the skin (if circumstances permit).
- Make a transverse incision through the skin, and using artery forceps spread the skin to display the vein which should be visible lying at right angles to the line of the incision.
- Mobilise the vein by using the forceps for blunt dissection.
- Grasp a suture with the forceps, pull it back under the vein and cut the top of the loop, so that there are two sutures, each one having one end each side of the vein. Separate these sutures so that there is approximately half to one inch between them.
- Tie off the distal part of the vein with the distal suture.
- Elevate and stabilise the vein using the proximal suture.
- Nick the vein transversely with sharp-pointed scissors (use the scalpel, if these are not available).
- Insert the intravenous cannula and secure it by tying the proximal suture.
- Suture the skin (if circumstances permit) and tape the giving set and cannula firmly in place.

Femoral vein venipuncture/cut down

Method
- Position yourself on the same side of the patient as the vein that you are going to use (avoid leaning across them).
- Identify the femoral artery about two finger-breadths below the mid-point of the inguinal ligament, and using two fingers over the artery pull the artery slightly laterally to tighten the skin.

Femoral venous cannulation
- Enter the skin over the femoral vein, with the point of the cannula pointed towards the head and at an angle of about 45° to the skin.
- Advance the tip of the cannula, until there is a flashback of blood, following which reduce the angle of the cannula to the skin to about 15-20° and advance it further up to the hilt.
- Connect the giving set and secure both in position with tape or a suture.

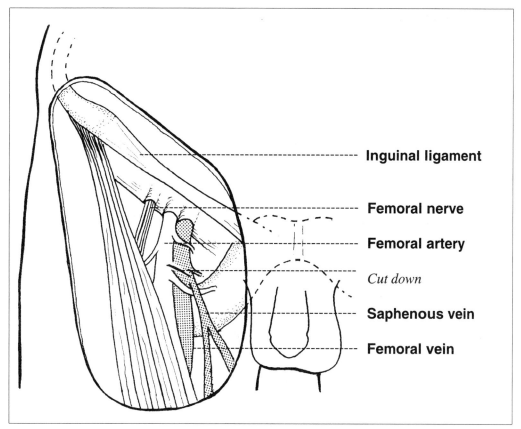

Figure 4-6 Sites for femoral cannulation and cutdown

Femoral vein cutdown
- Make an incision approximately 5 cm long just medial to the pulsations of the femoral artery.
- Clear the subcutaneous fat and tissue with artery forceps using blunt dissection.
- Dissect the vein free (it lies just below Scarpa's fascia)
- Using the same technique as for long saphenous vein cut down, elevate the vein, insert the cannula and secure it and the giving set.

Note: - In patients requiring immediate high volume fluid replacement, the end of a sterile giving set may be cut off obliquely and then inserted directly into the vein instead of a cannula.
   - Infusion rates of up to 1 litre per minute may be obtained using this method.

Central venous cannulation

- A central vein may be used for the administration of cardiac drugs
- In the very shocked patient a central vein may be easier to cannulate.
- The usual sites used are:
    - The internal jugular vein
    - The subclavian vein.

Aids to cannulation

- Application of a PASG may aid venous cannulation of the central and upper limb veins in the very shocked hypovolaemic patient.
- In cold weather local application of a "Warm Pak" may help dilate the peripheral veins.

Internal jugular vein cannulation

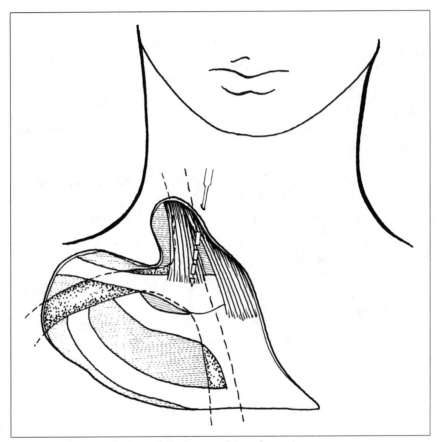

Figure 4-7 Cannulation of the internal jugular vein

Method
- Lie the patient down, head down and with the legs elevated (if possible), to reduce the risk of air embolism and help distend the neck veins.
- Approach the patient by standing at the head, facing towards the legs.
- Identify the sternal and clavicular heads of the sternocleidomastoid muscle.
- Identify the apex of the triangle that they form.
- Use a 10 ml syringe and a long 14G cannula.
- Insert the needle at the apex of the triangle (or at the middle of the anterior border of the sternal band of sternocleidomastoid) at an angle of 30° aiming towards the right nipple.

Note: The carotid artery is situated just medial to the vein.

- Withdraw the syringe plunger as soon as the needle is under the skin, and continue insertion and aspiration until there is a flashback of blood.
- Advance the cannula into the vein, withdrawing the syringe and needle as you do so.
- Attach the giving set to the cannula.

Complications
- Arterial puncture:
  - This is usually obvious.
  - Leave the cannula in situ, as withdrawal may result in an extensive haematoma.
- Pleural penetration.

Subclavian vein cannulation

Supraclavicular approach

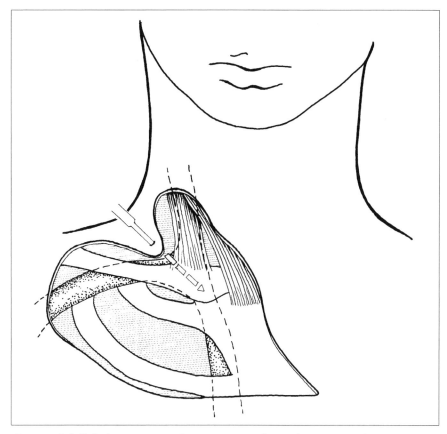

Figure 4-8 Subclavian cannulation: supraclavicular approach

Advantage
- Less likely than the infraclavicular approach to cause problems.

Method
- With the patient supine and the head down, elevate the legs to prevent the risk of air embolism, and to help distend the neck veins.
- Position yourself by the patient's right shoulder and turn the patient's head to the left.
- Identify the clavicle, the clavicular head of the sternocleido mastoid muscle, and the angle that they form.
- Insert the needle horizontally above the clavicle, bisecting the angle, and pass it directly behind the clavicle.
- Gently withdraw the plunger of the syringe until there is a flashback of blood.
- Proceed as for cannulation of the internal jugular vein.

Infraclavicular approach

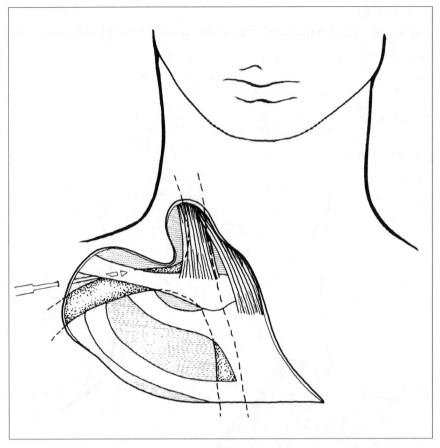

Figure 4-9 Subclavian cannulation: infraclavicular approach

Advantages
- Avoids moving the neck.
- Leaves both arms free.

Method
- With the patient supine, identify the clavicle, and find its mid point.
- Insert the cannula horizontally one finger's breadth below the clavicle, along the inferior border of the clavicle aiming for the opposite sternoclavicular joint.
- Gently withdraw the plunger of the syringe until there is a flashback of blood.
- Then proceed as for cannulation of the internal jugular vein.

Intraosseous infusion

- This is a simple and useful technique for emergency vascular access in children, especially those less than 6 years old, and in whom it is now considered to be the method of choice.
- In older children it should be used in preference to a venous cut down or central venous cannulation, when peripheral venous cannulation is difficult or unsuccessful.

Advantages
- Quick and easy to perform.
- Provides rapid access to the central circulation for fluid and/or drug administration (except bretylium).

Sites
- Proximal tibia:
    - 1-3 cm below the tibial tuberosity, on the antero-medial surface.
    - Only suitable for children up to the age of 5 years old (difficult to penetrate after this).

- Distal tibia:
    - Just proximal to the medial malleolus.
    - Suitable for all ages.

- Distal femur:
    - 2-3 cm above the lateral condyle.

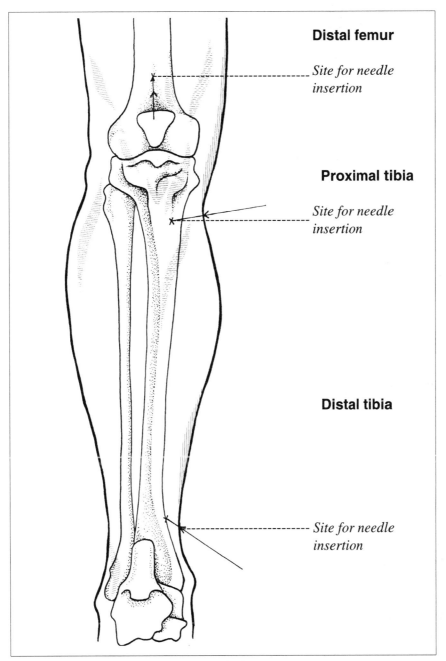

Figure 4-10 Sites for intraosseous infusion

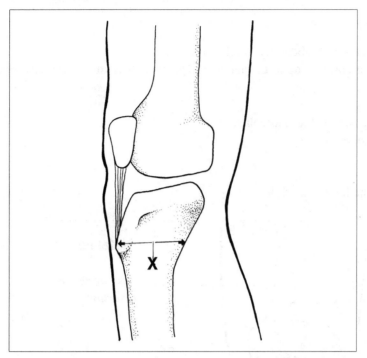

Figure 4-11 Intraosseous infusion: locating site for upper tibia

Method
- Identify the relevant anatomical landmarks.
- Using an intraosseous needle (if this is not available, a 16 or 18 gauge (babies under 8 months old) cannulation needle may suffice), and insert it perpendicularly into the bone to a depth of about 1.5-2.0 cm, if appropriate aiming away from the growth plate.

CAUTION: - Never insert an intraosseous needle distal to a fracture site.

- Needle entry into the marrow cavity is shown by:
    - A loss of resistance
    - Sustained positioning of the needle without support (in infants and small children, there may be very little support, and the device has to be held in place by hand or secured using the Molynar Disc (included with some devices).
    - Free flow of marrow aspirate or infusion fluid.
- Remove the stylet and attach a syringe. Withdraw the plunger and aspirate a little marrow to confirm correct placement.
- Administer blood replacement fluid by giving syringe boluses using minimal pressure or attach a giving set (although the rate of flow may be rather slow).
- Be careful not to over infuse!

Rate of infusion
- Gravity: 100 ml per hour.

Complications
- Osteomyelitis: 0.6%
- Skin infection: 0.7%
- Growth plate injury
- Subcutaneous infusion/oedema
- Subperiostal infusion
- Over penetration through to the other side of the bone.

Types of intravenous infusion fluid

Introduction

- The ideal infusion fluid/blood substitute should be:
    - Cheap, with a long storage life at any temperature.
    - Inert:
        - No risk of allergic, toxic, or incompatibility reaction
        - Does not interfere with grouping and cross matching
        - Has no effect on haemostasis or coagulation
        - No risk of electrolyte disturbance.
    - Isotonic with blood: low risk of fluid overload; both intravascular and interstitial.
- It should have:
    - A pH of 7.4 (similar to blood), but with a buffering effect
    - A relatively short half life, and be rapidly excreted
    - Good oxygen carrying capacity and oxygen release
    - No effect on renal function
    - No risk of disease transmission.
- The container should be:
    - Robust
    - A convenient shape
    - Squeezable
    - Fitted with a good integral hanging loop
    - Easy to connect to a giving set.

Crystalloids

Sodium chloride intravenous infusion 0.9%

Action
- Provides short term fluid replacement (30-60 minutes blood volume replacement) as rapid diffusion into the interstitial space occurs.
- Three times the blood loss must be infused to achieve full fluid replacement.

Advantages
- Low cost
- Long shelf life
- Low risk of infection or allergy
- Availability in convenient plastic containers.

Disadvantages
- The large volumes required to provide blood replacement.
- If large volumes are infused, the risk of causing:
    - Tissue oedema, especially cerebral and pulmonary oedema
    - Hypernatraemia.

CONCLUSION
- Only useful for short term fluid replacement.

Hartmann's/Ringer's lactate solution: sodium lactate intravenous compound

Description
- A buffered solution, similar to saline.

Advantages
- Lower sodium and chloride content than saline.
- Has some buffering action.

Disadvantage
- Lactate needs to be metabolised to bicarbonate in the liver. In the severely shocked patient, with an impaired hepatic circulation this may not take place, resulting in an increased accumulation of lactate, and a metabolic acidosis.

CONCLUSION
- The *crystalloid of choice* in Immediate Care.

Dextrose 5%: Glucose intravenous infusion 5%

Description
- 5% dextrose in 0.18% saline.

Action
- Dextrose is a readily utilisable energy source.

Disadvantages
- Prone to cause local venous thrombophlebitis.
- Low pH: usually about 3.0.

CONCLUSION
- Preferred by some for low volume intravenous infusions following myocardial infarction, and in paediatric resuscitation.

Colloids

Action
- Provide long term volume replacement.

Advantages
- There is a low risk of tissue oedema.
- Generally iso-oncotic with blood, which they replace on an equal volume basis.

Disadvantage
- Do not replace interstitial fluid loss.

Plasma substitutes

- Macromolecular substances, which are only slowly metabolised.

Gelatins/Bovine albumins

Haemaccel

Description
- A modified fluid gelatin, average molecular weight 30,000 4%, in sodium chloride 0.9%.

Action
- Promotes an osmotic diuresis and has a half life of several hours.

Advantages
- Relatively cheap.
- Is generally non toxic and does not affect the clotting mechanisms, except when large volumes are infused, which may result in haemodilution of clotting factors.
- Comes in convenient plastic containers.
- Is not affected by changes in storage temperature.
- Has a long shelf life of 5-8 years.

Disadvantages
- Prone to freezing in cold weather.
- There is a (low) risk of anaphylactic reactions: minor histamine release effect.
- Should not be mixed with citrated blood as the calcium ions in the colloidal solution will cause blood to clot in the giving set.

Gelofusine

Description
- Similar to Haemaccel (Polygelene: degraded and modified gelatin), average molecular weight 35,000, but with a lower potassium and calcium content, a higher sodium content and a slightly longer half life.

Disadvantages
- It is hyperoncotic with blood and therefore there is a greater risk of fluid overload, due to its fluid expanding effect.
- Gels below 3 °C.

CONCLUSION: The *intravenous fluids of choice* for initial blood replacement in Immediate Care.

Modified starches

Hydroxyethyl starch: Hetastarch: Hespan/Elohes 6%

Description
- Hetastarch 6%, in sodium chloride 0.9%.
- Similar to Dextran 70 physiologically.

Advantages
- Relatively cheap, compared to plasma, but is much more expensive than either colloid or crystalloid.
- Half life: long (12-14 hours).
- The shelf life is 2 years; it should be stored below 25 °C and above freezing.
- There is little risk of histamine release or anaphylactic reaction.

Disadvantages
- Tends to coat the platelets and has an anticoagulant effect; prolongs the clotting time.
- Should be used with caution in renal impairment.
- There is a small risk of allergic reactions; the mechanism is not known.
- Can fill the intravascular space and cause problems with getting an adequate blood volume infused and may cause fluid overload.

CONCLUSION: Only recently available in the UK, but gaining increasing acceptance in the USA. Should be *used with caution and only in small volumes.*

Dextrans

- Hydrolytic starch products, fractionated to produce solutions with molecules of a consistent size.
- Molecule sizes now available are 40,000 (40) and 70,000 (70).
- Coat the red cell membrane which may interfere with blood grouping and cross matching.
- Increase co-agulation times by impairing platelet function and fibrin formation.
- Stored in glass bottles, which are heavy, bulky, fragile and impractical for pre-hospital use.

Dextran 40: Gentran 40, Lomodex 40, Rheomacrodex 40

Description
- 10% dextrans of average molecular weight 40,000 in 5% glucose or 0.9% sodium chloride solution.

Advantages
- Promotes the microcirculation in small volumes.

Disadvantages
- May cause irreversible renal damage if it is used for resuscitation in acute hypovolaemic shock.

CONCLUSION
- *Not recommended* for the treatment of hypovolaemic shock.

Dextran 70: Gentran 70, Lomodex 70, Macrodex

Description
- 6% dextrans of average molecular weight 70,000 in 5% glucose or 0.9% sodium chloride solution.

Advantages
- An effective blood substitute.
- Long shelf life: 5 years.

Disadvantages
- Can interfere with coagulation (and hence with cross matching).
- Has a long half life of up to several days, which means that no more than 1 litre should be infused.
- There is a small risk of allergic reactions due to histamine release and other mechanisms.
- Should be stored at a steady room temperature; temperature variation may result in flaking.

Contraindications
- Congestive cardiac failure.
- Bleeding diatheses due to: thrombocytopaenia, hypofibrinogenaemia.

CONCLUSION: Not now used in Immediate Care in the UK.

Plasma

Albumin 5%

Description
- Freeze dried plasma; it is stored as a dry powder and has to be reconstituted.

Disadvantages
- It is expensive and in short supply.
- May cause serum homologous jaundice and has a high potassium content which can be dangerous in rapid transfusion.
- The shelf life is relatively short: 6 months.

CONCLUSION: Has now been *largely replaced by HPPF.*

HPPF (Human plasma protein fraction)

Description
- A 5% solution of protein, containing 88% albumin.

Advantages
- Does not carry the risk of producing either a serum homologous reaction or hyperkalaemia.
- Has a long shelf life of up to 5 years if stored between 2-25°C.
- The risk of disease transmission is very low.

Disadvantages
- It is in short supply, and is very expensive.

CONCLUSION: Physiologically perhaps the ideal blood replacement fluid.
Due to its cost, it is best reserved for replacement of plasma albumin in burns.
Not used in Immediate Care.

Whole blood

Disadvantages
- It needs careful storage between 3-6 °C.
- The shelf life is very short: between 21 and 35 days depending on the the preservative used.
- Allergic and incompatability "transfusion" reactions. There is a significant risk of this, even with unmatched O Rh NEG blood; therefore type specific blood should be requested at least.
- Contamination with pathogenic organisms, e.g. hepatitis, HIV. This risk is very low in the UK, as all blood is heat treated irrespective of screening.
- Hypothermia, and cardiac arrest may occur if the blood is not warmed sufficiently prior to infusion.
- It has a high viscosity (the microcirculation in shock may be improved by a reduction in the packed cell volume).
- If stored for more than a few days, platelets and white cells tend to fragment rapidly and lose their normal function, and there is a rise in the serum potassium.
- Overtransfusion with a consequent increase in viscosity, and pulmonary oedema may occur due to the difficulty of estimating blood loss accurately.
- There may be coagulation problems if more four units are infused (clotting factors, especially factor VIII, rapidly degrade in stored blood).

CONCLUSION
- Because of its short shelf life and special storage requirements, whole blood is not readily available and *not usually necessary* in Immediate Care, except for the patient with major blood loss, who is trapped for some time.

Choice of intravenous fluid

- Blood loss of up to 15% blood volume can safely be replaced by colloid or crystalloid alone. If the loss is greater than this, then 2 units (1,000 mls) of crystalloid should be used followed by one unit (500 mls) of colloid.
- In the Immediate Care situation, when treatment may be started shortly after blood loss, colloid is the fluid of choice. If there is more than about 30 minutes delay in starting the infusion, then there may be significant interstitial fluid loss. In this case the initial fluid should be crystalloid, followed by colloid.
- The correct volume to transfuse is difficult to assess, but a careful assessment of the patient's apparent and suspected injuries, together with measurement of the patient's vital signs, repeated at regular intervals, should give a very good guide.

PRACTICAL POINTS

Cold weather
- *Fluids, especially colloids, may thicken, freeze or form crystals, which can result in an increase in viscosity causing difficulty with infusing, patient cooling and cardiac dysrhythmias.*

Storage of intravenous fluids
- *Ideally intravenous fluids for immediate use should be kept in an insulated container at body temperature, e.g. the Transwarm intravenous fluid warming system. Alternatively:*
    - *At least one unit of each type of transfusion fluid should be kept in the passenger compartment of your vehicle, so as to keep it relatively warm.*
    - *The first bottles of fluid used should probably be those carried on the ambulance, as most ambulances are kept in centrally heated garages. Check with your local ambulance service!*

Warming intravenous fluids
- *Fluids can be warmed during infusion by wrapping the infusion bottle and drip chamber in a "hot pack", or using an Infupak which a purpose designed fluid warming device, consisting of an insulated bag into which a reusable hotpack and a bottle of infusion fluid can be inserted. An insulated sleeve for the giving set and line is also provided to reduce fluid cooling due to wind chill.*
- *Fluid warming is not only important for warming up cold infusion fluids, but also for administering warm fluids to warm up hypothermic and hypovolaemic patients.*

Grouping and cross matching whole blood

- If whole blood is going to be given, then blood samples should be obtained first for grouping and cross matching, and taken immediately to the laboratory, usually by the police.
- It is very important to supply clear and complete patient and doctor identification, preferably with a prearranged patient hospital number, as most laboratories will refuse to accept blood samples for grouping and cross matching without this information.
- At least one company can supply an armband with a unique patient number and a strip of numbered stickers for blood sample and other specimen containers for patients of unknown name or identity.

Monitoring

- Measurement/assessment of the patient's:
    - Respiratory rate
    - Oxygen saturation and pulse oximetry plethysmography
    - Pulse rate
    - Arterial pressure
    - Pulse pressure
    - Jugular venous pressure:
        - If this is raised in association with a low arterial pressure and tachycardia, it indicates:
            - Tension pneumothorax
            - Cardiac tamponade
            - Cardiogenic shock.
    - Temperature
    - Mental state.

Pain relief

- This is very important, as pain can precipitate and aggravate shock (see chapter on Pain Relief).

Complications

- Large volume transfusion of colloid/crystalloid followed by blood may result in:
    - Hypothermia
    - Acid/base disturbance
    - Hyperkalaemia
    - Hypocalcaemia
    - Clotting problems
    - ARDS.
- Rouleaux formation, if blood is administered through the same giving set as colloid.

Guidelines for provision of blood at the roadside

1 Introduction

1.1 On isolated occasions there is the need for blood transfusion at the roadside. Because of the dangers of mismatched blood, the most important factor is patient identification.

1.2 To achieve this it is necessary to hospital register the patient. With a patient identification number the risk can be kept to an absolute minimum.

1.3 Doctors in Immediate Care Schemes (and doctors in the Hospital, Flying Squads, or Hospital Surgical Teams) may on rare occasions need to give blood products at the roadside. Once the decision has been made that blood is required, it will be necessary to involve the Police or Ambulance Officers for transportation of specimens from the scene, and to bring blood products back.

1.4 Immediate Care Doctors must be aware that the recommended maximum of synthethic colloids, e.g. Haemmacel is 2 litres. They must note that a group of compatible cross match normally takes 30 minutes (from the time the specimen arrives in the laboratory).

2 Patient registration

2.1 Once the decision has been made that blood is required, the doctor or Ambulance Officer should contact the Accident Service using an Ambulance Officer's Cellnet phone to the Accident Service 'Red Phone'. A less accurate and less secure route is the radio telephone on the Ambulance Service radio frequency.

2.2 The person receiving the message in the Accident Service will require the following details:
   - The sex and ethnic origin of patient, approximate age, and location of accident.
   - The patient's first name, surname and date of birth if available.

2.3 With the minimum data of, e.g. "unknown male", an accident service number will be allocated to that patient. Further identification will be the location of the traffic accident, and the doctor requesting the blood. The Accident Service eight figure number will be given over the phone. It is unique to that patient.

2.4 The doctor at the scene should record the number. A blood specimen for cross match is taken. The specimen is labelled to include that number and as many details as possible. The date and time of taking the specimen *must* be put on the specimen bottle.

3   Transport

3.1   Specimens should be put in a polythene bag and given to the Police or Ambulance Officer, who will transport this to the Accident Department. The specimen should be given to a Casualty Officer (who will have been alerted in advance). The Casualty Officer will then check the details and write a blood transfusion form.

3.2   In the interim the Medical Records staff can, if details are known, identify whether the patient is known to the hospital and release an existing hospital number. Once the Casualty Officer has written the request for the cross match, the specimen will be conveyed to the Department of Haematology.

3.3   It is normal practice to order red cells in units of 6 for critical trauma.

4   Administration

4.1   Immediate Care Doctors should be aware that Infusion Sets should be for blood administration, and not a fluid infusion set. Ideally blood filters should be used.

4.2   If filters are not available at the scene they should be requested at the same time that the blood is ordered.

5   Summary

5.1   While this may appear a cumbersome system, it does work. The responsibility of the Immediate Care Doctor is to give accurate details to the Accident Service, who will carry out the patient registration to protect the patient against mismatched blood. If uncrossed group O Rh NEG blood is required, the same system would be used.

5.2   Doctors at the scene of an accident must note that the average time to get blood, from time of request, to time of arrival on scene, will be about 60 minutes. Therefore requests for blood should be made early rather than late.

5.3   If the patient's condition is critical, the Immediate Care Doctor may require extra assistance. Subject to availability it is probable that senior A&E staff can be transported to the scene, when the blood is delivered.

Cardiogenic shock

Incidence

- Commonly occurs following acute myocardial infarction (this is discussed in the chapter dealing with the management of acute myocardial infarction).
- Relatively rarely occurs following trauma.

Aetiology

- May occur as a result of:
    - Cardiac contusion caused by blunt chest injury
    - Cardiac tamponade due to penetrating injury
    - Tension pneumothorax
    - Air embolism.

Symptoms/signs

- These are similar to, but not identical, to those for hypovolaemic shock.
- The differences are:
    - Skin appearance:
        - Slightly pale in cardiogenic shock, very pale in hypovolaemic shock.
    - Jugular venous pressure:
        - Raised in cardiogenic shock, low in hypovolaemic shock.
    - ECG pattern: Injury pattern in cardiogenic shock, normal in hypovolaemic shock.

Management

- *Airway*
    - Airway maintenance, with cervical spine stabilisation if there is a history of recent trauma.
    - Oxygen.

- *Breathing*
    - Intubation and ventilation if the patient is unconscious.

- *Circulation*
    - Treatment of the cause.
    - Establish a slow intravenous infusion with crystalloid, if there is no associated hypovolaemic shock. This may also be used for intravenous drug administration if required.

Neurogenic shock

Incidence
- Commonly encountered, often in combination with other types of shock.
- More common in the young female and elderly.

Aetiology

- Head or spinal cord injury.

Pathophysiology

- Autonomic stimulation or disruption of the sympathetic pathways descending in the cervical and upper thoracic spine, results in loss of vasomotor tone and vascular pooling without any reflex cardiac stimulation.

Symptoms/signs

- Hypotension.
- Bradycardia.

Management

- Leg elevation.
- Atropine:
    - Incremental doses of 0.5-0.6 mg, administered intravenously over 5 minutes, up to a maximum of 2 mg.

Bacteriological shock

Introduction

- This is a condition which is very rarely encountered in Immediate Care, but is nonetheless an acute medical emergency. It may be sub-divided according to the aetiology and causative organism.

Septic shock

Incidence

- Very rarely encountered in the Immediate Care situation.
- Streptococcal septicaemia:
    - 600 cases per year in the UK
    - 30% are fatal
    - 5% are associated with chickenpox.

Aetiology

- May occur if:
    - There is a penetrating abdominal injury with contamination of the abdominal cavity with intestinal contents.
    - The patient cannot be conveyed from the scene of their accident for many hours, e.g. in prolonged or complicated entrapment.
    - The travelling time to hospital is very long, e.g. in remote areas or at sea.

Pathophysiology

- The causative organism is usually a Gram negative enterococcus, but may be a β-haemolytic streptococcus or staphlococcus.
- Due to severe infection, the cells have impaired ability to absorb oxygen, and the capillary walls at the site of infection are damaged and leak albumin and water.
- There may also be disseminated intravascular coagulation leading to consumptive coagulopathy, generalised bleeding and resulting hypovolaemia.
- The cardiac output is increased, while the systemic vascular resistance is low due to peripheral vasodilation secondary to pyrexia, and vasoactive mediators.
- The cardiac output may later fall due to hypovolaemia, and vascular resistance which rises due to the sympathetic response.
- The cardiac preload falls as hypovolaemia develops.
- A vicious cycle may then develop with a reduction in blood pressure and myocardial function still further.

Symptoms/signs

- Patients with a combination of septic shock and hypovolaemia are difficult to distinguish clinically from those who have hypovolaemia alone.
- Patients who have septic shock with a normal blood volume will have:
    - A pyrexia with warm pink skin
    - A modest tachycardia and tachypnoea
    - A near normal systolic pressure
    - A *wide pulse pressure.*

Management

- Initial treatment may include:
    - Oxygen
    - Intravenous infusion
    - Parenteral antibiotics, e.g. penicillin and a third generation cephalosporin such as cefotaxime
    - Possibly application of a PASG.

Toxic shock/Toxic shock syndrome

Incidence
- This is a rare, but potentially lethal condition, with a mortality of about 10% (20-50% when the causative organism is a *Streptococcus*) which may present to the General Practitioner or Accident and Emergency department, but may also be encountered by Ambulance crews and Immediate Care doctors.
- According to the UK Public Health Laboratory, there is an averaage of 18 cases each year in the UK.

Aetiology
- Infection associated with the following:
    - Childbirth:
        - Due to abortion or the retained products of conception.
    - Vaginal tampon use in menstruating women.
    - Any injury (accidental or iatrogenic) or illness, e.g. minor wounds, burns, abscesses and sinuses, and areas affected by postinfluenzal bronchopneumonia, tracheitis and empyema.

Pathophysiology
- The causative organism is usually a toxin producing *Staphlococcus aureus* or rarely a group A haemolytic streptococcus, which produces an endotoxin.
- The physiological response is similar to septic shock.

Symptoms/signs
- Influenza-like symptoms:
    - Myalgia.
    - Diarrhoea and vomiting.
    - Blotchy macular erythema: may be patchy, localised or generalised.
    - Sudden onset of high pyrexia: >38.9 °C.
    - Dizziness/postural syncope due to hypotension:
        - Systolic BP <90 mmHg
        - A postural drop in diastolic pressure of at least 15 mmHg
    - Confusion, drowsiness, without focal neurological signs when the fever and hypotension have been corrected.

Management
- Prevention of further production or absorption of toxin:
    - Removal of tampon, etc.
- Intravenous fluid replacement with crystalloid/colloid.
- Steroids.
- Intravenous antibiotics:
    - Flucloxacillin and/or benzylpenicillin (or erythromycin).
- Consider inotropic support.
- If circulatory collapse is profound, consider use of a pneumatic ant-shock garment (PASG).

Anaphylactic shock

Introduction

- This is one of the most acute medical emergencies, and requires immediate and aggressive management as the patient can die in minutes.

Definition: Anaphylactic shock is a state of immediate hypersensitivity, following exposure to a foreign protein or drug.

Incidence

- Relatively uncommon.

Aetiology

- Caused by exposure to or ingestion of specific allergens:
    - Pollens, insect stings, specific foods and hyposensitising (allergen) preparations.
    - "Foreign" serum, vaccines.
    - Therapeutic agents:
        - Antibiotics, iron injections, anti-inflammatory analgesics, heparin, and neuromuscular blocking agents.
    - Diagnostic agents:
        - Radio-opaque dyes.
- More likely to occur after parentral administration and in atopic individuals.

Pathophysiology

- Anaphylactic shock is an acute generalised allergic reaction with histamine release, resulting in:
    - Laryngeal oedema.
    - Bronchial constriction with mucous secretion, similar to acute severe asthma.
    - An allergic rash.
    - Severe hypotension:
        - This is secondary to peripheral vasodilation, with a drop in cardiac preload, an increase in heart rate, and an increase in systemic vascular resistance.
        - Later there may be bradycardia, followed by cardiac arrest.
- The onset may be extremely rapid, especially when the patient has become presensitised, e.g. insect sting, or relatively slow, when there has been no prior exposure and the route of administration is the alimentary canal.

History

- There is usually a history of atopy with similar, but milder attacks.
- In practice there is usually little doubt over the diagnosis.

Symptoms/signs

- There may be the rapid development of pruritis and erythema and an urticarial rash, with a feeling of impending doom.
- Pallor, limpness and apnoea are the commonest signs in children.
- Laryngeal oedema with stridor and hoarseness.
- Retrosternal tightness and dyspnoea with bronchospasm, and an audible expiratory wheeze.
- There is a progression from an initial sinus tachycardia to profound hypotension with tachycardia, and finally to severe bradycardia, coma and cardiac arrest.
- Nausea, vomiting, abdominal cramps and diarrhoea.

Management

Position
- Lay the patient flat with the legs elevated:
    - This aids the venous return and reduces hypotension due to dependent venous pooling.
- If the patient is unconscious, but his condition is otherwise satisfactory:
    - He should be put into the recovery position.

Treatment of the cause

Adrenaline
- This should be administered as soon as possible, unless there is a strong central pulse and the patient's general condition is good.
- *Any delay may be fatal.*

Adrenaline 1:10,000

Presentation:
- 10 ml 1/10,000 preloaded syringe (IMS).

Administration:
- By *slow* intravenous injection, titrated against patient response.
- The dose may be repeated at 5-15 minute intervals up to three times as required, depending on response.

Dosage:	Age (yrs)	Dose (mg)
	1	0.1
	5	0.25
	10	0.5
	12	0.75
	Adults	1

Adrenaline 1:1000

Presentation:
- 1 ml 1/1000 solution in a preloaded syringe (IMS).

Administration:
- By deep intramuscular injection.
- In the case of reaction due to injections or stings, the injection should be given close to the site.

Dosage:

Age (yrs)	Dose (ml)
<1	0.05
1	0.1
2	0.2
3-4	0.3
5	0.4
6-10	0.5
Adults	0.5-1.0

Medihaler Epi metered dose aerosol spray

Presentation:
- Adrenaline acid tartrate: 280 µg/metered dose.

Dosage:
- Adults: a minimum of 20 puffs.
- Children: 10-15 puffs.

Administration:
- By inhalation.

Antihistamine: chlorpheniramine (Piriton)

Indications:
- Antihistamines are a useful adjunct to adrenaline, and should be continued for 24-48 hours to prevent relapse.
- Should be given after adrenaline.

Presentation:
- 1 ml ampoules 10 mg/ml.

Dosage:

Age (yrs)	Dose (mg)
1	2.5
7	5
12	10
Adults	10-20

Administration:
- Intravenously, diluted in the syringe with 5-10 ml of blood and injected slowly over 1 minute. (Any side effects (drowsiness, giddiness and hypotension) should then be transient).

Airway: laryngeal oedema

Airway maintainance
- If the patient is unconscious, insert a Guedel airway.
- If there is stridor, consider endotracheal intubation using a gum elastic bougie.

Note: - This should *only* be attempted by the experienced intubator, as a clumsy or failed intubation will only increase laryngeal oedema and precipitate complete airway obstruction.
- If there are signs of severe upper airway obstruction, due to laryngeal oedema, immediately perform a cricothyrotomy.

Breathing: bronchospasm

Oxygen
  - This should be administered early by face mask; in as high a concentration as possible.

Ventilation
  - If there is no spontaneous respiration.

Steroids
  - If used, these should be administered as soon as possible after adrenaline, as they are slow to take effect (up to several hours) and have a short duration of action. Their use and effectiveness is being increasingly questioned in Immediate Care, unless travelling time to definitive care is very long.

Hydrocortisone succinate/sodium phosphate

  - Presentation:
    - Ampoules of:
      - Dry powder which has to be mixed with water *or*
      - Solution: 100 mg/ml in 1, 5 ml.

  - Dosage:
    - 100-500 mg (approximately 5 mg/kg).

  - Administration:
    - By slow intravenous injection over 0.5-1 minute.

Prednisolone (the steroid of choice)

  - Presentation:
    - Tablets: 5, 25 mg.

  - Dosage:
    - 30-60 mg.

Nebulised β_2 adrenergic agonists } see under Management of Asthma
Intravenous aminophylline }

Cardiovascular collapse

Circulatory support
  - Basic life support if appropriate.
  - Put up an intravenous infusion of colloid.
  - Consider the application of a pneumatic anti-shock garment (PASG).

Local allergic reaction

Infiltration with adrenaline
  - This may be useful in cases of acute localised reactions to injections or insect bites.
  - Acts by causing local vasoconstriction, and hence reduces further systemic absorption.
  - Great care has to be taken not to administer adrenaline intra-arterially into the peripheral circulation, i.e. the limbs, and fingers or toes, as peripheral gangrene due to arterial spasm may result.

Guidelines for the management of anaphylactic shock

Position
- Lie the patient down, with their legs elevated.

Treatment of the cause

- Administer:
  - **Adrenaline**
    - by intravenous or deep intramuscular injection (unless the patient is well with a good pulse).
    - Should be repeated at 10 minute intervals if there is no improvement.
  - **Antihistamines** (chlorpheniramine) by slow intravenous injection.

Airway

- Check that the patient has a clear airway:
  - If the airway is clear:
    - Insert a Guedel airway.
  - If the airway is obstructed (due to laryngeal oedema):
    - Consider cricothyrotomy.
- Administer high-flow **oxygen**.

Note:- Do *not* attempt endotracheal intubation, unless you are very experienced (may make matters worse).

Breathing

- Check that the patient is breathing:
  - If there is no spontaneous breathing:
    - Ventilate the patient:
      - Expired air ventilation
      - Bag and mask
      - Oxygen driven ventilator.
- If there is a wheeze, consider:
  - **Salbutamol**
  - **Aminophylline**
  - **Steroids**.

Adrenaline dosage for intravenous administration:	
Age (yrs)	Dose (ml)
1	0.1
5	0.25
10	0.5
12	0.75
Adults	1

Circulation

- Check for a pulse (radial or carotid)
  - If there is no pulse:
    - Administer external chest compressions
- If there is evidence of hypotension:
  - Put up an **intravenous infusion** (colloid or crystalloid)
  - Consider application of a PASG.

Disability (neurological)

- If the patient is unconscious:
  - Put them into the recovery position.

5

Circulation care: arrhythmias

Arrhythmias

Introduction

- Arrhythmic deaths are preventable.
- The commonest cause of lethal arrhythmias is acute myocardial infarction, but they may also occur in patients who have no or only minimal myocardial damage:
    - 30% of arrhythmias are not due to an acute myocardial infarction
    - 20% of arrhythmias are not due to coronary artery disease.
- The risk of developing a lethal arrhythmia following an acute myocardial infarction is greatest immediately after the onset of symptoms, and falls during the following 24 hours, although up to 95% of patients may develop some kind of arrhythmia. The most common arrhythmia post infarction is frequent PVCs.
- Arrythmias are the usual mode of sudden cardiac death.

General principles of management

- Treat the patient rather than the rhythm. Any arrhythmia causing significant symptoms or haemo-dynamic compromise should be treated immediately, if practicable.
- No antiarrhythmic drugs should be administered without ECG monitoring.
- If the rhythm changes, go back to the beginning of the guidelines for the new rhythm.
- In general, the use of more than one arrhythmic drug is best avoided and may only cause additional problems. If first line therapy fails consider electrical treatment (DC version for tachycardias, pacing for bradycardias).

Electrocardiogram (ECG) and cardiac events

Introduction

- All cardiac cells exhibit excitability, whereby an electrical stimulus of sufficient strength will result in a rapid membrane depolarisation, followed by a slower repolarisation. Depolarisation in myocardial cells results in their contraction.
- Only specialised conducting tissue normally depolarises spontaneously "automaticity", although other cardiac cells will discharge spontaneously in some situations, if they are not stimulated frequently enough.
- The SA node has the highest intrinsic firing rate, and if this fails, the AV node/junction will usually provide a junctional escape rhythm at a slower rate.

Electrophysiology

- The impulse generated within the SA node spreads through the atria to the AV node, causing atrial contraction (atrial systole).
- There is a delay as the impulse then enters the AV node, before it is rapidly conveyed down the bundle of His to the Purkinje fibres, from where it is travels to the ventricular muscle, resulting in ventricular contraction (ventricular systole).
- If the SA node firing rate is too slow, i.e. <30-50 per minute, or if there is complete heart block, then an ectopic focus in the AV junction or a ventricle will take over, resulting in a ventricular escape rhythm.

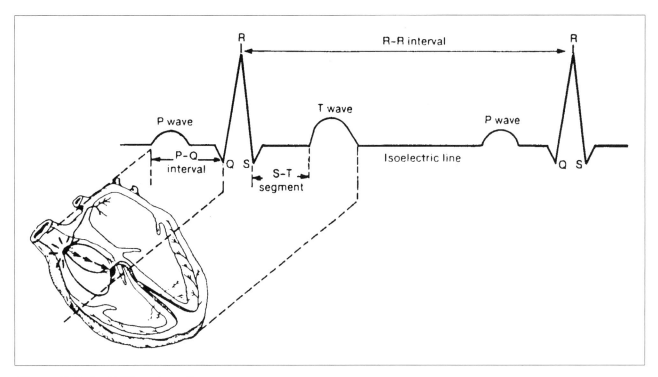

Figure 5-1 The ECG and cardiac events

- Conduction through the AV node is relatively slow and as a rule does not exceed 220 impulses per minute. This ensures that there is usually an adequate delay between atrial and ventricular contraction for optimum cardiac function and that the ventricles are protected from excessively rapid atrial rhythms.
- If the heart rate exceeds 120-140 beats per minute, then there may not be enough time for the ventricles to fill adequately, and the cardiac output may be reduced.
- Very rapid heart rates increase oxygen demand, reduce the strength of heart contractions and aggravate myocardial ischaemia, especially after a myocardial infarction, and may result in further infarction.

Obtaining an ECG recording

- In the emergency situation, an ECG rhythm recording may be obtained using either the defibrillator paddles or adhesive chest electrodes.

ECG electrode placement

Defibrillator paddle placement

- The paddles (with conductive pads or gel) or disposable electrodes should be placed below the right clavicle (-ve) just lateral to the sternal border and over the apex beat of the heart (+ve) covering the V4-5 positions of the ECG.
- If the positions are inadvertently reversed the tracing will appear upside down, which is of no consequence provided it is recognised.

Adhesive chest electrode placement

- Adhesive electrodes should be placed in the appropriate positions and connected to the ECG/ defibrillator leads:
    RED: Below the right clavicle
    YELLOW: Below the left clavicle   } avoiding areas where defibrillator paddles may be placed
    GREEN: Over the apex of the heart

ECG interpretation

Calculation of the heart rate
Time: Each small square = 0.04 seconds
          Each large square = 0.2 seconds = 5 small squares

QRS Rhythm: When normal is usually regular.

Regular QRS rhythm

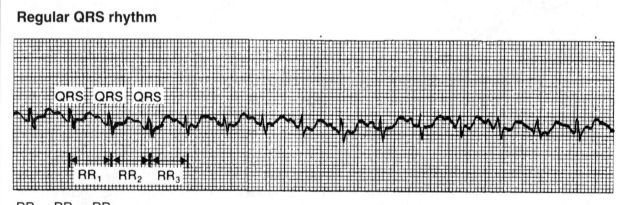

$RR_1 = RR_2 = RR_3$

Irregular QRS rhythm

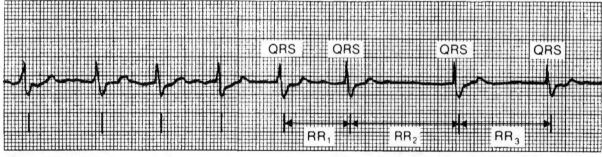

$RR_1 \neq RR_2 \neq RR_3$

Figure 5-2 QRS rhythm

Heart rate: $\dfrac{300}{\text{number of big squares between QRS complexes}}$

or $\dfrac{1{,}500}{\text{number of small squares between QRS complexes}}$

or   the number of QRS complexes in 6 secs x 10

Normal heart rate: 60-100 beats per minute (may be slower in athletes, faster in children).
Bradycardia: <60 beats per minute.
Sinus tachycardia: 100-160 beats per minute.
Supraventricular tachycardia: 140-220 beats per minute.
Ventricular tachycardia: 100-250 beats per minute.

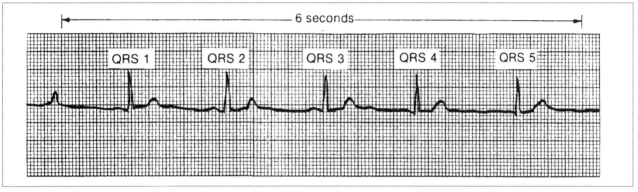

Figure 5-3 Calculation of heart rate: counting QRS complexes

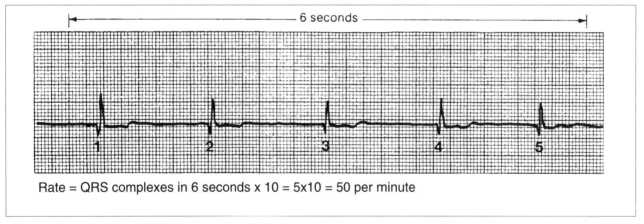

Rate = QRS complexes in 6 seconds x 10 = 5x10 = 50 per minute

Figure 5-4 Calculation of heart rate: bradycardia

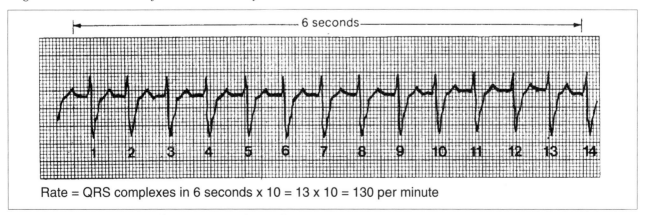

Rate = QRS complexes in 6 seconds x 10 = 13 x 10 = 130 per minute

Figure 5-5 Calculation of heart rate: tachycardia

ECG nomenclature

P waves
- Represent atrial depolarisation and therefore originate from the SA node, i.e. they are abnormal (and not strictly P waves) if they do not originate from the SA node, e.g. atrial ectopics, SVT.
- Usually precede the QRS complex.
- May be:
    - Bifid and broad (>3 small squares wide) in left atrial hypertrophy in leads II or III
    - Peaked (>3 small squares tall) in right atrial hypertrophy in leads II and III
    - Lost or inverted in ectopic rhythms and tachycardias
    - Lost in or dissociated from the QRS complex.

f waves
- Represent atrial depolarisation in atrial fibrillation:
    - Atrial rate: 350-600 per minute.
- May be fine or coarse.

F waves
- Represent atrial depolarisation in atrial flutter:
    - Atrial rate: 240-360 (usually about 300) per minute.
- Usually coarse: saw tooth.

PR interval
- Represents the time taken for excitation to spread from the SA node down over the atria to the AV node, down through the bundle of His, and to the ventricular muscle.
- Normally: >0.12 seconds (>3 small squares), but <0.20 seconds (<5 small squares).
- May be:
    - Short in Wolff Parkinson White syndrome and other pre-excitation syndromes
    - Prolonged in First Degree Heart Block (and often in Second Degree Heart Block)
    - Variable in Second Degree Heart Block type I
    - Irregular in Third Degree Heart Block (Complete Heart Block).

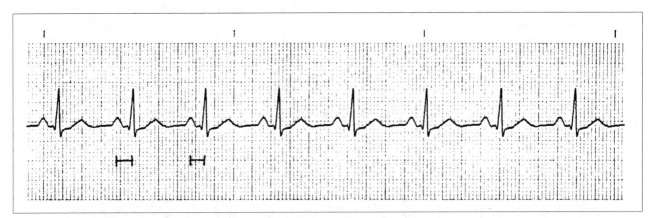

Figure 5-6 PR interval: normal

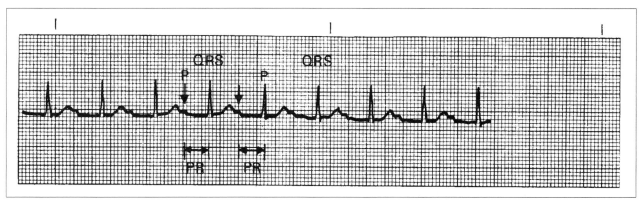

Figure 5-7 PR interval: prolonged - 0.28 sec

QRS complexes
-   Represents the time taken for excitation to spread through the ventricles.
-   In normal sinus rhythm should be:
    -   Preceded by a P wave
    -   < 0.12 seconds: < 3 small squares.
-   Will be:
    -   Wide (3 or more small squares) in bundle branch block and in ventricular ectopic beats or ventricular rhythms.
-   If abnormal, may be caused by:
    -   An ectopic ventricular focus causing premature ventricular contractions (PVCs).
    -   A ventricular tachycardia:
        - Broad complex: 0.12 seconds or more
        - Usually arise from a single ectopic focus.
    -   Ventricular escape beats/rhythm.
-   If abnormal and of variable morphology:
    - Arise from multiple (ventricular) foci.

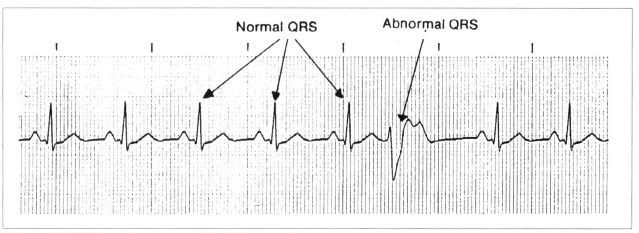

Figure 5-8 QRS complexes: normal and abnormal

Fibrillatory waves
-   Waves of random frequency, morphology and amplitude, representing totally disorganised electrical activity arising randomly in the myocardium, e.g. ventricular fibrillation.

R waves
-   Represent depolarisation in the ventricles.
-   Tall R waves in the left ventricular leads may indicate ventricular hypertrophy.
-   Loss of R wave progression in the chest leads may be an indication of myocardial infarction.

ST segment
- Represents the interval during which the myocardium remains at rest in a depolarised state.
- Should be isoelectric.
- There may be:
    - Convex elevation in myocardial infarction.
    - Concave elevation in pericarditis.
    - Depression: ischaemia, digoxin toxicity, and left ventricular hypertrophy.
- In acute myocardial infarction, the ST segment elevation (or reciprocal depression) occurs in the leads representing the site of the infarction (12 lead ECG):
    - Anterior, it will show in leads V2-5 (and often in I and AVL)
    - Inferior, it will show in leads II, III, AVF
    - Septal, it will show in leads V 1-4
    - Lateral, it will show in leads I, AVL, V 4-6.

T waves
- Represent ventricular repolarisation.
- These should usually be in the same direction as the QRS complex.
- If inverted they may be a sign of infarction or ventricular hypertrophy, but are often non specific.

ECG rhythm interpretation

Normal sinus rhythm

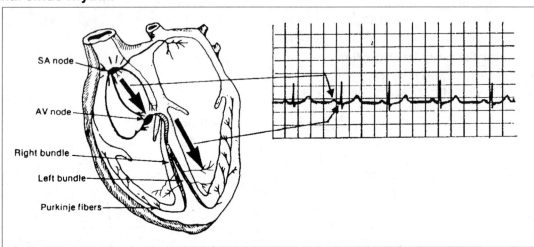

Figure 5-9 Normal sinus rhythm

ECG features

Rhythm: Regular.

Rate: 60-100 beats per minute.

P waves: Normal, each preceding a QRS complex.

Pacemaker site: SA node.

PR interval: Normal: 0.12-0.2 sec.

QRS complex: Normal, each preceded by a P wave.

Arrhythmias associated with cardiac arrest

Ventricular fibrillation

Incidence

- Most treatable and most common cause of sudden cardiac arrest following acute myocardial infarction.
- Responsible for 90% of early cardiac deaths.

Aetiology

- Occurs in 20% of patients with AMI (50% of these occur in first hour).
- May be preceded by other arrhythmias, or may occur without any previous rhythm disturbance.

Pathophysiology

- Condition of electrical anarchy; the chaotic electrical activity results in individual ventricular muscle fibres beating in a totally unco-ordinated fashion.
- Cardiac output is completely lost and the patient becomes unconscious.

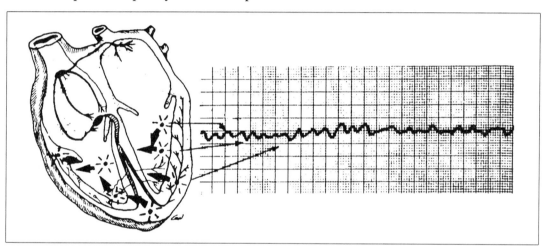

Figure 5-10 Ventricular fibrillation

ECG features

QRS rhythm: There is no true QRS rhythm, the complexes are totally irregular in frequency and amplitude.

Rate: Not usually possible to measure, usually >300 unco-ordinated waves per minute.

P waves: Not visible.

Pacemaker site: None.

PR interval: None.

QRS complex: None:
- There are numerous random fibrillatory waves of differing amplitude, morphology and duration.
- Initially the waves are often relatively coarse, but become finer until eventually there is asystole.

Precordial thump (delivers up to 8 joules of energy)

- A precordial thump should be administerd immediately. This may convert ventricular fibrillation, the most likely arrhythmia, or ventricular tachycardia into sinus rhythm, and is unlikely to be harmful.
- Reported success rates: ventricular fibrillation: 2%, ventricular tachycardia: 11-40%.
- A thump may exceptionally convert ventricular tachycardia into asystole, which is a much less favourable rhythm, and so it is therefore *not considered to be part of bystander BLS.*
- A thump may also be give in confirmed ventricular fibrillation when there is no defibrillator at hand.
- A cough may work as well as a thump, so monitored patients who develop ventricular fibrillation or pulseless ventricular tachycardia, should be encouraged to cough.

Method
- Give a moderately hard blow with a clenched fist to the sternum at the same point as chest compressions

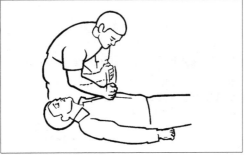
Figure 5-11a Administering a precordial thump

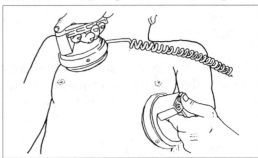
Figure 5-11b Defibrillation: paddle positions

Defibrillation (the only effective treatment for ventricular fibrillation).

- The chance of success is greatest if the defibrillation is given within 90 seconds of the arrest and declines rapidly thereafter.
- If no ECG monitoring is available, it is best to assume that the patient with a cardiac arrest is in VF.

Equipment
- Gel pads or disposable stick-on paddles are preferred because gel may be spread over the chest during the chest compressions and cause electrical arcing during defibrillation. They also reduce the trans-thoracic impedance, thus increasing the energy reaching the heart.
- Ideal paddle sizes: adults 13 cm, children 8 cm, and infants: 4.5 cm.
- Automatic external defibrillators (AEDs) may have difficulty recognising fine ventricular fibrillation and refuse to shock.

Method
- Remove any GTN patches (may explode as the shock is given), and make sure everything is dry.
- Place the paddles/pads below the outer half of the right clavicle, and just outside the apex of the heart, covering the V4-5 positions of the ECG. Some machines have paddles which fit over the precordium and under the left scapula (anteroposterior). The polarity of the paddles is probably not important.
- Do *not* place the paddles near the chest electrodes or within 12.5 cm of a pacemaker.
- Exert firm downwards pressure (about 12 Kg) on the paddles. This reduces trans-thoracic impedance.
- Before defibrillation shout "Stand by to defibrillate: Stand clear" and make certain that nobody is touching the patient or any attached equipment.
- Give the shock at the end of the expiratory phase of respiration (reduces trans-thoracic impedance).
- The defibrillator should be recharged immediately after each defibrillation, without removing the paddles from the chest, and the next shock given immediately, if the post defibrillation pulse/rhythm shows no improvement. Do not interrupt the shock sequence for chest compressions/ventilations (CPR), unless the defibrillator is slow to recharge.

Guidelines

- The first defibrillation should be given immediately after the precordial thump and before Basic Life Support is started (Basic Life Support by itself does not improve the situation and only slows down further deterioration).
- The first shock should be of 200 Joules. If this is unsuccessful, give another shock of 200 Joules, and if again unsuccessful, give a further shock of 360 Joules (trans-thoracic impedance is reduced with successive shocks, which is why a second shock of the same energy may be successful).
- In most instances of successful defibrillation, this is achieved within the first three shocks.
- If the third shock is unsuccessful, the patient should be intubated, an intravenous line established, and chest electrodes put in place. Take no more than about 15 seconds for this (if unsuccessful, try again next cycle).
- Administer adrenaline 1 mg intravenously (or 2-3 times this via an endotracheal tube), followed by ten cycles of chest compressions/ventilations (to allow for the drug to circulate) and three shocks 360 Joules.
- If this is not successful, repeat the loop, administering adrenaline 1 mg. with each cycle of shocks.
- Each cycle of shocks should take about 2 minutes (this may be difficult with limited personnel).
- After three loops, consider administering:
    - Sodium bicarbonate (50 mls of 8.4%).
    - An antiarrhythmic, e.g. lignocaine 100 mg, bretylium or amiodarone.
- If further defibrillation is unsuccessful, then the position of the paddles, e.g. to anteroposterior, or the defibrillator should be changed. The pads may also need to be replaced.

Ventricular asystole

Incidence

- Less common than ventricular fibrillation following AMI accounting for:
    - 10% of arrests outside hospital
    - 25% of arrests in hospital.
- Has an extremely poor prognosis except in trifascicular block (where P waves may be seen), extreme bradycardia or where it is a transient rhythm following defibrillation.

Aetiology

- Occurs as:
    - The end stage of ventricular fibrillation and electromechanical dissociation and other terminal cardiac events and indicates cardiac death.
    - The terminal mode of death in most cases of prolonged profound hypoxia following:
        - Respiratory arrest
        - Respiratory obstruction
        - Drowning
        - Fatal pulmonary oedema.

Pathophysiology

- Total loss of electrical and mechanical activity in the ventricles with failure of myocardial contraction:
    - May be either a primary arrhythmia or as a secondary arrhythmia following other rhythm disorders in myocardial ischaemia.
    - Due to complete loss of electrical activity in the heart.
    - Due to failure of the SA node to initiate a cardiac impulse.

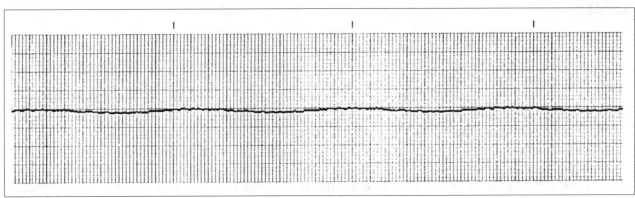

Figure 5-12 Asystole

ECG features

QRS rhythm: None: straight line, although in ventricular standstill, some atrial activity may persist briefly until complete asystole ensues (as may artefact, baseline wander and electrical interference).

Rate: None.

P waves: None usually, but may be present immediately after arrest.

Pacemaker site: None: no ventricular or junctional escape pacemaker and no escape rhythm is present.

PR interval: None.

QRS complex: None.

Management

- Check that there is clinical cardiac arrest.
- Check that the leads, connections, gain and brilliance of the monitor are correct.
- If hypoxia is the cause:
    - Administer oxygen, and intubate for efficient ventilation.
- If fine ventricular fibrillation cannot be excluded:
    - Give a precordial thump.
    - Defibrillate at 200 Joules
    - Defibrillate at 200 Joules
    - Defibrillate at 360 Joules.
- If fine ventricular fibrillation can be excluded or defibrillation is ineffective:
    - Intubate and/or establish intravenous access and immediately administer:
        - Adrenaline: 1/10,000: 1mg in 10 mls intravenously (or 2-3 times the dose via ET tube).
    - Perform 10 cycles of chest compressions/ventilations
    - Administer:
        - Atropine 3 mg (*once only*, as this should be sufficient to produce complete vagal block).
- If there is no response, but P waves or any other electrical activity is present:
    - Consider pacing.
- If there is no response, perform three further loops (on second loop, perform other proceedure: obtain intravenous access, intubate), after which give high dose adrenaline (5 mg administered intravenously).
- Recovery of patients with primary cardiac disease after 15 minutes is very unlikely, except in hypothermia, near drowning, or poisoning, which must be excluded before resuscitation is abandoned.

Note: Ventricular standstill:
- There is no ventricular activity, but atrial activity is normal.
- There are P waves, but no QRS complexes.
- May occur in complete heart block or as an agonal rhythm.

Electromechanical dissociation (EMD)

Incidence

- Outside hospital:
    - Uncommon: accounts for less than 3% of cardiac deaths
    - Commonest cause is trauma.
- Common in hospital: 30-70% of cardiac deaths.
- Treatment is only rarely successful.

Aetiology

Primary EMD: (failure of excitation-contraction coupling)
- Myocardial infarction (especially inferior wall).
- Drugs (beta blockers, calcium antagonists) and poisoning (overdosage of tricyclics).
- Electrolyte abnormalities (hypocalcaemia, hyperkalaemia).
- Atrial thrombus or myxoma.
- Hypothermia.

Secondary EMD: (mechanical embarrassment to cardiac output)
- Hypovolaemia due to trauma, concealed haemorrhage, etc
- Tension pneumothorax
- Pericardial tamponade after ventricular rupture or trauma
- Cardiac rupture
- Pulmonary embolism
- Prosthetic heart valve occlusion.

Pathophysiology

- Loss of effective myocardial contraction inspite of co-ordinated electrical activity.

ECG diagnosis

- May be normal sinus rhythm or other rhythm, e.g. atrial fibrillation (but no effective cardiac output).

Management

- Treatment of the underlying cause if possible:
    - Intravenous infusion for hypovolaemia
    - Pericardiocentesis for cardiac tamponade
    - Needle thoracocentesis for tension pneumothorax.
- Consider calcium chloride (10 ml of 10%) for:
    - Known or suspected hyperkalaemia
    - Known or suspected hypocalcaemia
    - Calcium antagonist use or overdose
    - Wide QRS complex EMD.

Guidelines for the management of life threatening arrhythmias

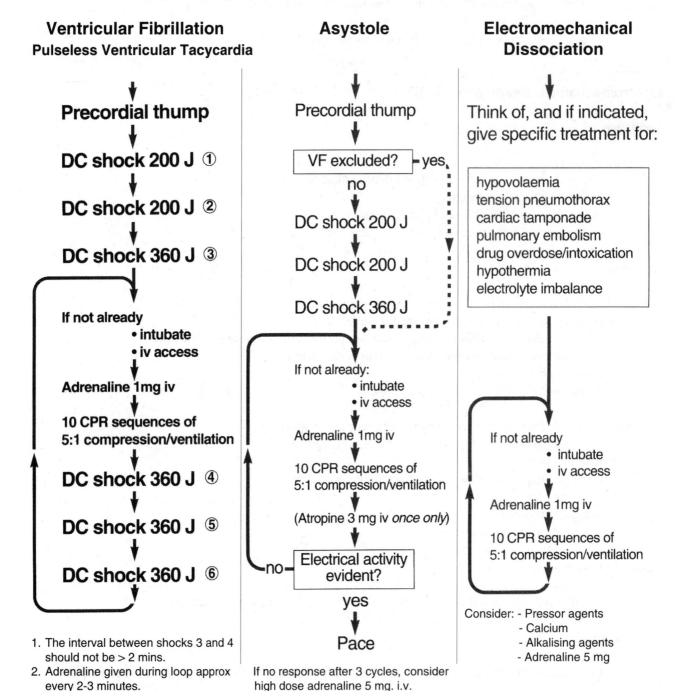

Ventricular Fibrillation
Pulseless Ventricular Tacycardia

Precordial thump

DC shock 200 J ①

DC shock 200 J ②

DC shock 360 J ③

If not already
- **intubate**
- **iv access**

Adrenaline 1mg iv

**10 CPR sequences of
5:1 compression/ventilation**

DC shock 360 J ④

DC shock 360 J ⑤

DC shock 360 J ⑥

1. The interval between shocks 3 and 4 should not be > 2 mins.
2. Adrenaline given during loop approx every 2-3 minutes.
3. Continue loops as long as defibrillation is indicated.
4. After 3 loops consider: alkalising agent antiarrhythmics

Asystole

Precordial thump

VF excluded? —yes
no

DC shock 200 J

DC shock 200 J

DC shock 360 J

If not already:
- intubate
- iv access

Adrenaline 1mg iv

10 CPR sequences of
5:1 compression/ventilation

(Atropine 3 mg iv *once only*)

—no— Electrical activity evident?

yes

Pace

If no response after 3 cycles, consider high dose adrenaline 5 mg. i.v.

Electromechanical Dissociation

Think of, and if indicated, give specific treatment for:

hypovolaemia
tension pneumothorax
cardiac tamponade
pulmonary embolism
drug overdose/intoxication
hypothermia
electrolyte imbalance

If not already
- intubate
- iv access

Adrenaline 1mg iv

10 CPR sequences of
5:1 compression/ventilation

Consider: - Pressor agents
- Calcium
- Alkalising agents
- Adrenaline 5 mg

Following successful defibrillation consider a lignocaine infusion of 3 mg/minute.

Note:-   Adrenaline and atropine should be given by the intravenous route, but if this is not possible they may be given by the endotracheal route, when the dose should be doubled or trebled. The intracardiac route is not recommended, except when there is no alternative.
-   All doses are based on a 70 kg man.
-   Both asystole and electromechanical dissociation can occur transiently after defibrillation for ventricular fibrillation, when the prospects for recovery are much better. The appropriate treatment is continued chest compressions and adrenaline.

Tachyarrhythmias:
Narrow complex tachycardias: supraventricular tachyarrhythmias

Sinus tachycardia

Incidence
- Very common after/during AMI occurring in up to 15% of patients.

Aetiology
- May be caused by:
    - AMI
    - Pain, pyrexia, hypoxia, shock and left ventricular failure
    - Drugs: adrenaline, atropine and isoprenaline.

Pathophysiology
- A very fast heart rate results in:
    - An increase in cardiac work, which results in further ischaemia and infarction
    - Inadequate ventricular filling and reduced cardiac output resulting in a fall in blood pressure
    - Cardiac failure.
- The rate is often related to the severity of the infarct.

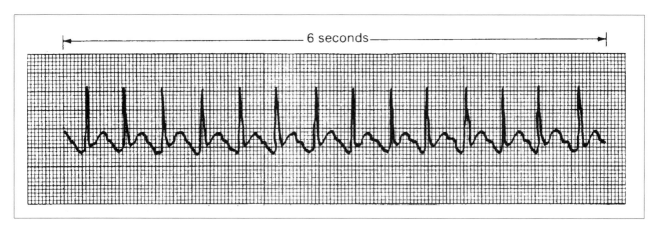

Figure 5-13 Sinus tachycardia

ECG features

QRS rhythm: Regular.

Rate: 100-160 beats per minute.

P waves: Normal preceeding each QRS complex. Very rapid rates may result in the P waves being lost in the previous T wave.

Pacemaker site: SA node.

PR interval: Normal (0.12-0.2 sec).

QRS complex: Normal: each preceded by a P wave.

Management
- Treatment of the underlying cause: pain, hypoxia, congestive cardiac failure.

Premature atrial contractions (PAC)

Incidence
- Common after acute myocardial infarction.
- May also occur in normal individuals, especially with increasing age.

Aetiology
- Tends to occur in organic heart disease.

Pathophysiology
- Causes no haemodynamic upset.
- May be associated with atrial tachycardia.

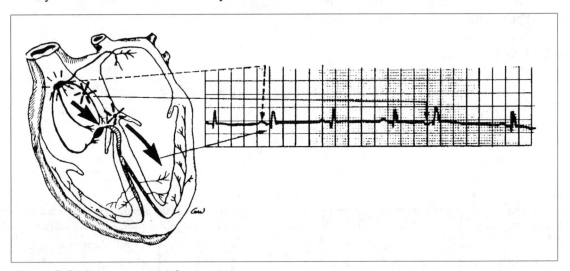

Figure 5-14 Premature atrial contractions

ECG features

- Abnormal premature P waves, often with a narrow QRS complex, but the QRS complex may sometimes be broad when aberrant conduction is present or absent, if conduction through the AV junction is blocked - the "blocked" PAC.

QRS rhythm: Irregular (regular basic rhythm, with occasional superimposed extra complexes).

Rate: Depends on the number of premature supraventricular beats and the underlying rate.

P waves: The premature P waves are often different from the normal P waves in size and shape.

Pacemaker site: The pacemaker for the supraventricular beat is an ectopic focus in some part of the atria or AV junction (junctional ectopic focus) other than the SA node.

PR interval: Variable depending on the rate of conduction between the ectopic pacemaker and the ventricular myocardium.

QRS complex: Usually normal, but aberrant conduction may occur.
              May be absent, if there is a failure of AV conduction.

Management
- Active treatment is not usually indicated.

Atrial fibrillation

Incidence
- This is a common arrhythmia especially over the age of 55 and after myocardial infarction, and may be transient and self limiting.

Aetiology
- Associated with increasing age, underlying heart disease, including mitral valve disease, thyrotoxicosis and in the context of AMI indicates ischaemia of the SA node or atria.

Pathophysiology
- Irregular atrial impulses occur at rates over 300 beats per minute.
- Almost always there is some degree of AV block, making the ventricular rate slower than the atrial rate, but it may still be fast and is always irregular (unless complete AV block is present).
- Atrial fibrillation may be paroxysmal, lasting minutes or hours, or may be continuous.
- Due to the lack of co-ordination between atrial and ventricular contractions, the atria and ventricles do not contract in a co-ordinated fashion. This may result in incomplete ventricular filling, which in turn may result in up to a 25% reduction in cardiac output and a lowered blood pressure.
- If the ventricular response is rapid, cardiac output is still further reduced, and the cardiac workload increased.

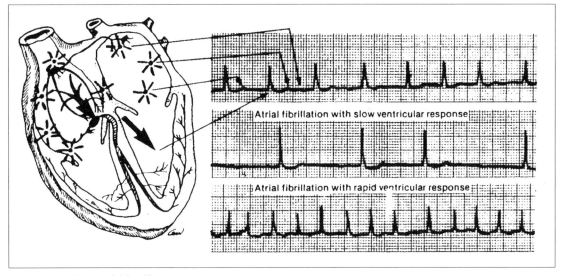

Figure 5-15 Atrial fibrillation

ECG features
- Irregular usually narrow (but may be broad) complex rhythm, with absent P waves.

QRS rhythm: Irregularly irregular.

Rate: Atrial rate is 350-600 per minute, but this is not measurable on the rhythm strip.
   The ventricular rate is 100-160 (or more) beats per minute if untreated, but may be slower if the patient is taking digoxin or other drugs active at the AV node, e.g. β-blockers, verapamil.

P waves: Absent. Instead there are fibrillatory (f) waves, which may be coarse or so fine that atrial activity is not apparent.

Pacemaker site: Multiple ectopic pacemaker sites throughout the atria.

PR interval: Not measurable.

QRS complex: Usually normal (but may be broad), but not preceded by P waves.

Management of acute arrhythmia

- If the patient is well:
    - Asymptomatic, with a ventricular (pulse) rate below 130 bpm, and the systolic BP is above 100 mmHg: none.
- If the patient is unwell:
    - Oxygen
    - Digoxin: 0.5 mg stat. orally, repeated at 8 hourly intervals for 24 hrs, and 0.25 mg thereafter. (less for elderly patients or those with known renal dysfunction).
- If the patient is well, but has a ventricular rate above 130 bpm, a systolic BP above 100 mmHg and the rhythm disturbance persists more than 30 minutes, consider:
    - Digoxin.
- If systolic BP is 90-100 mmHg and the patient is asymptomatic:
    - Digoxin.
- If the patient is unwell and has a systolic BP below 90 mmHg:
    - Consider DC cardioversion.

Atrial flutter

Incidence
- Relatively uncommon, but increases with age.

Aetiology
- Usually caused by underlying organic heart disease or damage, or by metabolic abnormalities.

Pathophysiology
- Results most often in 2:1 or 4:1 block, but variable block may occur.
- If the ventricular response is rapid, the cardiac workload is increased and the cardiac output may be reduced.

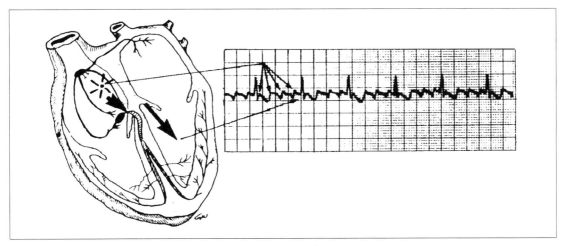

Figure 5-16 Atrial flutter

ECG features
- A regular narrow complex tachycardia, with a rate of 150 bpm should be considered to be atrial flutter until proven otherwise (consider carotid sinus massage to slow AV conduction as an aid to diagnosis).

QRS rhythm: Atrial rhythm is regular (or almost so).
The ventricular rhythm is usually fairly regular, with 2:1 - 4:1 block, but it will be irregular when the AV block is variable.

Rate: The atrial rate is often 240-360 per minute.
The ventricular rate is 140-160 per minute, but may be slower, especially if the patient is taking digoxin or β-blockers.

P waves: Absent. Instead there are flutter (F) waves, often in a jagged or "saw tooth" pattern.

Pacemaker site: An ectopic pacemaker in the atria.

PR interval: Not measurable.

QRS complex: Usually normal, following every second, third or fourth F wave.

Management
- As atrial fibrillation.
- Atrial flutter is often very responsive to low voltage DC cardioversion.

Paroxysmal supraventricular tachycardia

Incidence
- A fairly common arrhythmia, but uncommon following AMI.

Aetiology
- Paroxysmal atrial tachycardia (PAT) may occur in the young who have a history of similar attacks, and macroscopically structurally normal hearts, although in many cases a bypass track may exist between the atria and ventricles, e.g. in Wolff Parkinson White.
- May be precipitated in susceptible individuals by stress, coffee (caffeine), alcohol, heavy smoking, and hyperventilation.
- May be caused by structural damage to the SA or AV nodes, or digoxin overdosage.

Pathophysiology
- May also be due to:
    - A reciprocating AV junctional tachycardia.
    - Repetitive discharges from a single ectopic atrial focus.
- Persistent paroxysmal atrial tachycardia may result in left ventricular failure.

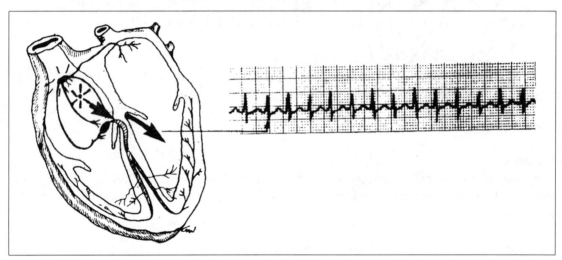

Figure 5-17 Paroxysmal supraventricular tachycardia

ECG features
- Regular narrow QRS complex.

QRS rhythm: Usually regular.

Rate: 140-220 beats per minute.

P waves: Absent or abnormal in morphology and position (usually present in some leads).

Pacemaker site: An ectopic focus in the atria or AV junction.
If there is a bypass tract between the atria and ventricles, a circus movement of excitation occurs between the atrial and ventricular myocardium and perpetuates the tachycardia (Wolff Parkinson White).

PR interval: May be none.

> If a P wave precedes a QRS complex, the PR interval is usually short. Where atrial depolarisation occurs from retrograde activation of the ventricles the P wave will usually follow the QRS complex and will be evident in the T wave.

QRS complex: Usually normal (depending on the heart rate).

Management

- Establish intravenous access.

- If the patient is *stable*:
    - Vagal stimulation:
        - Valsava manoeuvre
        - Carotid sinus massage
        - Face in cold water
        - Cough/deep breath.
    - Adenosine:
        - Initial intravenous bolus of 3 mg administered rapidly over 2 seconds.
        - If this does not terminate the rhythm within 1-2 minutes, this may be followed by 6 mg administered over 2 seconds.
        - If this does not terminate the rhythm within 1-2 minutes, a further bolus of 12 mg may be administered over 2 seconds.
    - Verapamil:
        - Initial intravenous bolus of 5 mg given rapidly over 20-30 seconds
        - Followed 15-20 min later by a further 10 mg,
    - *or -* Atenolol 2.5 mg. by slow intravenous injection, repeated 3-4 times at intervals of 10 minutes
    - Consider cardioversion (see below).

- If the patient is *unstable* (has adverse signs), administer:
    - Oxygen.
    - Consider sedation with diazepam/midazolam if the circumstances permit.
    - Synchronised DC cardioversion:
        - 75-100 Joules
        - 200 Joules
        - 360 Joules.
    - Amiodarone 900 mg over one hour and repeat cardioversion.

- If conversion is successful, but PSVT reoccurs, repeated cardioversion is not indicated.
    - Sedation

CAUTION: Verapamil can be dangerous in the elderly with ischaemic heart disease and impaired left ventricular function, and should *never* be given to patients taking high dose oral β-blockers.

Adverse signs

- Hypotension: systolic BP <90 mmHg
- Chest pain
- Heart failure
- Syncope
- heart rate >200 bpm.

Broad complex tachycardias

Premature ventricular contractions (PVCs)

Incidence
- May occur occasionally in normal people.
- Very common after acute myocardial infarction.

Aetiology
- Damage to the myocardium following AMI.
- Digoxin, hyperkalaemia
- Indicate increased ventricular excitability.

Pathophysiology
- If only occasional: of little importance.
- If frequent: they may compromise cardiac output.
- Some types are of particular importance, because if they occur following AMI, the rhythm may deteriorate to ventricular tachycardia or ventricular fibrillation:
  - In salvos
  - R on T phenomenon: important as this may initiate ventricular fibrillation.
  - Multifocal
  - Frequent PVCs (more than 6 per minute)
  - PVCs with every second beat: bigeminy (this rhythm may often be stable and benign).

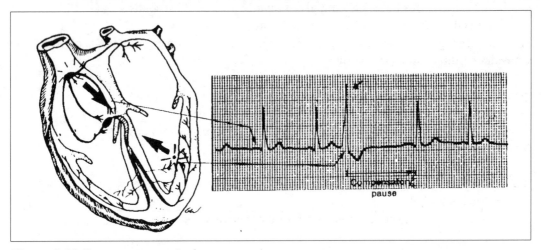

Figure 5-18 Premature ventricular contractions

ECG features

QRS rhythm: Irregular if the PVCs occur randomly, but may be regular with bigeminy, trigeminy, etc. The PVC is separated from the preceding normal QRS by a shorter than normal R-R interval.
Most PVCs are followed by a compensatory pause.

Rate: Determined by the frequency of the PVCs.

P waves: Absent before the PVC, but may follow a QRS if retrograde atrial activation occurs.

Pacemaker site: The pacemaker site for the PVC is an ectopic focus in one of the ventricles.

PR interval: None for the PVC, because it was not preceded by a P wave.

QRS complex: Distorted, bizarre and wide (0.12 seconds: three small squares or more). The T wave is usually in the opposite direction to the main QRS deflection.

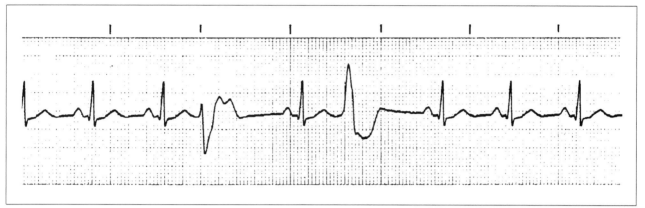

Figure 5-19 Multifocal PVCs: different sizes and shapes: indicate multiple ectopic ventricular foci

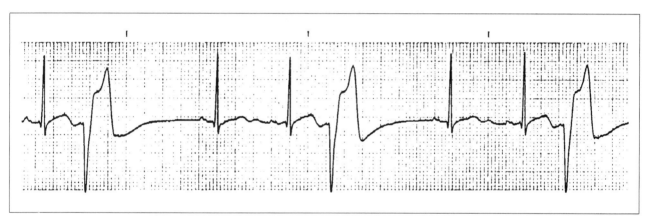

Figure 5-20 Frequent PVCs: Ventricular trigeminy (every third beat is a ventricular ectopic)

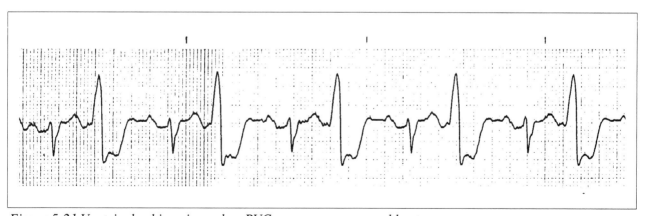

Figure 5-21 Ventricular bigeminy: when PVCs occur every second beat

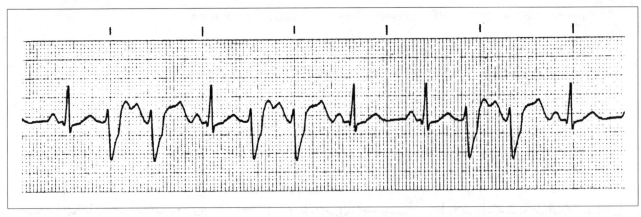

Figure 5-22 Two PVCs in a row (couplets) or more (salvos): may progress rapidly to ventricular tachycardia

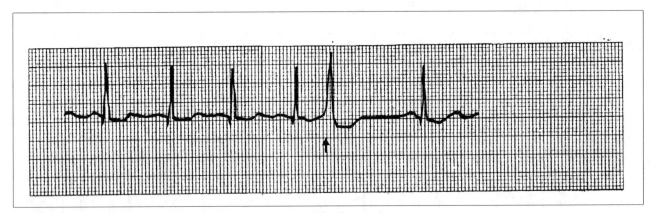

Figure 5-23 R on T pattern (a PVC falling on a T wave): may precipitate ventricular fibrillation

Management
- Occasional PVCs:
    - Observation only as these are unlikely to progress to VT.
- If it is one of the types likely to deteriorate to VT or VF:
    - Lignocaine hydrochloride:
        - 1 mg/kg (75-100 mg in the average adult) intravenously as a bolus.
        - If this is successful:
            - Lignocaine infusion: 2-3 mg/minute (lowest effective dose).
        - If unsuccessful consider:
            - Flecainide (0.05-0.1 mg/kg) intravenously
            - Amiodarone (5 mg/kg) intravenously over 20-120 minutes
- Bigeminy may respond to an increase in the heart rate, e.g. with atropine or pacing.

Note: Although some of these arrhythmias may deteriorate to ventricular fibrillation, it may appear without any prior arrhythmia.

Ventricular tachycardia

Incidence
- A common and life threatening arrhythmia after acute myocardial infarction.

Aetiology
- An ectopic focus in a ventricle.

Pathophysiology
- May progress rapidly to ventricular fibrillation.
- Slow VT (100-130 beats per minute):
    - May cause little haemodynamic compromise, unless there is impaired left ventricular function, e.g. in AMI.
- Rapid VT (160->250 beats per minute):
    - May result in collapse.

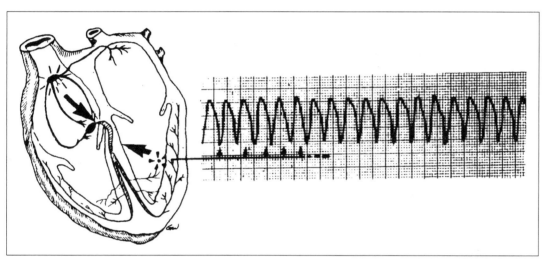

Figure 5-24 Ventricular tachycardia

ECG features
- In the context of ischaemic heart disease, a patient with a broad complex tachycardia should be presumed to have a VT.

Rhythm: Regular or slightly irregular.

Rate: 100-200 beats per minute or faster.

P waves: Often not seen as they are obscured by the QRS complexes.
When they are seen, they usually have no consistent relationship to the QRS complexes, i.e. there is AV dissociation (can be associated if retrograde activation of the atria occurs).

Pacemaker site: An ectopic focus in a ventricle.

PR interval: None.

QRS complex: Distorted, wide (0.12 seconds or more).

ECG criteria used to differentiate VT from SVT with aberrant conduction

Features which tend to indicate ventricular tachycardia, rather than supraventricular tachycardia:
- AV dissociation.
- Fusion or capture beats.
- RSR in V1 with the primary R wave being taller than the secondary R wave.
- Deep S wave in V6.
- Concordant pattern in the precordial leads, i.e. QRS vector in the same direction in leads V1-V6.
- Abnormal QRS axis, especially left axis (compare with a previous normal ECG, if available).

Any patient with a broad complex tachycardia should be presumed to have VT, if there is any doubt.

Management

- If there is no pulse:
    - Treat as ventricular fibrillation.
- If the patient is stable: i.e. the systolic BP is more than 100 mm Hg:
    - Administer oxygen
    - Administer analgesia (following AMI)
    - Establish an intravenous line and administer:
        - Lignocaine hydrochloride:
            - 100 mg intravenously over 1 minute
            - This converts the rhythm out of VT within 1 minute if it is going to work at all.
        - If successful:
            - A lignocaine infusion should be started beginning at a rate of 4 mg per minute for the first hour, reducing to a maintenance dose of 1-2 mg per minute for the next 24 hours.
        - If unsuccessful, consider:
            - Amiodarone: 5 mg/kg in 5% dextrose over 10-20 minutes } usually only in the
        - If this fails or the patient becomes unstable, consider: } hospital setting.
            - Cardioversion as in unstable patients }
- If the patient is haemodynamically unstable, i.e. systolic BP is less than 100 mmHg:
    - Administer oxygen
    - Establish intravenous access and administer analgesia.
    - Sedate if circumstances permit and the patient is conscious
    - Cardiovert at 50 Joules, 100 Joules, 200 Joules, 360 Joules.
    - If unsuccessful consider administration of lignocaine (as above).
- If the rhythm is recurrent:
    - Cardiovert again starting at the energy level previously successful; then consider amiodarone (see above).

Synchronised cardioversion

Synchronisation: Fires on the QRS complex avoiding the T wave.

Indications (in Immediate Care): Organised arrhythmias that are haemodynamically unstable. May be used to treat stable arrhythmias, e.g. atrial fibrillation in the hospital setting.

Management: Administer a sedative/hypnotic if the patient is conscious.

Power levels: Atrial fibrillation: 200 J (much lower if the patient is taking digoxin).
Atrial flutter: 10/50 J.

Bradyarrhythmias

Definition: Any arrhythmia where the heart (ventricular) rate is less than 60 beats per minute.

Incidence

- These arrhythmias are common after inferior myocardial infarction.

Aetiology

- If they occur after:
    - Inferior myocardial infarction:
        - The prognosis is good, as the treatment is usually simple and successful and the rhythm will usually revert to sinus rhythm, although temporary pacing may be necessary.
        - The arrhythmia is often transient and occurs as a result of reversible ischaemia or vagal overactivity.
    - Anterior myocardial infarction:
        - Bradycardia is a sign of extensive infarction involving the interventricular septum, and has a poor prognosis unless it is due to vagal overactivity alone.
        - Death is the usual outcome due to the development of cardiogenic shock as a result of the extensive muscle damage.
- May occur as a result of:
    - Previous treatment with β-blockers.
    - AV nodal and conduction system disease.

Electrophysiology

Aetiology
- Occurs most commonly after an inferior myocardial infarction (20% of all patients).

Incidence
- May be caused by:
    - Vaso-vagal slowing, or impairment of sino-atrial function, i.e. sinus bradycardia
    - First degree AV block (may not cause a bradycardia)
    - Second degree AV block (may not cause a bradycardia)
    - Third degree/complete AV block.

Symptoms/signs

- The patient's condition depends on the underlying aetiology and the rate, and may vary from their being:
    - Relatively well with little or no symptoms.
    - Very unwell with:
        - Chest pain due to cardiac ischaemia or even infarction
        - Dyspnoea
        - Confusion
        - Hypotension.

Principles of management

- The management of any patient depends basically on the clinical state.

  - Oxygen
  - Relief of pain
  - Anti-arrhythmic drugs

Relief of pain

  - Nitrates:
    - Sublinguallyor buccal preparations.
  - Morphine/diamorphine (with an anti-emetic):
    - Administered slowly and titrated to patient response to avoid respiratory depression.

Unstable angina (sudden increase in pain, etc.)
  - Management:
    - Stabilise:
      - Oxygen
      - Nitrates
      - Aspirin
      - Morphine/diamorphine.
    - Admit immediately.

Anti-arrhythmic drugs

Atropine sulphate: 0.5-2.0 mg administered intravenously in incremental doses of 0.3 mg, up to a maximum of 2 mg, over 5 minutes, is indicated if the patient is symptomatic.

- If the patient is still symptomatic then consider administration of:

Isoprenaline: 200 μg as an initial bolus, followed by an infusion of 2 mg in 250 ml of 5% dextrose, the infusion rate being titrated against heart rate.

Transcutaneous thoracic pacing

- Although this is not yet widely available in the pre-hospital situation, many new defibrillators incorporate a non-invasive pacing facility, using adhesive electrodes.
- If this is not available, it is recommended that the hospital to which the patient is being sent is forewarned if the patient has a bradyarrhythmia for which pacing is indicated:
    Second degree heart block type II.
    Third degree heart block.

  Note:- Hemiblock
       Bundle branch block
       First degree heart block   do not usually require pacing.
       Second degree heart block type I

Sinus bradycardia

Incidence
- Often found in normal fit young men, especially atheletes.
- Commonly occurs after inferior myocardial infarction.

Aetiology
- May be caused by normal doses of:
    - β-blockers
    - Digoxin
    - Opiates.
- Following AMI it indicates:
    - Increased vagal (para-sympathetic) tone.

Note:- If sinus bradycardia is present in a patient with an anterior infarction, it does not carry the same poor prognosis as the development of heart block).

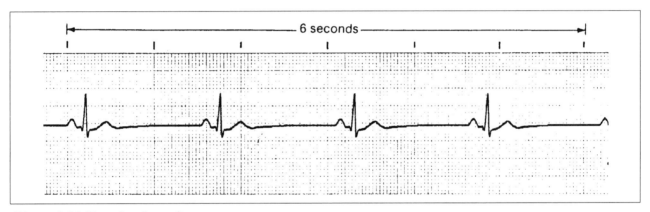

Figure 5-25 Sinus bradycardia

ECG features

Rhythm: Regular or very slightly irregular with a prolonged R-R interval between R waves.

Rate: <60 beats per minutes.

P waves: Normal: each followed by a QRS complex.

Pacemaker site: SA node.

PR interval: Normal (0.12-0.2 sec).

QRS complex: Normal: each preceded by a P wave.

Management
- No treatment is indicated if the patient is well.
- If the patient is symptomatic or hypotensive, then the initial treatment is with:
    - Atropine: 0.5-0.6 mg given intravenously in incremental doses up to 1.8-2.0 mg over 5 minutes.
    - Oxygen, nitrates, analgesia.
- Careful cardiac monitoring.

Sinus arrest

Incidence
- Relatively common.

Aetiology
- Commonest cause is sino-atrial disease.
- Often occurs as a result of ischaemic heart disease or rarely following AMI.

Pathophysiology:
- Caused by a defect in or damage to the SA node.

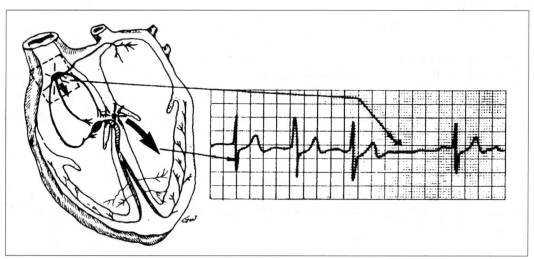

Figure 5-26 Sinus arrest

ECG features

Rhythm: Irregular (regular underlying rhythm with dropped beats).

Rate: Normal or slow.

P waves: Normal, when they are present, preceding a QRS complex (abnormal, if an atrial escape beat occurs)
However, if the SA node is blocked or does not discharge, the entire sequence of P-QRS-T is missed, unless an ectopic escape focus takes over and an escape beat occurs.

Pacemaker site: SA node.

PR interval: Usually normal (0.12-0.20 sec).

QRS complex: Normal, each preceded by a QRS complex.

} absent during SA block.

Management
- If the patient is well:
  - None.
- If the patient is unwell/haemodynamically compromised:
  - Administer atropine: 0.5-0.6 mg given intravenously in incremental doses up to a maximum of 1.8-2.0 mg over 5 minutes.

Heart block

Incidence
- Occurs in 5% of patients following AMI.

Aetiology
- Usually results from inferior infarction.

Pathophysiology
- Caused by a defect in the AV conducting system.

First degree AV block

Incidence
- Common after acute myocardial infarction.

Aetiology
- Damage to the AV junction.
- Increased vagal (parasympathetic) tone.
- Toxicity from cardiac drugs: β-blockers, digoxin, quinidine, procainamide.

Pathophysiology
- Following AMI, it may herald other more advanced degrees of heart block.

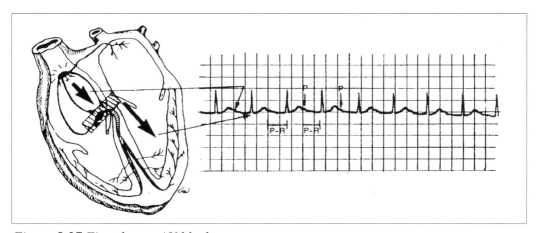

Figure 5-27 First degree AV block

ECG features

Rhythm: Regular.

Rate: Normal or slow.

P waves: Normal, preceding each QRS complex.

Pacemaker site: SA node.

PR interval: Prolonged PR interval: >0.2 seconds (5 small squares).

QRS complex: Usually normal each preceded by a P wave.

Management
- This rhythm is benign and requires no treatment, but the patient should be monitored in case the conduction disturbance deteriorates to a higher more serious degree of block.

Second degree AV block: Mobitz type I: Wenckebach phenomenon

Incidence
- A relatively common rhythm following acute myocardial infarction.

Pathophysiology
- This rhythm is usually transient and reversible and does not usually progress to a higher degree of block.

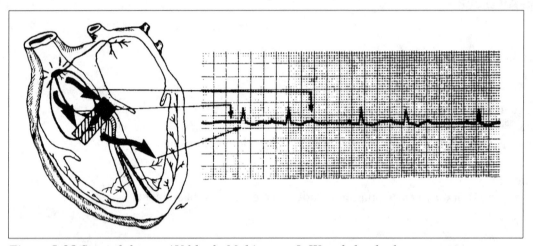

Figure 5-28 Second degree AV block: Mobitz type I: Wenckebach phenomenon

ECG features

Rhythm: Atrial (P wave) regular.
      Ventricular (QRS) rhythm irregular.

Rate: Atrial rate : Normal.
      Ventricular rate: May be normal or slow, depending on the degree of AV block.

P waves: Normal. A QRS complex is absent after every third, fourth or fifth P wave.
      There are more P waves than QRS complexes.

Pacemaker site: SA node.

PR interval: Progressively increases until a beat is dropped as AV conduction fails completely; the process is then repeated.

QRS complex: Normal: each preceded by a P wave, unless an escape beat occurs.

Management
- If the patient is well: no treatment other than close cardiac monitoring.
- If the patient is unwell:
    - Oxygen
    - Atropine: 0.5-0.6 mg given intravenously in incremental doses up to 1.8-2.0 mg over 5 minutes.
    - Consider isoprenaline if atropine is unsuccessful.

Second degree AV block: Mobitz type II

Aetiology
- May follow a large anterior AMI, and is caused by damage to the conducting system below the AV node and bundle of His.
- May be associated with bundle branch block or left axis deviation.
- Often *not* associated with ischaemic heart disease.

Pathophysiology
- An intermittent failure of AV conduction results in the dropping of beats. It may progress rapidly to complete heart block.

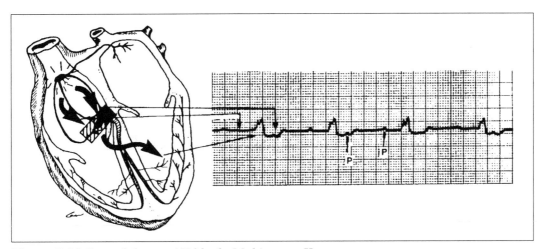

Figure 5-29 Second degree AV block: Mobitz type II

ECG features

Rhythm: Atrial (P wave) rhythm regular.
  Ventricular (QRS) rhythm may be regular or irregular.

Rate: Atrial rate normal.
  Ventricular rate may be normal or slow.

P waves: Normal, but not every P wave is followed by a QRS complex.
  There are more P waves than QRS complexes.
  The ratio of P waves to QRS complexes may be 2:1, 3:1, etc., or may follow no regular pattern.

Pacemaker site: SA node.

PR interval: Normal or prolonged, but constant.

QRS complex: Usually normal, but may be widened: each is preceded by a P wave.

Management
- If the patient is well: careful observation.
- If the patient is unwell with a bradycardia:
    - Oxygen
    - Atropine: 0.5-0.6 mg given intravenously in incremental doses up to 1.8-2.0 mg over 5 minutes
    - Consider isoprenaline if atropine is unsuccessful
    - Consider transthoracic cutaneous pacing.

Third degree AV block: complete heart block

Aetiology
- Usually occurs following acute myocardial infarction.
- Patients with an anterior infarction are often symptomatic.
- Often due to non-ischaemic causes.

Pathophysiology
- There is complete failure of AV conduction with no relationship between atrial and ventricular contractions.
- If the heart rate is below 35-50 beats per minute, the cardiac output may be significantly compromised.
- Additionally, occasionally there may be poor ventricular filling, due to the non co-ordination between atria and ventricles.

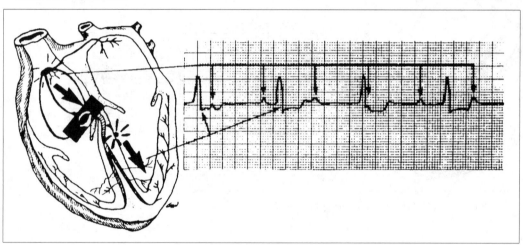

Figure 5-30 Third degree AV block

ECG features

Rhythm: Regular.

Rate: Atrial (P waves) rate: regular in sinus rhythm (may be atrial fibrillation or flutter).
Ventricular (QRS) rate: regular: 30-40 beats per minute.

P waves: Normal, but have no constant relationship to QRS complexes.

Pacemaker site: The SA node is usually the pacemaker for the atria (unless atrial fibrillation or other atrial arrhythmias are present), but impulses are blocked at the AV junction, and so do not reach the ventricles.
An ectopic focus in the AV junction or the ventricles then takes over.
The lower the focus in the ventricles, the slower the rhythm and the more abnormal the ventricular complexes.

PR interval: There is no true PR interval.

QRS complex: Usually wide and bizarre, although if the escape focus is in the AV node or junction they may look relatively normal.

Management
- If the patient is well:
    - Consider administration of atropine.
- If the patient is unwell, i.e. pale, sweaty, shocked and is haemodynamically compromised (pulse rate <55 bpm, systolic blood pressure <100 mmHg):
    - Atropine (more likely to be sucessful if the QRS complex is narrow): 0.5-0.6 mg given intravenously in incremental doses up to 1.8-2.0 mg over 5 minutes
    - Consider an isoprenaline bolus (50 µg), followed by an isoprenaline infusion (2-4 µg/min)
    - Transthoracic cutaneous pacing if available
    - Early evacuation to hospital.

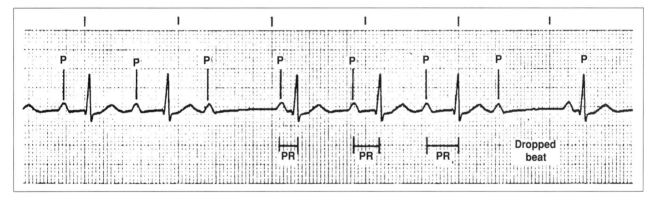

Figure 5-31 First degree AV block

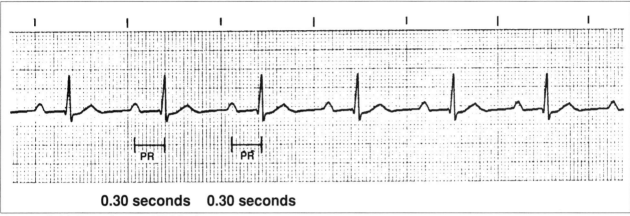

Figure 5-32 Second degree AV block: Mobitz I: Wenckebach

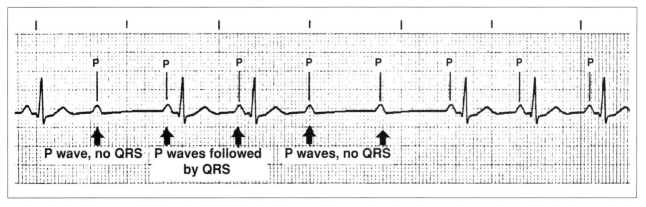

Figure 5-33 Second degree AV block: Mobitz type II

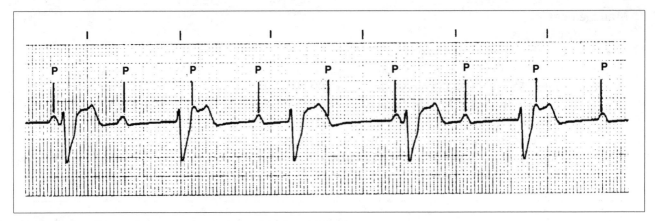

Figure 5-34 Third degree AV block: Complete heart block

Bifascicular block: right bundle branch block, and left or right axis deviation

Aetiology
- May occur in patients:
    - With an infarct
    - Asymptomatically.

Pathophysiology
- Associated with large infarcts which have a high mortality.
- May progress suddenly to more severe degrees of heart block.
- May often be an incidental finding.

Management
- Careful monitoring.

Note:- Trifasicular block:
- Has the features of bifasicular block with first degree AV block in addition (prolonged PR interval).
- Is a warning block and may progress to complete heart block.

Megacode

This is a method of team management of acute myocardial infarction involving cardiac arrest and/or life threatening arrhythmias first developed in the USA. It is also used for practising/testing performance.

The minumum number of people necessary to carry out effective Advanced Cardiac Life Support is three; four is better.

The whole situation is fluid and constantly changing as the initial response is replaced by more effective and efficient methods of patient management, which themselves change according to the patients need and the treatment carried out.

Team leader

- Manages the resuscitation team.
- Takes an overview of the resuscitation effort/monitors all pertinent information.
- Assesses the patient's condition.
- Monitors the team's performance.
- Monitors the ECG screen and provides the rhythm recognition.
- Is in control of defibrillation.
- Manages the post arrest care.

Team member 1: airway carer
- Maintains the airway:
    - Head tilt/chin lift
    - Jaw thrust
    - Oropharyngeal airway
    - Endotracheal intubation.
- Provides oxygenation and ventilation:
    - Mouth to mouth/nose
    - Mouth to mask
    - Bag and mask
    - Ventilator.

Team member 2: circulation carer
- Monitors a central pulse.
- Provides circulatory support:
    - External chest compressions.

Team member 3
- Establishes and maintains an intravenous infusion.
- May administer any cardiac drugs.
- Acts as a runner.
- Gets additional equipment as requested.
- Assists the other members of the team.
- Provides help with transport.
- Keeps record of:
    - Time elapsed
    - Shocks/drugs given.

Drugs used in the management of arrhythmias

Introduction

- This is a brief list of most of the drugs used in the early treatment of cardiac emergencies, together with a description of their basic pharmacology.
- Analgesics and sedating agents are described in the chapter on Pain Relief, and nitrates, β-blockers, diuretics, anti-platelet agents and thrombolytics in the chapter on Acute Myocardial Infarction.
- Not all the drugs listed are used in Immediate Care, but those that are not, are included so as to provide a reasonable overview of the subject.
- The two first line drugs: adrenaline and atropine, should be carried by all those involved in Immediate Cardiac Care.

Note:- Care should be exercised in the use of negatively inotropic drugs in patients with ischaemic heart disease as they may have impaired left ventricular function and their use may precipitate sudden heart failure (as they may in normal hearts if tachycardia conversion does not occur).

Adrenergic receptor agonists

Action
- Stimulate adrenoreceptors resulting in:
    - α_1 *and* α_2 *receptors:*
        - Arterial and arteriolar constriction: an increase in the systemic vascular resistance, resulting in an increase in cerebral and coronary perfusion during CPR.
        - Venoconstriction: a reduction in venous pooling and an increase in the venous return.
        - (Pupillary dilation).
    - β_1 *receptors:*
        - An increase in myocardial contractility and systolic pressure, i.e. a positive inotropic effect.
        - An increase in aortic diastolic pressure and blood flow, coronary perfusion pressure and coronary and cerebral blood flow.
        - An increase in pacemaker rates: increase in heart rate.
        - An increase in spontaneous electrical activity (converts fine ventricular fibrillation to coarse ventricular fibrillation).
        - An increase in myocardial oxygen demand.
    - β_2 *receptors:*
        - Smooth muscle vasodilation: bronchodilation, tremor.
        - Increased glycogenolysis and a subsequent increase in oxygen requirement, hypokalaemia.

Adrenaline
- A natural catecholamine, which acts as a neurotransmitter in the parasympathetic nervous system.

Action
- α, β_1, β_2 adrenoceptor agonist action.

Indications
- All forms of cardiac arrest because of its ability to preserve the cerebral and coronary blood supply;
    - VF and failed DC shock.
    - Electromechanical dissociation.
    - Asystole, when it may have the added advantage of coarsening and exposing fine VF.
- In anaphylaxis.

Presentation:
- Prefilled syringe (IMS): 10 ml of 1:10,000.

Dosage
- Adults: Intravenous injection: 0.5-1.00 mg
                Via endotracheal tube: 2.00-3.00 mg.
- Children: 10 μg/kg.
- Administration may be repeated every loop (at 2-3 minute intervals) during cardiac arrest according to the patient's response, until resuscitation is successful or abandoned.
- An increased dose of 5 mg may be given as a fourth dose in EMD or asystole.

Half life
- 1-2 minutes.

Side Effects
- Hypertension and cardiac arrhythmias (not a problem in cardiac arrest and unlikely to be a problem in the resuscitated patient due to its short half life).

Dopamine (Intropin)
- The naturally occuring precursor of adrenaline and noradrenaline.

Action
- Essentially sympathomimetic and inotropic: agonist effect on dopamine, α and β_1 receptors. The predominant action depends on the dosage.

Indications
- Drugs of choice for inotropic support in low output states, i.e., hypotension not due to simple hypovolaemia:
    - Cardiogenic shock
    - Infective shock.

Contraindications
- Tachyarrhythmia, marked increase in blood pressure.

Presentation
- Dopamine hydrochloride:
    - In 5% Dextrose: 250 ml containers of 200, 400, and 800 mg (800, 1,600 and 3,200 μg/ml).
    - IMS: 40 mg/ml: 5, 10, 20 ml.

Dosage
- 1-4 μg/kg/min:
    - Dopamine receptor effects:
        - Renal and gut vasodilation and increased urinary output.
- 4-10 μg/kg/min:
    - Above + β_1 effects:
        - Increase myocardial contractility resulting in an increase in cardiac output and heart rate.
- >10 μg/kg/min:
    - Above + α effects:
        - Vasoconstriction and may exacerbate cardiac failure and precipitate arrhythmias.
- Paediatric: 2-10 μg/kg/min

Administration
  - This should be by intravenous infusion and the dose adjusted according to the patient's response.
  - Must be given via a central line, and therefore not usually used in Immediate Care.

Half life
  - A few minutes.

Side effects
  - Nausea and vomiting
  - Hypertension, tachycardia.

Dobutamine (Dobutrex)
  - A synthetic analogue of dopamine.

Action
  - Positive inotrope, mainly affecting β_1 receptors.
  - Increases myocardial contractility, raising cardiac output, stroke volume and at higher doses pulse rate.
  - Overall it improves the myocardial oxygen supply and demand balance, if tachycardia is avoided.

Indications
  - As dopamine.

Presentation
  - Dobutamine hydrochloride: 12.5 mg/ml: 20 ml vials.

Dosage
  - 2.5 µg/kg, titrated to patient response.

Administration
  - As dopamine, but may be given via a peripheral line.

Advantages
  - Tends to lower the cardiac filling pressure, and usually reduces the peripheral resistance.

Note:- Often a combination of these two drugs (dopamine 5 µg and dobutamine 5-20 µg/kg) are given to maintain urine output and blood pressure.

Isoprenaline (Saventrine)
  - A synthetic catecholamine

Action:
  - Potent β_1 and β_2 effects with no α effects.
  - More cronotropic than inotropic, reduces the systemic vascular resistance, resulting in a drop in the systemic and diastolic blood pressures.
  - Results in improved myocardial contractility and a marked rise in heart rate and cardiac output.
  - Diverts blood supply from cerebral and coronary vessels to gut, muscle and skin.

Indications
  - second line arrhythmic when atropine has not been effective:
      - AV heart block
      - Symptomatic sinus bradycardia.

Presentation
  - Prefilled syringe (IMS): 10 ml: 20 µg/ml.

Dosage
  - Intravenous injection: 0.2 mg.
  - Intravenous infusion: 2-10 µg/minute.

Half Life
  - 2 minutes

Side effects
  - May convert bradycardia to a fast tachycardia.
  - Increases myocardial excitability resulting in arrhythmias, hypotension.
  - Sweating, headache.

Atropine sulphate

Action
  - Competitive muscarinic antagonist, which causes vagal inhibition at the SA and AV nodes.
      - SA node: increase in automaticity, resulting in a rise in heart rate (and rate related cardiac output). Blood pressure may rise as a result.
      - AV node: Facilitates conduction by blocking inhibitory effects.

Indications
  - Symptomatic bradycardia: sinus and nodal.
  - Asystole (after failure of adrenaline).
  - Symptomatic AV block.
  - Bradycardia related ventricular ectopics.
  - Hypotension: If the cardiac rate is slow.
  - Overdosage: neostigmine, physostigmine, organophosphates.

Presentation
  - Prefilled syringe (IMS): 1 mg/10 ml.

Dosage
  - Bradycardia:
      - Incremental doses of 0.5-0.6 mg over 5 minutes up to a maximum of 2 mg repeated as required.
  - Asystole:
      - 3 mg intravenously, 6-9 mg via endotracheal tube.

Half life
  - A few hours.

Side effects
  - Pupillary dilation (making interpretation of pupil sizes difficult), blurred vision, acute glaucoma.
  - Dry mouth, urinary retention, flushed, dry skin.

Calcium chloride

Action
- Increases cardiac muscle contractility.
- (Cerebral and coronary artery vasoconstriction).
- May slow the heart rate and precipitate arrhythmias.

Indications
- Cardiac arrest in patients with hypocalcaemia, hyperkalaemia or overdosage of calcium antagonists.

Presentation
- Prefilled syringe (IMS): 10%: 1 g/10 ml.

Dose
- 10 ml as a bolus every 5-10 min intravenously.

CAUTION
- Calcium chloride should *never* be mixed with sodium bicarbonate.
- A high serum calcium will aggravate digoxin toxicity.

Sodium bicarbonate

Indications
- Used to try to correct metabolic and respiratory acidosis in the prolonged resuscitation situation (after 20 minutes).
- It is much more important to ensure that oxygenation and ventilation are adequate.

Presentation
- Prefilled syringe (IMS): 8.4% in 50 ml: 1 mEq/ml.

Dosage
- 50 ml 8.4% intravenously (*never* by endotracheal tube).

CAUTION
- Central venous pH should be monitored as soon as possible after administration.

Antiarrhythmic drugs

Introduction

- Amiodarone and digoxin are the only antiarrhythmics which are not negatively inotropic, and are therefore the only drugs that can be safely given in patients who are hypotensive or have impaired left ventricular function.

Class 1: Membrane stabilising drugs

Introduction
- These are negatively inotropic and should be avoided in patients with impaired left ventricular function and a systolic blood pressure less than 95 mmHg.

- Usually divided into three classes according to their effect on the duration of the action potential, which is increased by impeding the transport of sodium ions across the cell membrane during activation and decrease phase 0 of the rapid depolarisation of action potential (rapid sodium channel)

Class 1a: Antiarrhythmic effects are confined to the atria.

Class 1b: Antiarrhythmic effects on ventricles.

Class 1c: No effect on the action potential, antiarrhythmic effect on atria and ventricles.

Class 1a

Disopyramide (Rythmodan)

Action
- May also have an anticholinergic effect (causing an increase in AV conduction rate).

Indications
- Paroxysmal atrial fibrillation.
- Ventricular arrhythmias (VT) especially after myocardial infarction, not responsive to lignocaine.

Presentation
- 50 mg/5 ml ampoules.

Dosage
- 2 mg/kg by slow intravenous injection over 5 minutes; maximum 150 mg regardless of body weight.

Side effects
- May impair cardiac contractility, and aggravate heart failure.

CONCLUSION: Class Ia *drug of choice.*

Procainamide

Indications
- Ventricular and supraventricular arrhythmias.

Presentation
- 100 mg/ml ampoules.

Dosage
- 20-50 mg/min to 1 g maximum in first hour.
- Has a short half life, and therefore needs to be topped up frequently.

Side effects
- Myocardial depression, heart failure.
- Nausea, diarrhoea.

Contraindications
- Heart block, heart failure, hypotension.

Mexilitine (Mexitil)

Indications
  - Ventricular arrhythmias (VT) resistant to lignocaine.

Contraindications
  - Heart block.

Side effects
  - Nausea, vomiting and tremor.

Presentation
  - 10 ml ampoules 25 mg/ml.

Dosage
  - Intravenous bolus of 250 mg or 5-10 ml, followed by 250 mg/hour for the first hour and 125 mg/hour for the second hour.

Class 1b

Lignocaine (Xylocard)

Action
  - Stabilises cell membranes reducing the rate of diastolic depolarisation. This decreases ventricular automaticity, suppresses ventricular ectopic activity, and raises the threshold for VF (this may reduce the incidence of primary VF following AMI, but does not alter the overall mortality).
  - Acts selectively in diseased and ischaemic muscle interrupting and preventing re-entry circuits.
  - Good local anaesthetic, but may cause serious myocardial depression.

Indications
  - Ventricular tachycardia
  - Frequent symptomatic PVCs
  - After successful defibrillation

  especially after myocardial infarction, but is no longer indicated for the routine prevention of VF.

Contraindications (relative)
  - Should not be given in all degrees of AV block
  - SA disorders.

Advantages
  - Very few proarrhythmic effects.

Presentation
  - IMS prefilled syringe: 2% lignocaine hydrochloride, 100 mg/5 ml.

Dosage
  - Rapidly metabolised and initial dose may only last 10 minutes, half life is then 2 hours.
  - Give an initial bolus of 100 mg (10 ml of 10 mg/ml) over 2-3 minutes followed by a repeat bolus of 50-100 mg after 5-10 minutes, and an infusion of 2-4 mg/min for 24 hours (maximum 3 mg/kg).
  - Paediatric: 1mg/kg.

Side effects (more marked in the elderly and those with hepatic impairement)
  - Parasthesiae, dysphasia, drowsiness, dizziness, hypotension, confusion, muscle twitching and fits.

Class Ic

Flecainide (Tambocor)

Indications
- Ventricular and supraventricular tachycardias.
- Ventricular extra systoles.
- Arrhythmias associated with the Wolff Parkinson White syndrome.
- Ventricular fibrillation refractory to lignocaine and electricity.

Contraindications (relative)
- Heart failure.
- PVCs following AMI.
- SA disorders.
- AV block.

Presentation
- 15 ml ampoules of 10 mg/ml.

Dosage
- 2 mg/kg intravenously over 10-30 minutes (max. 150 mg) with ECG monitoring, then as required by intravenous infusion.

Side effects
- May aggravate cardiac failure and has proarrhythmic effects, especially if administered with other drugs which prolong the QT interval..

Class II: β-blockers: See under chapter on Acute Myocardial Infarction

Action
- β adrenergic receptor blockers.

Class III: Repolarisation inhibitors

Action: Widen the action potential duration, and therefore the QT interval.

Bretylium tosylate (Bretylate)

Action
- Adrenergic neurone blocking agent.
- Initial action is to cause the release of noradrenaline stored in adrenergic neurones, which may result in transient hypertension and tachycardia. This is followed about 20 minutes later by full adrenergic blockade.
- The only drug to have a direct beneficial effect on VF by raising the fibrillation threshold.

Indications
- Recurrent or refractory VF or VT after lignocaine and DC version/defibrillation.

Presentation
- 50 mg/ml: 2 and 10 ml ampoules.

Dosage
- 5-10 mg/kg by slow intravenous injection over 8-10 minutes; may take 20-30 minutes to work.
- If successful; may be repeated after 1-2 hours or followed by an infusion of 1-2 mg/kg/hr.

Half life
- 7-9 hours.

Side effects
- Severe postural hypotension, nausea, vomiting.

Disadvantage
- If used, commits the rescuer to 30 minutes further resuscitation.

Amiodarone (Cordorone)

Action
- As well as Class III effects, it also has some Class I activity (inhibits the fast sodium channel)
- Mild negative inotropic effect and is a coronary artery dilator.

Indications
- Arrhythmias associated with the Wolff Parkinson White Syndrome.
- For serious arrhythmias when other drugs have been ineffective or are contraindicated for:
    - Supraventricular and ventricular tachycardia.
    - Atrial fibrillation and flutter, recurrent ventricular fibrillation.

Contraindications
- Sinus bradycardia, AV block, (thyroid problems).
- If administered concurrently with other drugs which prolong the QT interval, amiodarone may paradoxically become arrhythmogenic.

Side effects
- Skin photosensativity, pulmonary fibrosis, thyroid dysfunction, peripheral neuropathy, hepatotoxicity (with long term use only).
- Nausea (even at low doses).
- Concurrent administration of β-blockers or verapamil may result in an increased degree of nodal block.

Presentation
- 150 mg/3 ml ampoules.

Dosage
- Up to 5 mg/kg in 100 mls 5% dextrose (not saline) intravenously over 1-4 hours (onset of full action may take several hours).
- For Wolff Parkinson White Syndrome: may be given orally.

Half life
- Long.

Class IV: calcium channel blockers/calcium antagonists

Action:
- Inhibit the slow calcium channel in the AV node.
- Reduce myocardial oxygen consumption.

Verapamil (Cordilox)

Action
- Inhibits the action potential in the SA and AV nodes, resulting in an increase in AV block and an increase in the refractory period of the AV node.
- Arteriolar vasodilation and reduces cardiac contractility (has a significant negative inotropic effect)

Indications
- Atrial fibrillation and flutter.
- Paroxysmal supraventricular tachycardia (drug of choice if adenosine is not available).
- Relief of cardiac ischaemic pain: angina (orally).
- Hypertension.

Contraindications
- Bradycardia, sick sinus syndrome, pre-existing AV nodal disease, heart block, heart failure, atrial flutter or fibrillation complicating the Wolff Parkinson White syndrome.
- Patients taking:
  - High doses of β-blockers (may precipitate severe refractory hypertension)
  - Digoxin (may cause asystole), quinidine or disopyramide.

Presentation
- 5 mg/2 ml ampoules.

Dosage
- SVT: 5-10 mg intravenously rapidly over 30 seconds initially, followed 15-20 minutes later by a further 5-10 mg intravenously if required.

Side effects
- Headache, flushing.
- Hypotension, bradycardia, heart block, asystole.
- May precipitate heart failure and exacerbate conduction disorders especially in children.

Note: - The negative inotropic effects of these antiarrhythmic drugs tend to be cumulative, so care should be exercised if they are used together.
- Their tendency to cause as well as treat arrhythmias may be aggravated by hypokalaemia.

Adenosine
- A naturally occuring purine nucleotide found throughout the body; formed by the breakdown of adenosine triphosphate (ATP) and S-adenosylhomocysteine.

Action
- When given intravenously, it acts at the adenosine A_1 (myocardial) and A_2 (coronary artery) receptors.
- At the A_1 receptors this interaction results in an outward shift of intracellular potassium and hyperpolarisation of the cardiac cell membranes, resulting in depression of the AV node and the

blocking of conduction.
- Effective at terminating episodes of paroxysmal supraventricular tachycardia including those involving the AV node in a re-entry pathway.
- Half-life is 10-15 seconds, so that a blocked arrhythmia may re-emerge .

Indications
- Paroxysmal supraventricular tachycardias including those associated with the Wolff Parkinson White syndrome.
- As an aid to the diagnosis of broad complex tachycardias:
    - If it stops a tachycardia, it is likely to be junctional in origin and involve the AV node.
    - If there is transient AV block with specific ECG changes (Pwaves, f waves of F waves), the arrhythmia is likely to be due to atrial tachycardia, flutter, or fibrillation.
    - If there is no effect, the arrhythmia is likely to be ventricular fibrillation.

Contraindications
- Asthma
- Second or third degree AV block.
- Sick sinus syndrome (unless pacemaker is fitted).

Side effects (occur in about 20-25% of patients and last less than one minute)
- Most common:
    - Transient facial flushing, dyspnoea, bronchospasm, a chocking sensation, nausea, light-headedness, chest pain and a peculiar unpleasant feeling.
- Less common:
    - Sweating, palpitations, hyperventilation, headache, blurred vision, burning sensation.
    - Severe bradycardia requiring pacing.
    - Transient ECG rhythm disturbances.
- Potentiated by dipyrimadole.
- Antagonised by methylxanthenes, e.g. aminophylline, theophylline and caffeine.

Presentation
- 3mg/ml: 2 ml ampoules.

Dosage
- Initial intravenous bolus of 3 mg administered rapidly over 2 seconds into a large vein, e.g.: antecubital fossa, followed by a saline flush.
- If this does not terminate the rhythm within 1-2 minutes, this may be followed by 6 mg administered over 2 seconds.
- If this does not terminate the rhythm within 1-2 minutes, a further bolus of 12 mg may be administered over 2 seconds.
- Additional or higher doses are not generally recommended.

Advantages
- It is safe to administer to patients with a broad complex tachycardia (unlike verapamil).
- It exhibits no negative inotropic effects.
- It is safe to administer to patients on β-blockers (unlike verapamil).
- It is safe in children (unlike verapamil): dosage: 0.0375 mg/kg.

*CONCLUSION: Drug of choice for the management of supraventricular tachycardias.
Useful as an aid in the diagnosis of tachycardias of unknown type.
Should only be administered to monitored patients with full resuscitation facilities available. Not licensed (yet) for pre-hospital use.*

6

Pain relief

Pain relief

Introduction

- Apart from any humanitarian reasons, the relief of pain has a high priority in Immediate Care following the preservation of life and the treatment of major injuries, as pain by itself may result in a significant deterioration in the patient's condition.
- The requirement for analgesia may vary from one individual to another.

Pathophysiology

- Pain causes an increase in circulating catecholamines resulting in vasoconstriction, tachycardia and hypertension.
- This may cause reduced tissue perfusion and cellular damage, an increase in intracranial pressure, and myocardial ischaemia.
- Pain may also cause an increase in muscle tone and metabolism, and can precipitate or exacerbate shock.

Management

Physical

- Treatment of the cause of the pain should be attempted where appropriate, e.g. removal of caustic substances, and splinting and reduction of fractures, which may itself require prophylactic analgesia.

Systemic analgesia/analgesics

Introduction

As a general rule, the best drugs are those with which you are familiar, and are happy and confident to use.

Administration

- Most analgesics should only be given *intravenously* in the Immediate Care situation, and *not intramuscularly*. In the shocked patient, they may be poorly absorbed initially and thus be ineffective, but later as the patient's tissue perfusion improves, they may enter the circulation as a bolus, causing relative overdosage. In addition, if drugs are administered intramuscularly following AMI, they may cause a rise in muscle enzymes, which may cause diagnostic problems, and bruising if the patient is subsequently given thrombolytics.
- It should be borne in mind when administering analgesics, that many patients suffering trauma may also have consumed alcohol, which may interreact with the analgesic you are using, and that many others, especially the elderly, may not be medically fit, and will require a smaller dosage.
- Some analgesic, e.g. opiates and buprenorphine may cause hypotension and should therefore not be given to patients who are sitting, but only to those who are horizontal.

The ideal pre-hospital analgesic

- Effective.
- Rapid onset.
- Easily administered.
- Packaging: Small, tough, easily portable.
- Short duration of action: 1-2 hours.
- Cause minimal respiratory depression.
- Have no negative inotropic effects.
- Cause some sedation, without psychomimetic effects.

Opiates/opiate analogues

- Opiates are effective and are widely used, being the analgesics of choice for the relief of cardiac pain.

Action
- Strong analgesic effect
- Relieve anxiety and fear
- Vasodilation
- (The above properties make them especially useful in the management of acute pulmonary oedema).

Administration
- By slow intravenous injection. The elderly require a smaller dose.

Major problems
- They are controlled drugs and have to be kept securely and there are special regulations regarding their prescribing and stock control.

Disadvantages
- They may cause nausea and vomiting, especially during ambulance transportation, and although these symptoms are rarely seen in the patient with very severe pain, they should be given with an anti-emetic such as metoclopramide.
- They may also cause depression of respiration, hypotension, drowsiness and constricted pupils, and can precipitate shock.
- Their use is *not recommended in the head injured patient*, and they should be used with caution when there is respiratory embarrassment or shock, or where there is a known history of chest disease or asthma.

Morphine sulphate injection

- A potent and effective analgesic, with anxiolytic properties.

Action
- It has a rapid onset and relatively long duration of action of several hours, which may cause prolonged masking of the vital signs.

Presentation
- 10, 15, 30 mg/ml in 1 and 2 ml ampoules.

Dosage
- Best given in small incremental doses, so as to avoid overdosage.

Disadvantages
- Prone to cause nausea and vomiting.
- May also cause respiratory depression.

Morphine sulphate/cyclizine (Cyclimorph)

Presentation
- Cyclimorph 10: 10 mg morphine tartrate, cyclizine 50 mg in 1 ml ampoule.
- Cyclimorph 15: 15 mg morphine tartrate, cyclizine 50 mg in 1 ml ampoule.

Disadvantages
- In AMI, cyclizine may aggravate severe heart failure, and counteract the benefit of opioids.

Dosage
- Adult: 10-15 mg initially.

CONCLUSION: A convenient combination preparation that is *widely used* in Immediate Care.

Diamorphine

Action
- More potent than morphine with a more rapid onset and shorter duration of action (2 hours).
- Possibly more sedative and less likely to cause nausea/vomiting than morphine.

Presentation
- 5 mg or 10 mg as a dry powder.

Dosage
- Adult: 5-10 mg.

Disadvantage
- Comes as a powder and has to be made up, just prior to administration.
- May cause respiratory depression

CONCLUSION: Effective and is *the opiate of choice for the relief of cardiac pain (in combination with an anti-emetic).*

Pethidine hydrochloride

Action
- This is less effective as an analgesic than morphine/diamorphine, and is more likely to increase the heart rate.
- Rapid onset of action (5 minutes) and relatively short acting (2-3+ hours).
- It has anti-spasmodic properties (useful in renal and biliary colic).

Presentation
- 50 mg/ml in 1 and 2 ml ampoules.

Dosage
- Adult: 50-100 mg intravenously.

Disadvantages
- Prone to cause respiratory depression, nausea/vomiting and marked hypotension.

CONCLUSION: *Not widely used* in Immediate Care.

Synthetic opiate analogues

Pentazocine (Fortral)

- A mixed opiate agonist/antagonist.
- It is much less effective as an analgesic than morphine.

Presentation
- 30 mg/ml in 1 and 2 ml ampoules.

Dosage
- Adults: 30-60 mg.

Disadvantages
- Hallucinogenic and should not be used in the patient with respiratory depression or a head injury.
- May cause an increase in heart rate, blood pressure and cardiac work and should not be used following a myocardial infarction.
- Now a controlled drug.

CONCLUSION: Not widely used in Immediate Care, and *not particularly effective.*

Alfentanil hydrochloride (Rapifen)

- A new potent narcotic analgesic, with a rapid onset of action and a very short half life.
- Opiate agonist reversible by naloxone.

Presentation
- 500 μg in 2 and 10 ml ampoules.
- It is also available as:
    - Rapifen dilute: 100 μg/ml in 5 ml ampoules (500 μg).
    - Rapifen concentrate: 5 mg/ml in 1 ml ampoules.

Dosage
- Adults: a 500 µg initial bolus given over 30 seconds.
- Children: 30-50 µg/kg initially followed by increments of 15 µg/kg (children metabolise alfentanil more rapidly than adults).
- The peak effect takes about 90 seconds, giving profound analgesia for 5-10 minutes. Further increments of 250 µg may be given as required.

Disadvantages
- Causes respiratory depression, and is contra-indicated where there are respiratory problems.
- Transient hypotension, and bradycardia leading to asystole reversible by atropine (so the pulse must be carefully monitored).
- May cause muscle spasms (rigidity), so ideally a muscle relaxant should be given first (not often practical in Immediate Care).
- Concomitant medication with erythromycin may result in impaired metabolism (of alfentanil).

CONCLUSION: Not recommended for use in Immediate Care at present.

Buprenorphine (Temgesic)

- Long acting mixed opiate agonist/antagonist.
- Only partially reversible by naloxone. This may cause problems if the patient requires stronger (opiate) analgesia, as it competes with opiates and may block them from receptor sites.

Presentation
- 200/400 µg: small sublingual tablet.
- 300 mg/ml in 1 and 2 ml ampoules.

Dosage
- Sublingually: 200-400 µg initially.
- Intravenously: 300-600 µg.

Disadvantages
- Can cause drowsiness, dizziness, confusion and psychomimetic symptoms, nausea/vomiting (in 15-20% of patients, more marked in the elderly) and occasionally severe respiratory depression.

CONCLUSION: Not recommended for use in Immediate Care.

Nalbuphine hydrochloride (Nubain)

- A long acting semi-synthetic opiod analgesic, with mixed opiate agonist/antagonist properties, fully or partially reversible by naloxone, indicated for moderate to severe pain, including cardiac pain.
- Rapid onset of action after intravenous administration (2-3 minutes), long duration of action (3-6 hours).

Presentation
- 10 mg/ml: 1 and 2 ml ampoules.

Dosage
- 20 mg of nalbuphine administered intravenously has equivilent potency to 5 mg of diamorphine.
- Pain: 10-60 mg
- Acute myocardial infarction: 10-30 mg slowly intravenously (may be repeated after 30 minutes).

Advantages
- An effective analgesic which causes less nausea and vomiting than other opioids.
- It does not have any cardiovascular effects in patients with a healthy cardiovascular system.
- It is not a controlled drug.

Disadvantages
- It can cause comparable respiratory depression to morphine.
- It may also cause sedation and less frequently, sweating, nausea, vomiting, dizziness, dry mouth, vertigo and headache.

CONCLUSION: Although at present there has been *relatively little experience* of the use of this drug in Immediate Care, it is *considered by some to be the best of the synthetic opioids, and is gaining increasing acceptance, especially for use by ambulance personnel.*

Naloxone (Narcan)

Action
- A pure opiate antagonist used to treat opiate overdosage, especially respiratory depression induced by synthetic or natural opioids, and the mixed opiate agonists/antagonists Pentazocine and Buprenorphine.

Presentation
- Naloxone hydrochloride 400 μg/ml: 1 and 2 ml ampoules.
- Narcan Neonatal: 20 μg/ml: 2 ml ampoule.

Dosage
- Adults:
    - 800 μg as an intravenous bolus, repeated at 2-3 minute intervals if there is no improvement in respiratory function up to a maximum of 10 mg.
    - Larger doses are required for the treatment of overdosage with mixed opiate agonists/antagonists than for pure agonists.
    - It has a short duration of action (half life: 1 hour), and further increments may therefore need to be given.
- Children:
    - 10 μg/kg intravenously initially up to a maximum of 100 μg.

CONCLUSION: An *essential* drug for the Immediate Care doctor.

Anaesthetic analgesic

Ketamine (Ketalar)

Action
- This is an anaesthetic induction agent unrelated to other anaesthetic agents, with analgesic properties in sub-anaesthetic doses.
- Does not cause significant depression of the pharyngeal reflexes.

Presentation
- 10 mg/ml: 20 ml vials, 50 mg/ml: 10 ml vials, 100 mg/ml: 5 ml vials.

Dosage
- Analgesia: 20-25 mg intravenously by slow injection, 50-100 mg intramuscularly.
- Anaesthesia:
    - Intravenously: 2 mg/kg over at least 60 seconds gives good anaesthesia lasting for 5-10 minutes.
    - Intramuscularly: 8-10 mg/kg gives surgical anaesthesia in 3-4 minutes, lasting 15-25 minutes (but absorption may be poor in the hypovolaemic).

Contraindications
- Hypertension.

Disadvantages
- May induce dose related nightmares with or without psychomotor activity manifest by confusion and irrational behaviour. These can be minimised by concurrent administration of diazepam or midazolam
- May not be effective in the alcoholic.
- May cause respiratory depression if administered too quickly intravenously.

Advantages
- Has a hypertensive action and is particularly useful in amputations, but it can exacerbate hypotension in the already shocked patient.

CONCLUSION: Its use in immediate care is *underrated*.

Other analgesics

- There has been little experience in the use of the newer analgesics, and what little use there has been has failed to show that they offer any significant advantages over opiates.

Diclofenac (Voltarol)

Action
- A NSAID with marked analgesic and anti-inflammatory properties, which has been used for pain relief in renal or biliary colic, and may potentiate the effects of opiates in orthopaedic injuries.
- It has a relatively slow onset of action and lasts for 6-10 hours.

Presentation
- 25 mg/ml: 3 ml ampoule.

Dosage
- 75 mg.
- May be repeated after 30 minutes depending on response.

Administration
- By deep *intramuscular* (intragluteal) injection, which can cause induration and local pain. In the shocked patient, it may only be poorly absorbed.

Advantages
- Causes little sedation or respiratory depression.

Disadvantages
- Can cause gastrointestinal problems including ulceration.

CONCLUSION: Gaining increasing acceptance as a useful analgesic in Immediate Care, especially for providing pain relief for patients with fractures.

Nefopam (Acupan)

Action
- A new analgesic unrelated to either opiates or NSAIDs, which does not affect the vital signs, and is less likely than narcotics to cause sedation.

Presentation
- 20 mg/ml: 1 ml ampoule.

Dosage
- 20 mg.

Administration
- Given *intramuscularly* and takes 15-20 minutes for its onset of action and lasts up to 6 hours.

Disadvantages
- Contraindicated in patients with a history of epilepsy, and those taking monoamine-oxidase inhibitors (MAOIs).

CONCLUSION: It should not be used for analgesia in myocardial infarction, as there is no clinical experience of its use in this situation.
It is best used for musculoskeletal pain and can be used in the head injured patient. Its value in Immediate Care is *UNPROVEN*.

Inhalational analgesics

Nitrous oxide/oxygen (Entonox/Nitronox)

- This is a 50% mixture of nitrous oxide and oxygen.

Presentation
- Blue cylinders (usually size D for pre-hospital use) with a white and blue quartered collar.

Action
- Causes little sedation.
- It is an effective analgesic, with pain relief, equivalent to that obtained with morphine, being obtained with nitrous oxide concentrations as low as 20%.

Administration
- It is usually self administered by mask or mouthpiece (which can be easier to use in the fully conscious patient).
- Some of the more recent giving sets are more compact than the original BOC set, and have the demand valve with the mouthpiece enabling greater separation of cylinder and patient, and require a lower triggering pressure.

Advantages
- It is rapidly effective and reversible (it can take 2-5 minutes to be fully effective).
- It contains 50% oxygen which is also of benefit to the shocked patient.

Disadvantages
  - The two gases can separate out at very low temperatures (below -6 °C) and the cylinders should thus be stored horizontally and shaken before use, in cold weather.
  - The apparatus is relatively heavy (6 kg), cumbersome, and expensive.
  - Portable cylinders only last about 20 minutes.
  - There is a danger of further depressing left ventricular function resulting in hypotension and heart failure if it is combined with high doses of morphine in patients with impaired cardiac function. However, it may be used in addition to morphine if heart failure can be excluded.

Contraindications
  - Chest injuries, where there is a risk of pneumothorax (nitrous oxide is more soluble than nitrogen and diffuses into air filled body cavities faster than nitrogen can diffuse out, resulting in a build up of pressure causing a pneumothorax to become a tension pneumothorax).
  - Use at high or low altitudes or after diving.
  - In cardiac failure.

Precautions
  - Due to its oxygen component, it should be used with care where there is a risk of combustion, e.g. where cutting equipment is being used.

CONCLUSION: It is still the *analgesic of choice* for relief of mild to moderate pain in the prehospital situation.

Sedating agents

Benzodiazepines

  - These have anxiolytic, muscle relaxant and anti-convulsant properties, and can potentiate the effect of analgesics.
  - Retrograde amnesia may occur.

Diazepam

Action
  - Relatively long acting, and fat soluble.

Presentation
  - Intravenous injection:
    - Valium (aqueous solution, which is highly irritant, causes local pain, inflammation and phlebitis).
    - Diazemuls (an oil in emulsion which causes no inflammation):
      - 5 mg/ml: 2 ml ampoules.
  - Rectal infusion (Stesolid): 2 mg/ml, 4 mg/ml: tubes of 2.5 ml (5, 10 mg).

Dosage
  - Intravenously:
    - 10-30 mg:
      - Initially give a 10 mg bolus then administer the next 10 mg in 2 mg boluses over 30 seconds, titrated to the patient's response, e.g. ptosis.

- Rectally:
    - Adults: 10 mg.
    - Children (1-3 yrs): 5 mg, over 3 yrs: 10 mg.
    - The elderly: 5 mg.

Disadvantages
- Valium is highly irritant and should always be given into a large vein (or rectally in children).
- Can cause apnoea and more rarely hypotension.

CONCLUSION: There are better benzodiazepines for use in Immediate Care.

Midazolam (Hypnovel)

Description/action
- A short acting water soluble benzodiazepine with a half life of about 2 hours.
- It is used mainly as an induction agent.

Presentation
- 10 mg/2 ml 10 mg/5ml ampoules.

Dosage
- 10 µ/kg initially, i.e. 7 mg for a 70 kg man.

Administration
- It is given intravenously and the dose should be carefully titrated against the patient's response, as apnoea can occur.

CONCLUSION: In Immediate Care it can be *very useful* for sedating the head injured patient who is hypoxic and violent, and for tranquilising the very anxious.

Note: - Midazolam is often used with Ketamine.

Flumazenil (Anexate)

Description
- The first specific benzodiazepine antagonist.

Action
- A benzodiazepine itself, it acts by competing for, and then blocking benzodiazepine receptors.

Presentation
- 100 µg/ml: 5 ml ampoule.

Dosage
- Administer by slow intravenous infusion, and titrate against patient response.
- Initially 200 µg should be given over 15 seconds, with a further 100 µg every 60 seconds as necessary. Usual dose 300-600 µg, the maximum dose is 1 mg.
- It has a rapid onset of action, and a short duration of action, which can result in re-emergence of the effects of the original benzodiazepine after several hours.
- Should be administered with care as cardiac arrhythmias may be precipitated.

Indications
- Reversal of benzodiazepine induced central sedative effects.

Uses
- Benzodiazepine overdosage.

Local anaesthesia

- This has advantages, when the patient may be medically unfit, due to its relative lack of systemic effects. In Immediate Care, there may however, be problems due to lack of operator expertise, access and local complications.

Local anaesthetic agents

Lignocaine hydrochloride (Xylocaine/Lidocaine)

Presentation
- 0.5, 1, 1.5 or 2% solutions with or without adrenaline, in a large variety of sizes, and containers:
    - Ampoules, vials and pre-filled syringes.

Dosage
- Adults: 200 mg maximum or 500 mg with adrenaline.
- "Lignocaine with adrenaline" is best avoided in Immediate Care as intra-arterial injection or injection into digits results in severe vasoconstriction and may lead to gangrene.

Side effects
- Restlessness.
- Tremors and convulsions.
- Cardiac and respiratory depression.

CONCLUSION: The *most widely used* local anaesthetic.

Bupivacaine (Marcaine)

- A newer more potent and longer acting local anaesthetic than lignocaine.

Presentation
- 0.25, 0.5% solutions with or without adrenaline and 0.75% plain solution, in 10 ml ampoules.

Dosage
- Adults:
    - 0.5% up to 30 ml for a peripheral block.
    - 0.25% up to 60 ml for local infiltration.

Disadvantages
- Can have a depressant effect on the myocardium.

CONCLUSION: Its use is *best avoided in the patient who is shocked.*

Nerve blocks

Femoral nerve block

- Probably the most useful block in Immediate Care, as it is relatively easy to give.
- It produces deep anaesthesia over the medial part of the thigh and lower leg, including the periosteum, which can be beneficial to the patient with a fractured shaft of femur.
- The nerve lies just lateral to and slightly deeper than the femoral artery.

Method:
- Identify the anterior superior iliac crest, the pubic tubercle, and the inguinal ligament.
- The injection is given 1-2 cm lateral to the femoral pulse, just below the inguinal ligament at a depth of about 3-4 cm.
- About 20 ml of 1% lignocaine, *without adrenaline*, or 10 ml of 0.5% plain bupivacaine should be given fanwise.
- Withdraw regularly to make sure the needle is not in the femoral artery.

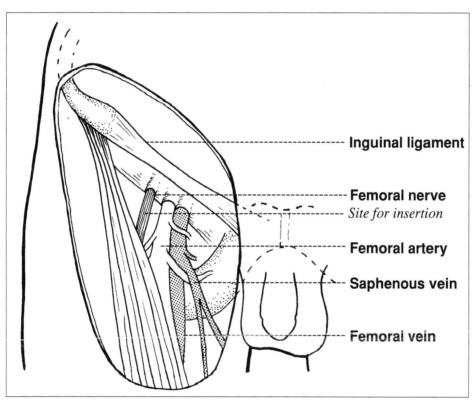

Figure 6-1 Femoral nerve block

Brachial plexus nerve block

- May be very difficult to perform and is best left to the expert!

Wrist nerve block

- Blocks of the radial, ulnar or median nerves are possible, but are of limited use in Immediate Care.

Digital nerve block

- Blocks of fingers and toes may be useful where these are trapped in machinery.

Ankle nerve block

- Similar to the wrist.

Intercostal nerve block

- May be of use in the patient with a flail chest, but there is a risk of pneumothorax.
- The block is given just beneath the ribs, about 6-7 cm lateral to the spinous process of the vertebra.

Controlled drugs: regulations

The law

- The basic law governing the supply and use of controlled drugs is the Misuse of Drugs Act 1971.
- In 1985 the drugs were reclassified into schedules 1 to 5 by the Misuse of Drugs Regulations 1985.

Schedule 2 drugs
- Opiates and some opiate analogues (controlled drugs) including: morphine, diamorphine, pethidine, and amphetamines in medical use.
- Subject to the full controlled drugs regulations relating to prescriptions, safe custody, registers, etc.

Schedule 3 drugs
- Barbiturates, pentazocine and buprenorphine.
- Subject to the special prescription requirements (except phenobarbitone), but not to the safe custody requirements (except buprenorphine) nor the need to keep registers, although there are requirements to keep receipts for 2 years.

Schedule 4 drugs
- Benzodiazepines.
- Subject to minimal control regulations; not subject to control drug prescriptions or safe custody regulations.

Schedule 5 drugs
- This exempts those medicines which contain small quantities of the drugs mentioned in schedule 4, from control, e.g. those containing codeine, dihydocodeine, pholcodeine and dextropropoxyphene.

Possession and supply of controlled drugs

- Doctors, acting in their professional capacity, have authority to possess and supply these drugs.
- They may administer or direct any other qualified person to administer such drugs.

Safe custody of controlled drugs

- Doctors must keep Schedule 2 controlled drugs and buprenorphine in a locked receptacle that can only be opened by them or somebody authorised by them.

Note:- A locked car is not considered to be a locked receptacle, but a locked case inside a locked car is acceptable. A locked glove compartment in a locked car is not acceptable.
  - This can present a considerable problem especially to doctors involved in Immediate Care, as they need to keep their emergency drugs including opiates ready for instant use. It is suggested that they carry the minimum quantity of controlled drugs, and ideally keep them in a locked car safe, with good access for an emergency. It may cause problems if emergency equipment is always kept locked up.

Controlled drug registers

- Doctors must keep a register of schedule 2 drugs and buprenorphine, which must be bound, rather than loose leaf, for recording all transactions relating to these drugs. There should be an "in" and "out" page for each separate drug, and each different strength of each drug.
- All entries must be in chronological order, made within 24 hrs of supplying or obtaining a drug. The "in" page must show the date of purchase, the supplier, the name, quantity and strength of the drug supplied. The "out" page must state the date of supply of the drug together with the name and address of the patient to whom the drug was supplied, and the strength and quantity of the drug.
- Entries must be in ink and no entries may be cancelled, obliterated or altered. Any correction must be made with an explanatory marginal note or footnote, which must be dated.
- Registers must be preserved for 2 years since the last entry, and should be available for Home Office inspectors (who have the right of entry) to examine them without warning (they may also inspect a doctor's stock of controlled drugs).

Destruction of controlled drugs

- Doctors may not destroy opiates in their stock, except in the presence of someone authorised by the Secretary of State. Such persons include Home Office Inspectors, Regional Medical Officers, FHSA Medical Advisors and all police officers.
- A record must be made of the quantity destroyed, together with the date on which they were destroyed, and must be signed by the authorised person.

Prescriptions for controlled drugs: Drugs in schedules 2 and 3

- These must be hand written in indelible ink by the prescriber in full, including their usual signature and the date (which alone may be stamped), and must contain:
  - The name and address of the patient.
  - The form of the preparation: tablets, capsules and description if appropriate, e.g. s/r (slow release)
  - The strength.
  - The dose to be taken.
  - The total number of tablets, capsules or ampoules (or the total volume of a liquid) in both words and figures.

Importation/exportation of controlled drugs

- Patients may only carry 15 days supply of any Schedule 2 or 3 controlled drugs for their own personal use.
- If especially high doses are prescribed or the treatment is for more than 15 days a Home Office licence may be required.

Licence for importation of controlled drugs

- Doctors importing schedule 2 and 3 drugs into the UK must have a personal valid Home Office licence.
- This is renewable annually.
- This is of particular importance for doctors doing aeromedical work, who may wish to carry these drugs with them on flights to treat patients and bring them back into the country if not used.

7

Resuscitation in pregnancy

Resuscitation in pregnancy

Introduction

- When the pregnant patient is seriously ill or injured, two lives are at risk: the mother and the fetus.
- Efficient and effective Immediate Care may make all the difference between saving or losing one or two patients. In rare circumstances a decision may have to be made as to which life has the higher priority. This may place an almost intolerable burden on those involved in their Immediate Care.
- The management of the seriously ill or injured pregnant patient is essentially the same as that for any patient but should take into consideration differences in anatomy and physiology.

Incidence

- Cardiac arrest in late pregnancy is rare (and recovery even rarer) occuring about 1:30,000 pregnancies.
- Trauma occurring during pregnancy is much more common.

Aetiology

- Acute causes of maternal death in pregnancy include (in descending order of frequency):
    - Haemorrhage :
        - Uteroplacental
        - Cerebrovascular.
    - Embolism:
        - Pulmonary
        - Amniotic fluid.
    - Cardiac.
    - Status epilepticus.

Pathophysiology

- In pregnancy both the anatomy and the physiology of the mother change, especially towards the end of the pregnancy.
- These changes have a significant effect both on the mother's response to life threatening conditions and on the techniques required for successful resuscitation.

Anatomical changes in pregnancy

Features predisposing to difficult resuscitation management
Intubation
- Full dentition
- Oedema or obesity of the neck
- Supraglottic oedema.

Ventilation
- Greater oxygen requirement
- Reduced chest compliance
- More difficult to observe the rise and fall of the chest with ventilations

Chest compressions
- Enlarged breasts
- Vena caval compression by gravid uterus
- Flared rib cage
- Raised diaphragm.

Heart
- Increases in size and may be displaced slightly upwards and to the left as the uterus enlarges.

Uterus
- In the first trimester of pregnancy the uterus is thick walled and is protected by the bony pelvis.
- During the course of the pregnancy the uterus grows out of the pelvis and becomes an intra-abdominal organ. As such it is also more susceptible to injury.
- In later pregnancy the wall of the uterus becomes progressively thinner, and there is relatively less amniotic fluid offering less protection for the fetus.
- The placenta, because of its lack of elastic tissue, is particularly vulnerable to shearing forces, especially those caused by blunt injury, which may result in placental abruption.

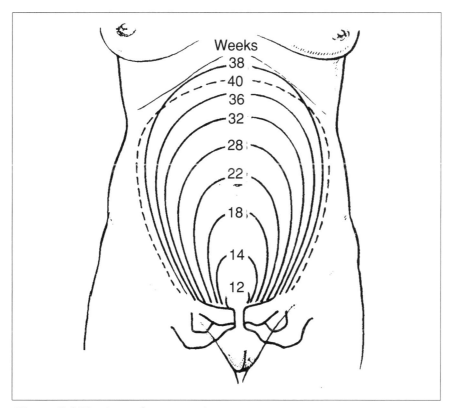

Figure 7-1 Uterine enlargement in pregnancy

Physiological changes in pregnancy

Airway
- There is relaxation of the gastro-oesophageal junction and delayed gastric emptying which results in an increased risk of oesophageal reflux and aspiration of gastric contents.
- Intubation is therefore advisable in the unconscious pregnant patient.

Respiratory system
- Increased oxygen requirement.
- Increased ventilation:
    - The tidal volume is increased by 40%, without an increase in respiratory rate.
    - There is a relative respiratory alkalosis.
- Reduced chest compliance.
- Reduced functional residual capacity.

Cardiovascular system
- *Cardiac output:*
    - Increased by 30% (40% at term)
- *Plasma volume:*
    - This is increased by up to 50%, without a corresponding increase in total oxygen carrying capacity (red blood cells).
    - This results in a relatively low haemoglobin level (true anaemia is also common).
- *Pulse rate:*
    - The resting pulse rate increases: 84-92 bpm.
- *Blood pressure:*
    - The systolic and diastolic blood pressure falls by 5-15 mmHg.
- *Hypovolaemia:*
    - The pregnant patient is able to tolerate greater blood and plasma loss than the non pregnant patient before showing signs of hypovolaemia (see chapter on Shock), but this is at the cost of shunting blood away from the uterus and placenta.
- *The Supine Hypotension syndrome:*
    - The gravid uterus may cause pressure on the inferior vena cava when the pregnant patient is supine, resulting in impairment of the venous return and a fall in the cardiac output of up to 40%. This in turn can result in a fall in blood pressure.

Neurological system
- There is a risk of eclampsia in the third trimester. This may mimic the fits due to severe head injury and should always be borne in mind especially if hyper-reflexia is present.

Skeletal system
- The sacro-iliac and pubic ligaments relax.

Gastrointestinal system
- Incompetent gastro-oesophageal (cardiac) sphincter
- Increased intra-abdominal pressure, leading to increased intragastric pressure

results in an increased risk of gastric aspiration

Assessment of the pregnant patient

The mother
- This should be the same as for the non pregnant adult and should be as rapid as possible.
- Hypotension may be due to placental abruption.

The fetus
- This should *only* take place after the mother has been assessed *and resuscitated* if necessary.
- Determine the date of the mother's last menstrual period and calculate the duration of the pregnancy.
- Measure the fundal height and see if this corresponds with the dates. If it is higher than expected, this may indicate placental abruption.
- Examine the uterus looking for:
  - Uterine contractions
  - Uterine tenderness
  - Fetal movement
  - Abnormal fetal parts palpable:
    - Indication of uterine rupture.
- Monitor the fetal heart rate (if possible). This depends on the age of the fetus and the monitoring aids available:
  - Pinard fetal stethoscope.
  - Doppler ultrasound device
    - Normal heart rate: 120-160 bpm
    - Fetal distress: Bradycardia: <110 bpm
- Look for vaginal loss of bood or fluid (do *not* do a vaginal examination).

Management of the pregnant patient

- The prime objective in managing the seriously ill or injured pregnant patient is to assess, manage and stabilise the mother first, and then the fetus.
- Only in exceptional circumstances, e.g. when the mother is about to die or has just died should the assessment and management of the fetus come first.
- The outcome of resuscitation required following following serious illness or injury is more favourable after delivery of the fetus (immediate surgical delivey should be considered if feasible, if there is no improvemrnt in the condition of the moribund pregnant patient within 5 minutes).

Basic life support in pregnancy

Airway
- Maintain the airway (with cervical spine stabilisation in trauma).
- Apply cricoid pressure if the patient is unconscious, because of the increased risk of gastric regurgitation.

Breathing
- Effective ventilation may be relatively difficult because of the patient's:
  - Increased oxygen requirement
  - Reduced chest compliance
  - Rib flaring and diaphragmatic splinting.
- In pregnancy, it may also be more difficult to see if the patient's chest is expanding during ventilation.

Circulation

Position
- The pregnant patient should be placed on her left side so as to reduce the effects of the Supine Hypotension syndrome.

Method
- If there is *no possibility of cervical spine injury:*
  - With the patient lying on her back, elevate the right hip, flex the right knee, and displace the right leg to the left and put the patient into the left lateral position.
  - Displace the uterus manually to the left.
- If there *is a possibility of cervical spine injury:*
  - Apply effective cervical splintage.
  - Elevate the right hip by putting a pillow under the right buttock (being careful not to move the cervical spine).
  - Manually displace the uterus to the left.

Cardiac arrest
- This may be more difficult in the pregnant patient due to the flared ribs, raised diaphragm, enlarged breasts, and obesity.
- Vena caval compression *must* be relieved by positioning the patiently correctly, *otherwise all attempts at effective resuscitation will be futile.*

Hypovolaemia
- If a PASG is applied, only inflate the leg compartments.

Advanced life support in pregnancy

Airway

Oxygen
- Administer high flow oxygen: important due to the increased oxygen requirement of mother and fetus.

Intubation
- This should be performed early if the patient is unconscious because of the increased risk of aspiration
- This may be more difficult in the pregnant patient.
  - In particular laryngoscope insertion may be more difficult if the patient has a short obese neck and large full breasts.

Circulation

Arrhythmia management
- This is as for non-pregnant adults, except that bretylium should be used before lignocaine.

Hypovolaemia - a major cause of fetal death
- Establish intravenous access using two large bore intravenous cannulae if major trauma.
- Rapid fluid replacement should be started using colloid.

Trauma in pregnancy

Blunt trauma in pregnancy

Aetiology
- The most common causes of blunt trauma in pregnancy are:
    - Road traffic accidents: seat belt injury, abdominal trauma.
    - Falls
    - Assaults.

Placental abruption
- A common cause of fetal death.
- May occur up to 48 hrs after injury.

Signs
- Vaginal bleeding
- Uterine irritability
- Abdominal tenderness
- Increasing fundal height
- Maternal hypovolaemic shock
- Fetal distress.

Traumatic uterine rupture
- Occurs in late pregnancy.

Signs
- May range from massive haemorrhage and hypovolaemic shock to minimal symptoms/signs.
- A separately palpable uterus and fetus is pathognomonic.

Penetrating trauma in pregnancy

- As the uterus enlarges it becomes increasingly vulnerable to penetrating trauma, when its presence can protect the other intra-abdominal organs from injury.
- Gunshot and stab wounds often result in fetal death, but maternal survival is usually good.

Burns in pregnancy

- Burns of >50% occurring in the second or third trimesters are associated with a high mortality rate.

Management:
- Immediate delivery:
    - Maternal death is certain unless she is delivered and the fetal prognosis is not improved by waiting.

Notes

8

Neonatal resuscitation

Neonatal resuscitation

Introduction

- Basic resuscitation of the newborn is a technique that all those involved in domiciliary obstetrics should be trained in and competent at performing, whilst those practising Immediate Care should be competent in performing advanced resuscitation of the newborn. This is becoming increasingly important with the proposed run down in hospital based obstetric flying squads and their replacement by extended trained ambulancemen supported by appropriately trained general practitioners.

Incidence

- The number of newborn babies requiring resuscitation outside hospital is very small, but will probably increase in the United Kingdom, if the trend away from managed hospital obstetrics and towards more home confinement continues.
- One third of all resuscitations of neonates occur in babies born after normal uneventful pregnancies and labours and have no apparent risk factors.

Aetiology

- Babies born outside hospital fall into two groups:
    - Planned home confinements:
        - These are nearly all carefully selected beforehand and in particular the mothers are usually multiparous and have an uncomplicated previous obstetric history.
        - The incidence of babies requiring resuscitation is very small in this group.
    - Accidental pre-hospital delivery:
        - This usually occurs due to:
            - Failure or refusal to recognise pregnancy, or concealed pregnancy.
            - Poor recognition of the beginning of the second stage of labour.
            - Very rapid labour.
            - Transport or geographical delay.
        - The incidence of babies requiring resuscitation in this group is rather higher.

Pathophysiology

Normal
- At birth the baby's lungs are full of fluid.
- The baby's first few breaths are vigorous so that the surface tension from the fluid is overcome. and it is driven out of the alveoli and into the circulation, and the lungs begin to fill with air. Subsequent breaths do not need to be so forceful.
- Blood flow through the lungs increases as the pulmonary capillaries open up and oxygenation improves.
- The median time from delivery to the onset of spontaneous respiration is only 10 seconds.

Asphyxia
- If the newborn baby has never tried to breathe, it is more difficult to expand the lungs with air, as the lungs are still full of fluid, and more pressure than is usually necessary for normal ventilation will have to be applied initially to fill the alveoli "opening pressure". This is easier if the initial inflation/ventilation/inspiration is slightly prolonged.
- If a baby stops breathing after having taken its first few breaths, less pressure will be required to ventilate it, than if it had never breathed.
- Hypoxia or acidosis results in narrowing of the pulmonary arterioles, which results in a further reduction in the blood supply to the lungs, and a further increase in hypoxia.
- Prolonged asphyxia results in apnoea, poor perfusion, poor tone, no movement and bradycardia.

Hypothermia
- If newborn babies are not kept warm and dry:
    - Their temperature will fall rapidly (10°C every 5 minutes) and they will become hypothermic, which in turn will result in hypoglycaemia, respiratory distress and acidosis.

Management
- The principal of management must be to prevent problems arising, and to recognise and treat those problems that do so as rapidly as possible.

Heat loss
- Immediately after birth:
    - Dry the infant, quickly, but thoroughly, using a warm towel.
    - Having done this remove the now wet towel and replace it with a fresh warm towel.

Position
    - Place the baby supine on a flat surface, head down.
    - If active resuscitation is necessary:
        - Slightly extend the neck, if necessary using a small pad under the shoulders.
        - Do *not* overextend or flex the head, which may result in kinking of the trachea and airway obstruction. If ventilation is unsatisfactory: reposition the head.

Airway/breathing

Tactile stimulation
- Some infants with mild asphyxia, who fail to breathe, can be stimulated to do so by:
    - Gently flicking the soles of their feet.
    - Rubbing the back for a few seconds.
- If this succeeds, subsequent gentle stimulation may help these infants to keep breathing.
- If there is not a rapid response, proceed to active resuscitation.

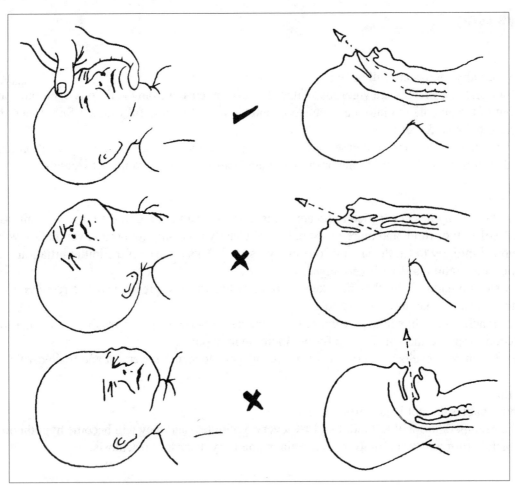

Figure 8-1 Positioning the neonate to maintain the airway

Suctioning

- The use of oral powered mucous extractors should be avoided, as congenital contamination with the human immunodeficiency virus (HIV) has been shown to occur.
- Catheter size: 4, 6 and 8 F.G.
- In the healthy baby, suctioning is not usually necessary.
- It may be necessary gently to suck out the oropharynx by inserting a catheter no more than 5 cm, if the amniotic fluid is:
    - Bloodstained
    - Meconium stained
    - Excessive.

Note:- Rough and deep suctioning may cause:
- Laryngeal spasm or vagal stimulation which may result in bradycardia.
- Delay in the onset of spontaneous respiration.

- If the nose is blocked, suck it out gently (babies are obligatory nose breathers).

Oxygen

- If respiration is inadequate or the baby is cyanosed:
    - Administer oxygen by face mask or funnel (if available), which should have perforations or a side vent to prevent a build-up of pressure.
    - If the breathing is persistently shallow or irregular, or if there is apnoea, especially with cyanosis: start artificial ventilation.

Neonatal mask
- - The mask should be soft, transparent and is usually circular.
- - It should cover the baby's mouth and nose.
- - It should be well fitting, so that when it is tightly applied it does not press on the eyes or overhang the chin.

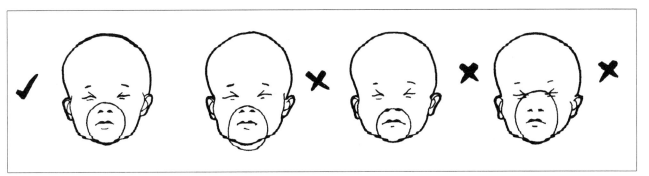

Figure 8-2 Position of mask

Basic neonatal life support

Airway
- - Check for respiratory effort.
- - If this is present and perhaps vigorous, but doesn't result in chest expansion, there is probably airway obstruction.

Clearing the airway

Method
- - Open the airway by slightly extending the neck.
- - Hold the chin gently forward using the finger on the mandible, being careful not to compress the soft tissues of the neck.

Ventilation

Method
- - Hold the mask firmly in place and give intermittent ventilations by squeezing the bag gently with your fingertips. If compression is too forceful, it may cause excessive pressure in spite of the pressure relief valve.
- - Rate: 30-40 ventilations/minute.

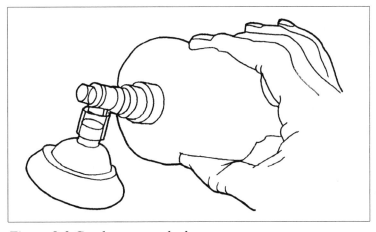

Figure 8-3 Gently squeeze the bag

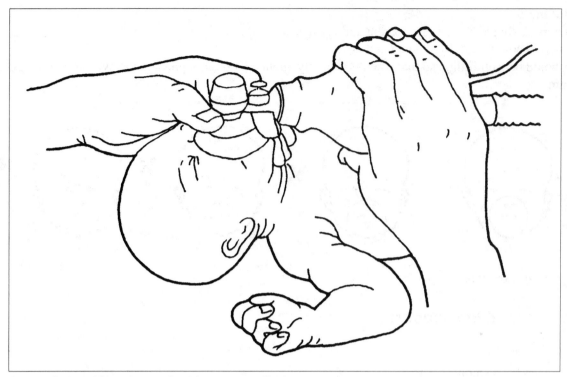

Figure 8-4 Holding the mask and squeezing the bag

- Oxygen:
    - Concentration: as high as possible.
    - Flow: 4-6 litres/minute.
- Watch the chest rise and fall with each ventilation.
- If synchronous chest movement does not occur:
    - Readjust the the head position to ensure that the neck is adequately extended and the airway is not obstructed.
    - Check that the mask makes an adequate seal.
- If necessary, clear the airway again by suctioning the mouth and nose.
- If in doubt gently insert an infant airway, making certain that it passes over the tongue to reach the pharynx.
- If the lungs are particularly difficult to inflate and the chest does not move: intubation is indicated.

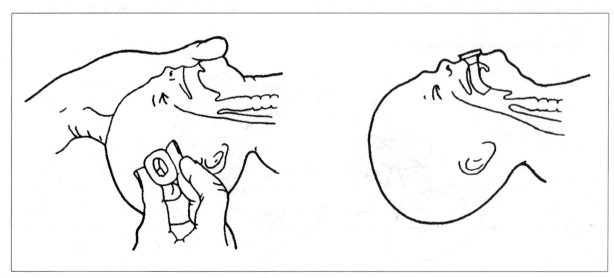

Figure 8-5 Insertion of an airway

Circulation

External chest compression
- Administer external chest compression if the baby has a bradycardia (<60 beats per minute) or if the pulse is absent or is difficult to palpate. There is usually associated pallor.

Method 1
- Grasp the chest with both hands, placing the thumbs over the junction of the middle and lower third of the sternum. Apply pressure by pressing down with both thumbs.

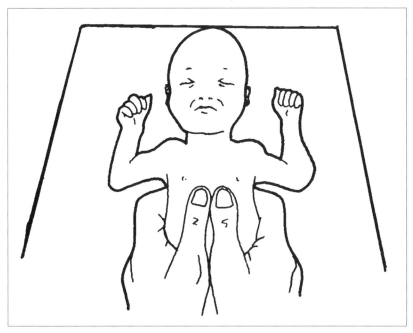

Figure 8-6 External chest compressions: method 1

Method 2 (less effective, but more commonly used as thumbs become fatigued quickly with method 1)
- Place two fingers:
  - 1-2 cm below a line joining the nipples *or* 1-2 cm above the xiphisternum
- One hand may support the back, while the other applies rhythmic sternal pressure.
- During the relaxation phase, do not lift the fingers or thumbs off the chest.

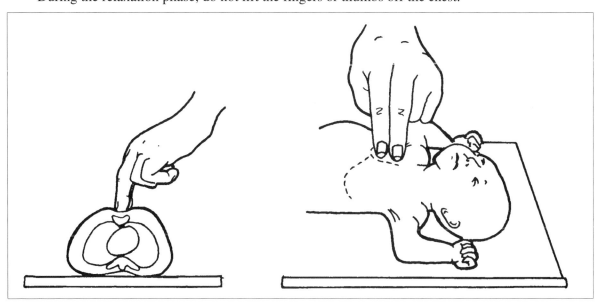

Figure 8-7 External chest compressions: method 2

Note: - Damage to the liver and other viscera, and fractured ribs may be caused:
- If the finger or thumb positions are too low over the sternum or liver.
- If the compressions are too forceful.

- Rate: >100 compressions/minute.

Co-ordination of inflations and chest compressions

- Following the initial ventilations, the ratio of ventilations to compressions should be 1:3
- Check the heart rate after 30-60 seconds and thereafter about every 2 minutes.

Naloxone (see chapter on Pain Relief)
- This should be considered if the baby's mother has had Pethidine administered during labour.
- The intramuscular route is preferred as it is as effective as the intravenous route, but the effect lasts longer.

APGAR score

Apgar Score	0	1	3
Heart rate	Absent	< 100	> 100
Respiratory effort	Absent	Weak, cry or shallow	Good
Muscle tone	Limp	Some flexion	Active, well flexed
Reflex/ Irritability	None	Grimace	Cry
Colour	Pale/ Blue	Body pink Extremities blue	Pink

- The APGAR scoring system at 1 and 5 minutes gives information about the degree and severity and prognosis of asphyxia.
- The time taken from birth to the baby's first gasp and the onset of regular respiration should also be recorded.

Advanced neonatal life support

Neonatal intubation

Endotracheal tube size
- This depends on the weight and gestation of the baby:

Endotracheal tube sizes in neonates		
Size	Weight	Gestation
2.0-2.5	< 750 g	< 26 weeks
2.5-3.0	750-2000 g	26-34 weeks
3.0-3.5	> 2000g	34+ weeks

Type of tube
- Plain uncuffed tubes are best (Coles tubes, which have a shoulder near the tip can cause glottic injury and are no longer recommended).
- A stylet may aid intubation, but it should be moulded to the same shape as the tube and should not protrude beyond the end of the tube.

Laryngoscope
- A straight bladed laryngoscope is probably best for use in Immediate Care.
- Blade size:
    - Small preterm baby: size 0
    - Usual sized baby: size 1

Method
- Place the baby on a flat surface, covered with a warm sheet or towel (if not already done).
- Position the baby, keeping the head in the midline, and slightly extend the head in relation to the body.
- Before intubating, try to ventilate the baby several times with a bag and mask.
- To intubate:
    - Gently insert a straight bladed laryngoscope into the mouth with the left hand, holding the lips apart with the fingers of the right hand.

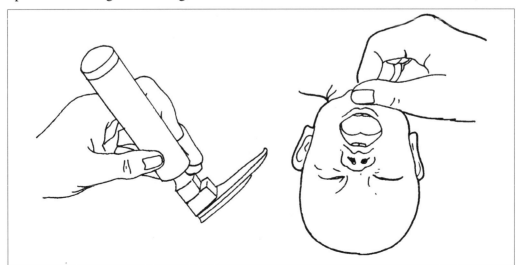

Figure 8-8 Neonatal intubation 1: Preparing to intubate

- Guide the blade over the surface of the tongue, which is pushed to the left as the blade is advanced until the uvula is seen and continued until the epiglottis is visualised.
- The tip of the blade may be advanced by lifting the epiglottis gently.

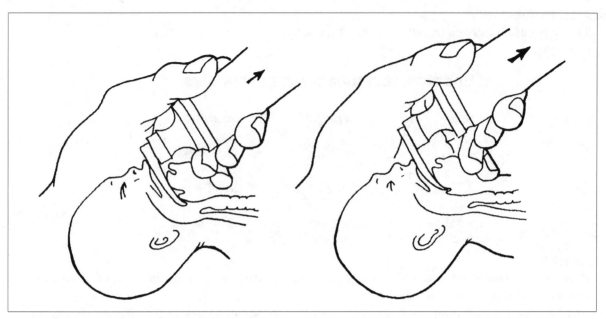

Figure 8-9 Neonatal intubation 2: Positioning the laryngoscope blade

- Use the laryngoscope blade to lift the tongue forward gently to view the larynx (if the blade is inserted too far and enters the oesophagus, withdraw it gradually until the larynx is seen).

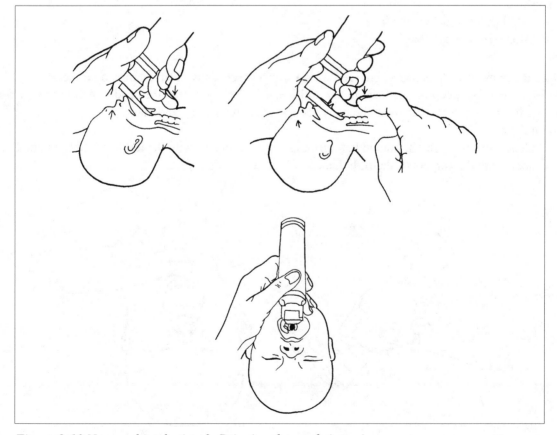

Figure 8-10 Neonatal intubation 3: Bringing the cords into view

- Clear the cords and posterior pharynx with a sucker.
- Apply gentle pressure to the trachea with your fifth finger to bring the cords into view, ensuring that the trachea remains central.
- Holding the endotracheal tube in your right hand, pass it down from the right side of the mouth towards the larynx, insert the tip between the cords, and advance it until the mark is just above the cords.
- Resting the right hand lightly on the baby's face, hold the tube firmly, and gently remove the laryngoscope (and stylet if one has been used).

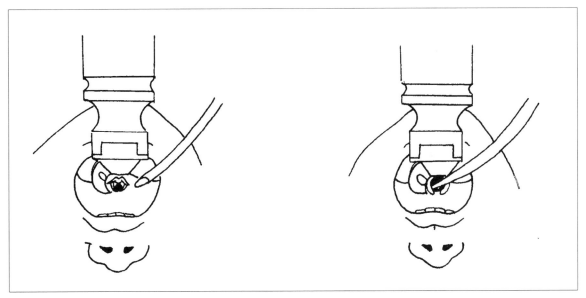

Figure 8-11 Neonatal intubation 4: Passing the endotracheal tube

- Connect the oxygen tubing with blow-off valve set (at 345 kPa or 50 p.s.i.), to deliver 4-6 litres of oxygen per minute and connect it to a self inflating bag (usually 240 ml) .
- Ventilate the baby at a rate of about 30 breaths per minute.
- Watch the baby's chest for lung expansion, and monitor the pulse rate and colour. Auscultate the chest for breath sounds and check that air entry is equal.
- Secure the tube with tape.
- Continue ventilation until the baby is breathing spontaneously.
- Remove any secretions by suctioning down the tube.
- Once the baby is breathing normally and has a good colour, normal pulse rate, good muscle tone and movement, allow it to breathe spontaneously through the tube, and if breathing is unobstructed, remove the tube during inspiration.
- If ventilation has to be continued, secure the endotracheal tube more securely prior to transportation.

Note:- Intubation should not take more than seconds. If you are not successful within this time: withdraw the tube and ventilate the baby with a bag and mask before attempting intubation again.
- If chest movement is poor after intubating, the tube is probably in the oesophagus, so withdraw the tube and after ventilating the baby, try to intubate again.
- If breath sounds and chest movement are not symmetrical: the endotracheal tube is probably in one of the main bronchi, so withdraw the tube slowly, listening for the restoration of equal air entry.
- If the baby's condition does not improve and chest movement remains inadequate: increase the inflation pressure.

Guidelines for resuscitation of the newborn

During delivery

- Suck out the mouth and nose of the baby *only* if:
    - The amniotic fluid is copious, or blood or meconium stained.

Normal breathing

- If the baby is breathing normally and crying and has a good heart rate, with normal colour and good muscle tone:
    - Dry the infant and prevent heat loss.
- If there are copious secretions or blood in the mouth:
    - Gently suck out the oropharynx.
- If the nose is blocked:
    - Gently suck out the nose.
- Rapidly inspect the baby to make sure that there are no gross abnormalities.
- Severe asphyxia will be indicated most rapidly by the absence of breathing and by poor circulation.
- The initial and 5 minute APGAR score should be recorded if possible.

Shallow/irregular breathing

- Dry the infant.
- Place on warm dry towels.
- Estimate the heart rate by either:
    - Auscultation *or*
    - Taking the brachial pulse or
    - Observing umbilical cord pulsations.
- If the heart rate >100 beats/minute and the baby is well perfused with good tone:
    - Gently clear the oro- and naso-pharynx.
- Administer oxygen.
- Apply tactile stimulation.
- If the baby fails to improve, consider ventilation.

If breathing has started, but then stopped

- Dry, keep the infant warm.
- If the heart rate >100 bpm, perfusion is maintained and tone is normal:
    - Apply tactile stimulation.
- Check airway patency.
- If the baby does not respond immediately:
    - Ventilate.
    - If the mother has had pethidine during labour, consider administration of:

Naloxone (Narcan Neonatal)

Dosage
- 10 μg/kg repeated every 2-3 minutes intravenously, or 200 μg (60 μg/kg) intramuscularly.

If the baby has never breathed

- If the heart rate is >100 bpm, the baby is not pale (well perfused) and movement and tone are present:
  - Give tactile stimulation.
  - Apply suction as necessary.
  - If there is a gasp:
    - Administer oxygen.
  - If there is no response or the baby's condition is deteriorating:
    - Consider intubation.
    - Ventilate.
- If the heart rate is slow (<100 bpm) (the baby is usually pale and limp):
  - Apply suction briefly.
  - Ventilate immediately.
  - Give external chest compressions if the heart rate is persistently < 60 bpm and the perfusion is poor (pale baby).
  - If mask ventilation fails, consider intubation.

Meconium

- If meconium is unexpectedly present as the head is delivered, suck out the mouth before delivery.
- Dry and warm the baby.
- Suck out the mouth and nose again.
- Administer oxygen.
- If the meconium was very thick, inspect the oropharynx and vocal cords under direct vision:
  - If meconium is present in small quantities in the trachea:
    - Intubate and apply suction.
    - Continue to aspirate until the meconium is cleared unless there is a bradycardia.
    - If the tube becomes blocked, replace it rapidly with another.

Guidelines for resuscitation of the newborn (summary)

	Normal breathing	**Breathing impaired**		**Not breathing**	
Signs in first minute ⬇	Breathing regular	Breathing shallow or irregular	Breathing stopped after first breath	Not breathing	
First breath	Within seconds	Usually in the first few seconds		Never breathed	
Heart rate	>100	>100		>100	<100
Peripheral perfusion	Well perfused ⬇	Usually normal ⬇		Variable often reduced ⬇	Poor ⬇

Suction only if necessary ⬇

Dry, wrap up in warm towels suction mouth and nose ⬇

Dry, wrap up in warm towels suction mouth and nose ⬇

Give oxygen by funnel
Tactile stimulation ⬇

⬇

Dry, wrap in warm dry towel ⬅ Improvement   If no immediate ➡ **Start resuscitation** improvement ⬇

⬇

Hand to mother

Position the baby

Ventilate with face mask

Apply external chest compressions if heart rate <60 bpm or pulses poor or absent

⬇

Unexpected meconium

- Suck out as soon as head is delivered

- Place baby in head down position

- Suck out mouth and nose

- Administer oxygen by funnel

Intubate and ventilate with 100% O_2

9

Paediatric resuscitation

Paediatric resuscitation

Introduction

- Large numbers of fit and healthy children die every year as a result of trauma and a smaller, but nonetheless a significant number die as a result of serious, but transient illnesses.
- The importance of the efficient and effective practice of Immediate Care skills on children has been under-rated in the past, but this has now been recognised and the differences in the management of children and adults requiring Immediate Care defined, so that appropriate training and expertise can be developed for the benefit of these children.

Life threatening illness/serious accidents in children

Incidence

- The type of problem encountered in children depends on age and to a lesser extent on sex.
  - Infants prior to toddling:
    - Mostly respiratory disease
    - Few accidents (including non-accidental injury).
  - Younger children (up to 8 years): prone to injury: adventurous and relatively oblivious of danger.
    - Burns
    - RTAs
    - Ingestion of foreign bodies/dangerous chemicals.
  - Older children/adolescents (8-14 years):
    - Accidents
    - Respiratory disease.

Aetiology

- Hypoxia is the commonest cause of cardiac arrest in infants and children.
- Other causes of death include:
  - Sudden infant death syndrome (cause unknown).
  - Hypovolaemia:
    - Haemorrhage (trauma)
    - Loss of body fluids (burns, diarrhoea)
  - Congenital heart disease
  - Septicaemia.

Non-accidents/life threatening illness in children

Aetiology

- Sudden infant death syndrome "SIDS".
- Gastoenteritis: hypovolaemic shock.
- Congenital heart disease.
- Septicaemia.
- Laryngotracheal bronchitis.
- Asthma

Accidents/trauma in children

Incidence

- Accidents account for:
    - 11% of all deaths in children aged 28 days to 14 years.
    - 32% of all deaths in children aged 5-14 years.
- Trauma is:
    - The second most common cause of death in children aged 1-4 yrs (92 per million population per annum)
    - The most common cause of death in children aged 5-14 yrs (86 per million population per annum).
- Accidents involving children account for one fifth of all emergency hospital admissions:
    - Slightly more boys are admitted than girls.

Aetiology

Age
- 0-1 year: - Choking/suffocation
            - Burns
            - Drowning
            - Falls.

- 1-4 year: - Road taffic accidents (as vehicle occupants)
            - Burns
            - Drowning
            - Falls.

- 5-14 year: - Road traffic accidents (as vehicle occupants or pedestrians)
             - Bicycling accidents
             - Burns
             - Drowning.

Types of injury/accident
- Burns/scalds (most common)
- Falls (next most common)
- Drowning
- Smoke inhalation
- Non accidental injury (NAI)
- Electric shock
- Poisoning/solvent abuse
- Road traffic accidents.

Domestic accidents
- The 0-14 year age group accounts for 19% of all home accidents.
- 72% occur in children between the ages of 1 month and 4 years.
- The most dangerous rooms are:
    - The living room: 35%
    - The hall: 14%
    - The kitchen: 12%.

Road traffic accidents
- Pedal cyclists: 26% of all pedal cycle accidents involve children.
- Pedestrians: 17% of all pedestrian accidents occur in the 4-14 year age group.
- Boys are injured in 70% of all RTAs involving children.

Pathophysiology

- There are many differences between children and adults, in particular:

Anatomical differences between children and adults

- Greater relative surface area with less subcutaneous fat: greater heat loss.
- Relatively large head for body size, with a protuberant occiput.
- Shorter narrower airway:
    - Small oral cavity but a relatively large tongue which fills the oropharynx .
    - Large angle of the jaw:
        - Infants: 140°
        - Adults: 120°
    - The epiglottis is more U-shaped than in adults.
    - The larynx is conical and is situated further forward and higher up the neck in children:
        - The glottis is situated at the level of C3 in infants, C5-6 in adults.
        - The cricoid ring is the narrowest part of the airway
        - Relatively little laryngeal swelling may result in airway obstruction.
    - The trachea is relatively short:
        - Newborn: 4-5 cm
        - At 18 months: 7-8 cm.
- Relatively small blood volume and small veins.

Physiological differences between children and adults

- Small infants are obligatory nose breathers, because of the large tongue filling the oropharynx.
- Children have a relatively high metabolic rate and a high oxygen consumption, with a reduced functional residual capacity and a high closing capacity resulting in a (physiological) right to left shunt.
- In children, most breathing is diaphragmatic, and as children are unable to increase their tidal volume, they increase their respiratory rate in response to hypoxia.
- Young children have soft ribs, which deform easily. If they breathe rapidly and deeply, e.g. in response to hypoxia, they develop intercostal muscle recession and use their accessory muscles (sternomastoids).
- The pulse rate increases in response to hypoxia and hypercapnia.
- Relatively small volumes of blood or fluid loss can result in hypovolaemic shock due to the child's small total blood volume. Initial compensation, however is very effective and children tolerate fluid loss very well, before going into severe shock. Careful estimation of blood or fluid loss is therefore required, together with careful haemodynamic monitoring if over or under transfusion is to be avoided.
- Prone to dehydration.

Biochemistry
- Prone to hypoglycaemia due to relatively small glycogen stores.

Pharmacology
- Infants and children metabolise and react to drugs in a different way from adults, the difference depending on the drug.

Pathophysiology

Cardiac arrest
- Usually occurs secondary to hypoxia/hypoxaemia.
- The usual arrhythmia is asystole preceded by bradycardia.

Trauma
- Because children are small, multisystem injury is common.
- Major blunt injury usually results in thoracic and abdominal injury.
- Penetrating injury is unusual.
- Head injury is more common: children have a relatively large head.
- Significant internal injury may occur in the absence of bony injury.

Burns
- Relatively small burns may result in hypovolaemic shock.

Normal values for vital signs in children at rest

Age	Heart rate	Systolic blood Pressure	Respiratory rate	Blood volume
	(beats/minute)	(mmHg)	(breaths/min)	(ml/kg)
< 1 year	120-140	70-90	30-40	90
2-5 years	100-120	80-90	20-30	80
5-12 years	80-100	90-110	15-20	80

Basic paediatric life support: care of the unconscious child

General management

- Follow the same basic guidelines as adults:
    - Assessment and management of:
        - **A**irway (with cervical spine stabilisation in trauma)
        - **B**reathing
        - **C**irculation with haemorrhage control
        - **D**isability (neurological assessment and management)
        - **E**xposure (trauma only).

Assessment

- Assess the scene: look for out for any hazards, problems, etc.
- Assess the child's responsiveness:
    - If the child is unconscious:
        - Try to awaken with a loud voice and gentle, but firm, shaking or pinching.
    - If there *is* a response:
        - Put the child into the recovery position and monitor the pulse and respirations.
        - Keep warm as children are very prone to heat loss:
            - Use a space blanket, woollen blanket, etc. with a warming device, e.g. a "Hot pack", if appropriate, but beware of causing burns.
    - If there *is no response*:
        - Open the airway.

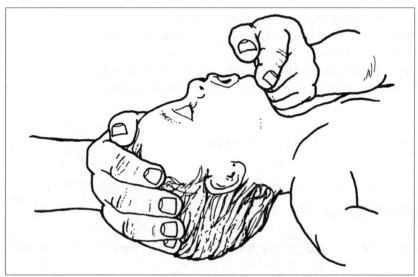

Figure 9-1 Airway maintenance

Airway care

- Open the airway

Method
- Tilt the head:
    - Apply gentle neck extension, but be careful not to hyperextend it as this may kink the trachea and obstruct the airway.
    - In small infants a support positioned under the shoulders may be helpful.
- Lift the chin, with your finger tips under the tip of the mandible. Do not press on the soft tissue under the chin with your fingers as you may push the tongue into the airway, obstructing it.
- The infant is an obligatory nose breather, and care should be taken to check and maintain the patency of the nasal passages.
- Jaw thrust is nearly always successful in clearing the airway in children if head tilt, chin lift are not.
- It may be necessary to try various positions before satisfactory airway control can be achieved.
- Check for airway patency by:
    - *Looking* for chest and abdominal movement.
    - *Listening* and *feeling* for the child's breath on your cheek or the back of your hand from their nose or mouth.
- Airway obstruction may be indicated by:
    - Increased respiratory effort and/or noisy breathing (stridor) or choking.

Airway obstruction

- Indicated by choking or stridor (noisy breathing):
    - Harsh high pitched inspiratory noise:
        - Usually due to an obstruction outside the thoracic cavity, i.e. in the larynx.

Note:- Expiratory noise (wheeze):
        - Usually due to a fixed airway obstruction or a problem in the chest, e.g. asthma.
    - Grunting (a noise at the end of expiration):
        - Usually caused by a cardiac problem.

Aetiology/management
- Tongue falling back into pharynx
    Aetiology:
        - Unconsciousness.
    Management:
        - Elevate the jaw further and/or change the child's position (only use an airway in the deeply unconscious child).
- Foreign body ingestion
    Aetiology:
        - This may be blood, loose teeth, food, a toy or vomit.
    Management:
        - Small objects: encourage to cough, suctioning
        - Large objects: *see management of choking below.*
- Tissue swelling
    Aetiology:
        - Croup
        - Laryngotracheobronchitis (LTB)
        - Epiglottitis
        - Hereditary angio-oedema (HANE).
    History:
        - This should be obtained from the parents, if possible, and may be useful in helping to distinguish between tissue swelling (infection), foreign body ingestion, asthma and other conditions.
    Management: See chapter on Medical Emergencies.

Foreign body ingestion/choking

Management
- This depends on the age of the child.
- If possible, encourage the child to cough.

Blind probing/finger sweeps
    - This is *not recommended, except for large objects* as it may cause:
        - Further impaction of the foreign body.
        - Damage to the upper airway, with resultant oedema and sometimes haemorrhage, and may even precipitate acute laryngeal spasm.

Abdominal thrusts
    - *Not advisaable* in infants (under the age of one) as it may cause severe intra-abdominal injury including rupture of the liver and spleen.

Back blows
- This should be attempted first.
- The method used depends on the size of the child.

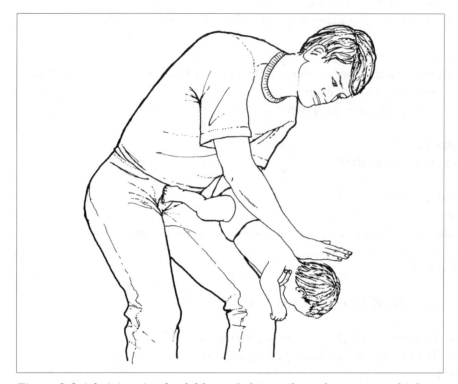

Figure 9-2 Administering back blows: Infants: along the rescuers thigh

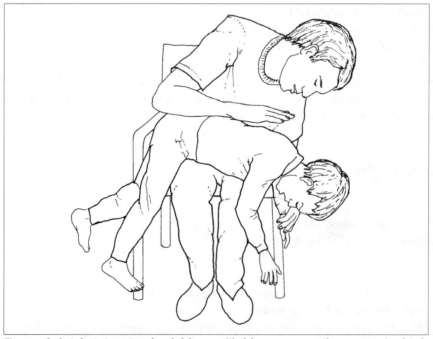

Figure 9-3 Administering back blows: Children: across the rescuer's thighs/knees

Method
- Position the child face down, with the head lower than the trunk.
- The method used depends on the child's size:
    - In infants this may be along the rescuer's thigh.
    - In older children this may be across the rescuer's thighs/knees.

- Deliver five firm back blows initially.
- If this is unsuccessful:
    - In infants (under one years old):
        - Administer five chest thrusts.
    - In children (over one year old):
        - Administer five abdominal thrusts (see chapter on Basic Life Support), *or* chest thrusts.

Abdominal thrusts
- Give five abdominal thrusts with the heel of one hand, taking care not to use excessive force.

Chest thrusts
- With the child's head pointing downwards, encircle the head with your hands and squeeze vigourously so as to cause a sudden rise in intrathoracic pressure.
- If it not possible to get your hands around the chest, apply pressure at the same point on the sternum as for chest compressions; one fingers breadth below the nipple line.

- If there is still no result:
    - Check the mouth for a foreign body, which by then may have become visible, and extract it.
- Open the airway.
- Administer expired air ventilations (see below).
- If there is no improvement:
    - Repeat the above cycle, but more forcibly.
    - Consider advanced airways management (see below):
        - Laryngoscopy: (*only* for experts, as instrumentation may make a bad situation worse).
        - Cricothyrotomy.
        - Ventilation.

CAUTION: - If one foreign body is present, there may be another!

Tissue swelling

Management
- Steam or humidity may be beneficial, especially in croup.
- Oxygen.
- If there is no improvement:
    - Administer expired air ventilation.
    - Consider:
        - Laryngoscopy
        - Cricothyrotomy
- Treat the cause: See chapter on Medical Emergencies.

Breathing (ventilation)

Management
- If the airway is clear:
    - Check that the child's ventilatory effort is normal by looking for normal chest expansion or abdominal movement.
    - If there is intercostal recession, see-saw movement of the chest and abdomen (indicating residual airway obstruction) *or* flaring of the nares in small children *or*
- If there is no air movement:
    - Clear the airway and start expired air ventilation immediately.

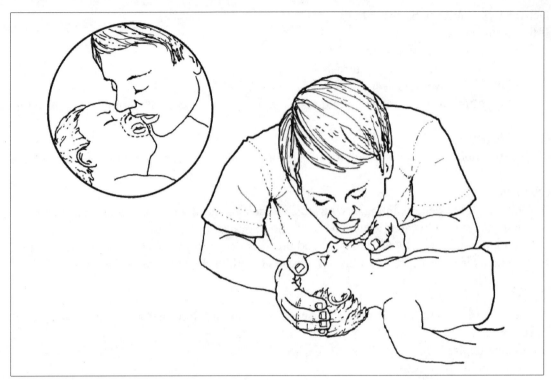

Figure 9-4 Mouth to mouth and nose expired air ventilation

Expired air ventilation

Method
- Hold the airway open.
- Infants under one year old: cover the child's mouth and nose with your mouth (babies are obligatory nose breathers and usually have a good nasal airway).
- Children over one year old: cover the mouth or nose with your mouth.
- Expire gently, watching for any movement of the child's chest and abdomen, indicating lung expansion:
  - Small airways and low compliance may occasionally necessitate more forceful expirations.
- Give five breaths initially.
- If the child requires ventilation only, adjust the rate to the size of the child:
  - Neonates: 20-30 breaths per minute.
  - Children: 15-20 breaths per minute.
  - Adolescents: 10-15 breaths per minute.
- Volume:
  - Neonates: 20-30 ml.
  - This can be adjusted by watching the child's chest movement.
- Any increase in ventilation should be achieved by raising the rate of delivery of expired air ventilations, rather than the airway pressure and tidal volume, which can cause a pneumothorax.
- Gastric distension:
  - This may occur resulting in splinting of the diaphragm.
  - If gastric distension does occur, consider decompressing the stomach by applying manual pressure to the upper abdomen, with the child in the lateral position (beware of causing aspiration of gastric contents!).

Circulation

- Treatment of airway or breathing problem should be attemped before any effort is made to treat cardiac arrest or circulatory problems (with the exception of severe haemorrhage).

Severe haemorrhage in children

Incidence
- Uncommon in children.

Aetiology
- Trauma.

Pathophysiology
- Small children tolerate large volume blood loss very badly (see above).

Symptoms/signs
- Rapid weak pulse.
- Monitor pulse rate, rhythm and volume in a large artery (see below).

Management
- Apply direct firm pressure over the bleeding point.

Cardiac arrest in children

Incidence
- Primary cardiac or circulatory arrest is rare in children except where there is congenital heart disease; the young heart is very resilient and will continue to beat for several minutes after respiratory arrest.

Aetiology
- Bradycardia is a common response to hypoxia, and is best treated by maintaining adequate ventilation.
- Restoration of alveolar ventilation with 100% oxygen will usually improve cardiac output and lead to recovery.

Note: - Bradycardia with a heart rate <60 bpm, should be treated as cardiac arrest.

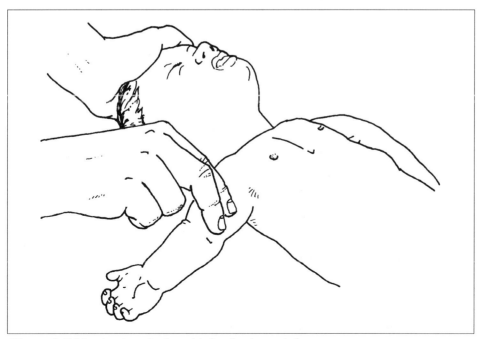

Figure 9-5 Monitoring the brachial pulse in an infant

Management
- Feel for the pulse in a large artery:
    - Infants under one year old: brachial artery.
    - Children over one year old: carotid artery.
    - Assess the volume, rate and rhythm.
- If these pulses are absent, try the femoral or axillary pulses or monitor the apex beat.
- In infants: if there is no pulse *or* the rate is less than 60 bpm, then start external chest compressions.
- In children over the age of one: start external chest compressions, if there is no pulse.

Note: - The right axillary artery is a common site for cardiac catheterisation, and operation scars should be looked for there (especially if there is an absent pulse).
  - Look for surgical scars in the chest or abdomen: may indicate congenital heart disease.

External chest compression

Method
- Apply firm, but gentle pressure over the lower sternum:
    - Small babies: treat as neonates.
    - Infants under one year old:
        - Use two fingers and depress the sternum about 2 cms.
    - Children over the age of one year:
        - Use the heel of one hand and depress the sternum about 3 cms.
- Rate:
    - 100 compressions per minute.

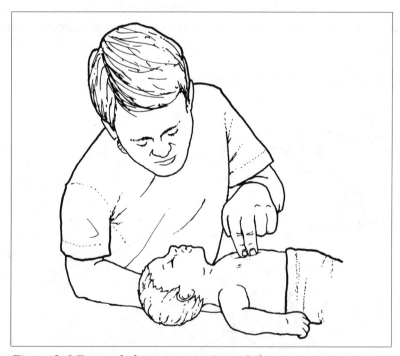

Figure 9-6 External chest compressions: Infants

- Compressions:
    - Should be smooth.
    - Compress up to one third of the AP diameter of the chest.
    - The compressive phase should last at least half the cycle.

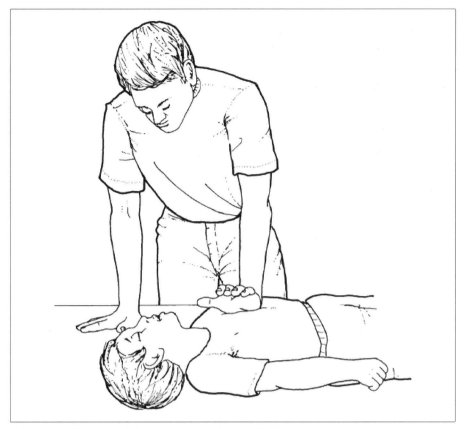

Figure 9-7 External chest compressions: Children

- Ratio of compressions to inflations for one rescuer:
    - Infants/young children: 5:1
    - Older children: 15:2.

Note:- It is very important that adequate ventilation be achieved.
    - Even with two rescuers, it may be necessary to pause in between chest compressions to achieve this.
    - Flexibility:
        - The rescuer(s) should adapt his/their technique to achieve an adequate pulse and ventilation.

- After about one minute, actvate emergency medical services by calling for an ambulance.

Advanced paediatric life support

- This is the use of artificial aids in the management of the acutely ill child, and usually comes after Basic Life Support.

Airways

Oropharyngeal airway (Guedel)

Indications
    - If the child is unconscious and has *no* gag reflex.
    - If used inappropriately, it may precipitate choking, laryngospasm and vomiting.

Size
- 000-4 depending on the size of the child
- The length is best estimated by measuring the distance from the lips to the angle of the jaw.
- Too small an airway may not overcome the obstruction of the tongue and may force it backwards blocking the airway.
- Too big an airway may press against and damage the posterior pharyngeal wall.

Insertion
- In infants and small children, this is done without rotating the device.

Nasopharyngeal airway

- Often a very useful and simple device to use in children.
- Tolerated better than oropharyngeal airways in the conscious or semicomatose child.

Size
- The largest size which passes easily through the external nares.

PRACTICAL POINT: An ET tube cut short and lubricated well, with a safety pin through the proximal end to prevent it slipping into the nose, makes a good substitute for a nasopharyngeal airway.

Endotracheal intubation in children

- This is the most reliable method of maintaining an adequate airway and ventilating infants and children.

Endotracheal tube sizes for children

Age	Internal diameter of ET tube (mm)	Length (cm) Oral	Nasal	Suction catheter (FG)
Premature	2.5-3.0	11.0	13.5	6
Newborn-8 weeks	3.5	12.0	14.0	8
2-24 months	4.0	13.0	15.0	8
2 years	4.5	14.0	16.0	8
4 years	5.0	15.0	17.0	10
6 years	5.5	17.0	19.0	10
8 years	6.0	19.0	21.0	10
10 years	6.5	20.0	22.0	10
12 years	7.0	21.0	22.0	10
14 years	7.5	22.0	23.0	10
16 years	8.0	23.0	24.0	12

- As a rough guide:
    - Endotracheal tubes: *Size:* $\underline{\text{Age of child}} + 4$ mm (*this gives a size 0.5 mm smaller than that*
        $$4 \qquad \textit{usually required for routine intubations)}$$
        or of similar external diameter to the child's little finger or nostril.

    Length: $\underline{\text{Age of child}} + 12$ cm
    $$2$$

- Croup:
    - Use a smaller endotracheal tube than usual (even so, intubation may be very difficult).

- Epiglottitis:
    - Intubation for epiglottitis is best avoided and should only be attempted by the experienced intubator in a hospital setting.
    - In Immediate Care cricothyrotomy is to be preferred and may be life saving.

Laryngoscopes
- For the inexperienced a straight blade is probably the best for use in young children.

Endotracheal intubation

Method
- See chapter on Neonatal resuscitation.
- After insertion:
    - Listen to the chest to ensure that air entry is adequate and equal on both sides and that the tube has not inadvertently entered the right main bronchus.
    - Secure the tube and attachments firmly with tape.
- Empty the stomach:
    - Insert a gastric tube to prevent aspiration and relieve any gastric distension.

Airway obstruction

Cricothyrotomy

- This should be considered in cases of severe upper airways obstruction by, e.g. foreign body, maxillofacial trauma, severe laryngeal oedema.
- Needle cricothyrotomy (a 14G intravenous cannula is preferred).
- Difficult to perform in very small children.

Method: See chapter on Airway Care.

Breathing (ventilation)

Oxygen therapy
- Very important in children owing to their high oxygen consumption. Their physiological right to left shunt may be exacerbated by, e.g. thoracic injury or diaphraghmatic splinting due to intra-abdominal injury.
- Supplemental oxygen (100% if possible) may be delivered by:
    - Facemask
    - Nasal cannulae (probably best for toddlers and pre-school children, but *not* for infants)
    - Endotracheal tube.

Ventilation
- If the child is not breathing, this must be achieved either by:
    - A bag and mask (preferably with an oropharyngeal or nasopharyngeal airway).
    - A bag and endotracheal tube.

Masks
- The Rendell-Baker facemask is recommended as it has minimal dead space.
- Soft circular plastic masks may also be useful.

Bags
- Sizes: infant, child or adult.
- Should:
    - Be self inflating.
    - Have a pressure limiting valve.
    - Be oxygen filled.

Automatic ventilators
- These are *not* recommended.

Ventilation bag sizes for children

Age and weight	Bag volume (ml)	Tidal volume (ml)
<2 yrs (<7 kg)	240	205
2-10 yrs (7-30 kg)	500	350
>10 yrs (>30 kg)	1600	1000

Circulation

- Children with hypovolaemia or fluid loss require rapid active management.
- The increased physiological reserve of children's circulation when compared to adults means that the vital signs may be only slightly abnormal in spite of significant blood loss.

Classification of hypovolaemic shock in children

Class of shock	I	II	III	V
Blood loss (%)	<15%	20-25%	30-35%	>40%
Pulse rate	raised 10-20%	tachycardia >150/min	tachycardia >150/min	tachycardia/ bradycardia
Blood pressure	normal	systolic pressure slightly reduced	systolic pressure reduced	severe hypotension
Pulse pressure	normal	slightly reduced	reduced	very low peripheral pulses absent
Respiratory rate	normal	tachypnoea (35-40)	tachypnoea	falls
Capillary refill	normal	slow	very slow	very slow
Extremeties	normal	cool, peripheries	cold, clammy cyanotic	pale, cold cyanotic
Mental state	normal	irritable, confused aggressive	lethargic	comatose

Assessment
- Heart rate and rhythm:
  - ECG.
- Heart sounds and breathing:
  - Stethoscope.
- Blood pressure:
  - Paediatric cuff with a width 2/3 length of child's upper arm.
- Temperature: rectal or axillary thermometer, or thermocouple.

PRACTICAL POINT: An adult cuff, folded over, is sufficient for all except small infants.

Management

Intravenous cannulation in children

- Access to the circulation for administration of drugs and fluid replacement is difficult in children.

Peripheral venous cannulation
- The peripheral veins are likely to be shut down, although more central veins, such as the femoral and external jugular are often dilated and may be easier to cannulate.
- In practice, any visible vein may be cannulated.
- If peripheral venous cannulation cannot be achieved within two or three minutes, another route for venous access needs to be established.

Central venous cannulation
- True central veins, i.e. the internal jugular and subclavian veins are probably the best routes for drug administration, although they are not of proven value in infants.
- Central venous cannulation has the disadvantage that it is difficult to perform in children, and should not be used by the inexperienced. In particular patient movement during chest compression makes central veins even more difficult to cannulate, and it can be difficult to differentiate between arteries and veins because of low arterial pressure and oxygen saturation. Accidental administration of calcium into a carotid or subclavian artery will have disastrous results.

Intraosseous infusion
- This is a useful route for drug and fluid administration, especially in children under 6 years old.
- For method, see chapter on Circulation care: shock.

Intravenous infusion fluids

- Beware of over-transfusion and administer fluids sparingly (total blood volume in children: 80 ml/kg).
- A careful record should be kept of the estimated blood loss and fluid transfused.
- Hypovolaemic shock:
  - Crystalloid
  - Colloids: Haemaccel, Gelofusine, Hetastarch.
  - Blood (if available).
  - Volume: 20 ml/kg crystalloid followed by 20 ml/kg colloid initially.
- In cardiopulmonary resuscitaion:
  - 10 ml/kg 0.9% sodium chloride solution, should be administered, as expansion of the circulating blood volume increases cardiac output.

- If resuscitation is delayed:
    - Small infants need at least 10% glucose, and may need boluses of 50% glucose as their glycogen stores are easily depleted.
- If possible all intravenous fluids should be warmed to body temperature prior to infusion.

Disability (neurological state)

- If the child is old enough and well enough to co-operate, the neurological status can be assessed using standard methods.
- Children change from being:
    - Happy/anxious
    - Miserable, crying: not too ill
    - Quiet, not interested in anything including parents: may be very ill
    - Restless: hypoxic
    - Exhausted: very ill, precedes respiratory arrest.

Exposure of the patient

- Removal of the child's clothing is necessary to allow adequate physical examination and the execution of practical procedures.
- Children and especially infants, lose heat very rapidly owing to their relatively large surface area, thin skin and lack of subcutaneous fat. A fall in body temperature results in a rise in oxygen consumption as compensatory metabolic processes start to provide an increase in heat production, peripheral vaso-constriction and a consequent lactic acidaemia.
- It is very important therefore that if the ambient temperatures are low:
    - The child is not exposed unnecessarily before being put in the ambulance, which itself should be kept as warm as possible.
    - The child should be kept warm, if exposure outside the ambulance is unavoidable, using:
        - Heat insulation
        - Warm or Hot packs *(being very careful not to burn the child)*.

Body weight in children

Estimation

- It can be extremely difficult to estimate an infant's or a child's weight in the Immediate Care situation, but the guides below may help. An alternative is to use the paediatric resuscitation chart (see below) obtainable from the *British Medical Journal*.
- Infants double their birthweight in 5 months.
- Infants treble their birthweight in 1 year.

Method 1
- Weight at 1 year: approximately 10 kg.
- Then, add 2 kg/year up to age 4 years (weight at 4 years: 16 kg).
- Then, add 3 kg/year up to age 10 years (weight at 10 years: 34 kg).

Method 2
- Between 1 and 9 years: (age + 4) x 2: (weight at 4 years: 16 kg).
- Between 7 and 12 years: age x 3: (weight at 10 years: 30 kg).

Arrhythmia management

Asystole and bradycardia

Incidence
- Most common arrest arrhythmia in children.

Aetiology
- Usually occurs secondary to hypoxia, due to an airway or breathing problem.
- Bradycardia (<60 bpm for infants <1 year, <40 bpm for children >1 year old), usually precedes asystole.

Management
- Perform basic life support, to maintain ventilation and the circulation (and hence myocardial/cerebral oxygenation). This may be all that is necessary to restore adequate cardiac output.
- Intubate and ventilate with 100% oxygen.
- Establish intravenous/introsseous access.
- Administer intravenous/intraosseous adrenaline: 10 μg/kg (0.1 ml/kg of 1:10,000 solution) *or* 10 x this dose via endotracheal tube if intravenous/introsseous access has not been established within 90 seconds.
- Perform cardiopulmonary resuscitation for about 3 minutes.
- Administer: adrenaline: 10 μg/kg, followed by cardiopulmonary resuscitation for about 3 minutes.
- Repeat the loop, administering fluids and alkalysing agents if resuscitation is prolonged.

Ventricular fibrillation

Incidence
- Uncommon in children, and is usually only seen as a terminal rhythm following cardiac arrest.

Aetiology
- May be caused by hypothermia or disturbances in calcium or potassium levels, and digoxin toxicity.

Management
- Administer a precordial thump.
- Defibrillate: administer 2 joules/kg initially, followerd again by 2 joules/kg, then increase to 4 joules/kg.
    - Paddle size (select those which provide the best contact with the child's chest wall):
        - Infants: 4.5 cm, children: 8.0 or 13 cm (if only large paddles are available; turn the child on its side, place the paddles on the front and back of the child and defibrillate through the chest).
- Intubate and ventilate with 100% oxygen.
- Establish intravenous/intraosseous access.
- Administer adrenaline: 10 μg/kg.
- Perform cardiopulmonary resuscitation for about one minute.
- Defibrillate: 4 joules/kg (repeated up to twice (three times in all), if there is no response).
- Consider the management of hypothermia, drug overdosage or electrolyte imbalance, if these are a likely cause.
- Administer adrenaline: 10 μg/kg, perform CPR for about one minute, and repeat the loop.
- After three loops: consider administration of an alkalysing agent and or an antiarrhythmic.

Electromechanical dissociation (EMD)

Incidence
- Rare.

Aetiology
- Hypovolaemia (commonest), tension pneumothorax, cardiac tamponade, drug overdosage, hypothermia.

Management
- Intubate and ventilate with 100% oxygen.
- Establish intravenous/intraosseous access.
- Administer adrenaline: 10 µg/kg.
- Administer intravenous fluid replacement: 20 mls/kg.
- Perform cardiopulmonary resuscitation for about 3 minutes.
- Treat the cause, if possible.
- Administer adrenaline: 10 µg/kg, perform CPR for three minutes, and repeat the loop, as necessary.

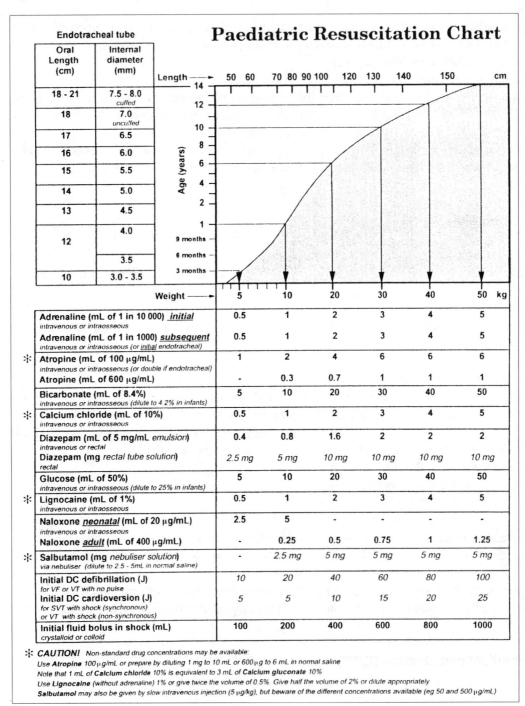

Figure 9-8 Paediatric resuscitation chart

Other cardiac drugs

- Lignocaine:
  - *Indication:* Ventricular arrhythmias
  - *Dosage:* 0.1 ml/kg of 1%, administered intravenously
        (This may be repeated after 5 minutes if necessary, followed by an infusion.)

- Frusemide:
  - *Indication:* Cardiac failure.
  - *Dosage:* 1-5 mg/kg administered intravenously.

Drug administration in children

- When drugs are administered by the peripheral venous or intraosseous routes, they should be flushed through with 0.9% sodium chloride solution to help them to reach their site of action.
- Access for drug administration may be difficult to achieve in children, and if intravenous or intraosseous access cannot be obtained within 90 seconds, then endotracheal/endobronchial administration should be considered.

Endotracheal/endobronchial administration
- This route may be used for: adrenaline, lignocaine and atropine (*never* bicarbonate).
- It should only be used in the very early stages of resuscitation, as drug absorption may be unpredictable and unreliable for this route.
- The dose should be double the intravenous dose (adrenaline ten times the intravenous dose), and the drug diluted in 2-3 ml of 0.9% sodium chloride solution.
- After drug administration, the child should be hyperventilated (five inflations) to help distribution and absorption of the drug by the pulmonary vascular bed.

Medical problems: life threatening illness in children

Heat loss in children

Pathophysiology
- Infants and young children can lose heat rapidly because of their relatively larger body surface, and may have difficulty generating enough heat to compensate for any heat loss. This is due to their relatively small glycogen stores and lack of body fat.

Management
- Insulation:
  - Warm blankets, space blankets.
- Heat:
  - Hot water bottles, but beware of causing burns!
  - Prewarming intravenous fluids.
- Energy:
  - Infusion of dextrose.

Sudden infant death syndrome (SIDS)

- The sudden death of any infant or young child between the age of one week and two years, which is unexpected by history and in which a thorough postmortem examination fails to demonstrate an adequate cause of death.
- The incidence has been dramatically reduced by a public education program encouraging mothers not to allow their babies to sleep in the prone position.

Incidence

- Affects 1:500 children.
- Age:
  - Most common cause of death in the post-neonatal period (28-364 days).
  - The majority of deaths occur between 4-20 weeks (peak incidence: 8-18 weeks), 80% of deaths occur before 8 months.
  - Rare over the age of 1 year.
- Responsible for:
  - >30% all cardiac arrests in children.
  - 20% of all infant deaths in England and Wales.

Aetiology

- At present the cause is unknown, but several mechanisms may be responsible.
- It may be due to a combination of:
  - Immature control of respiration and temperature (over wrapping and sleeping prone).
  - Carbon dioxide retention (sleeping prone on a soft mattress).
  - A minor respiratory infection.
- Other factors:
  - Intercurrent infection.
  - Bottle feeding.
  - Twins: especially if:
    - Delivered pre-term
    - Low birth weight.
  - Social and economic deprivation.
  - Low birth weight, short gestation period and reduced birth length.
  - Winter/cold weather.
  - Illegitimacy.
  - Single parent family.
  - Mothers:
    - Who have smoked, or taken opiates or barbiturates
    - From ethnic minorities.
  - The incidence increases with ascending birth order and reduced birth interval.

Management

- Basic/Advanced life support.
- Treatment of the cause, if this is obvious.

10

Acute myocardial infarction

Acute myocardial infarction (AMI)

Introduction

- The treatment of acute myocardial infarction is something with which every doctor should be familiar, both in General and in Hospital Practice, especially if he or she is involved in Immediate Care, as all will come across the patient with an acute myocardial infarction from time to time and be expected to institute immediate effective treatment, the objective of which is to minimise the mortality and morbidity following AMI.

Incidence

- Coronary artery/ischaemic heart disease is the commonest single cause of premature death in the UK, accounting for about 25% of all deaths, and results in an annual total of more than 175,000 deaths.
- Each year about 250,000 people will experience an acute myocardial infarction, of whom nearly 50% will die as a result. Of these, 80% will die within the first 4 hours: 25% within the first 15 minutes, 40% within the first hour.
- Two thirds of deaths occur out of hospital; between 3.5-21% of deaths occur in the presence of a General Practitioner and 5% occur during transport to hospital.
- On average a General Practitioner will be called to treat an AMI only twice a year.

Aetiology

- The cause of coronary heart disease is multifactorial and is not yet fully understood, but several risk factors are asssociated with an increased likelihood of developing the disease, which is characterised by the build up of atheromatous plaques in the coronary arteries.

Pathophysiology

Precipitating factors

- The build up of atheromatous plaques, covered by a thin, fibrous cap in the coronary arteries. This results in restriction and turbulence of the blood flow.
- Enlargement of these plaques then occurs due to further atheroma deposition and occasionally intra-plaque haemorrhage, which results in cracking, splitting and ulceration of the plaque's fibrous cap. This then forms a surface on which the platelets aggregate.

- Increased turbulence and restriction of the arterial flow occurs and with the platelet aggregation triggers coagulation, leading to local thrombus formation.
- This intraluminal thrombus may increase in size resulting in total arterial occlusion or it may be completely lysed following which the plaque fissure may be resealed.
- Arterial occlusion results in overactivation of the sympathetic nervous system. Consequent coronary constriction may also occur, but this is rarely the sole cause of AMI.

Mechanism

- Occlusion of a main coronary artery, usually (in over 90% of cases) by thrombus associated with atherosclerotic changes in the coronary arteries, results in infarction and necrosis of the heart muscle supplied by that artery.
- Myocardial damage usually starts in the subendocardial layer and spreads progressively outwards.
- Ischaemic changes begin to develop in the myocardium within 3-5 minutes, and myocardial necrosis begins within 20 minutes.
- This becomes irreversible in about 4-6 hrs (50% complete in 6 hrs, 100% complete in 24 hrs).

Severity

- The more proximal the infarction, the greater the amount of potential muscle damage.
- The better the collateral blood supply, the less the amount of damage.

Electrophysiology: ECG in AMI

- May be useful in confirming the diagnosis, locating the infarct and monitoring progress, but the correlation between the ECG tracing and the underlying pathology is poor, especially soon after AMI.
- The development of a Q-wave within a few hours of the infarction, indicates irreversible full thickness muscle damage.
- The absence of a Q-wave, indicates that the infarct has not caused full thickness muscle necrosis.
- Patients who are given thrombolytics early are less likely to have a full thickness infarct and are less likely to have Q-waves.
- Patients with non Q-wave infarctions have lower mortality rates in hospital, but are more likely to have recurrent angina ar a second infarction.
- There may be autonomic dysfunction:
    - Sympathetic overactivity resulting in tachycardia.
    - Parasympatheic (vagal) overactivity resulting in bradycardia and frequently in hypotension.

Location

- Usually, the left ventricle is affected, although in inferior infarction, right ventricular ischaemia and necrosis are relatively common.
- The correlation between ECG site and coronary artery anatomy is poor.

Anterior myocardial infarction
- Usually occurs due to occlusion of the left anterior descending coronary artery resulting in infarction of the anterior wall of the left ventricle and the intraventricular septum.
- May result in pump failure due to ventricular septal defect (VSD), aneurysm or rupture and arrhythmias.

Inferior myocardial infarction
- May occur due to occlusion of the right or left circumflex coronary arteries resulting in infarction of the inferior surface of the left ventricle. The right ventricle and the interventricular septum may also be damaged.
- Results in bradycardia due to damage to the AV node. Pump failure is less common.

Posterior or lateral myocardial infarction
- Usually occurs due to occlusion of the left circumflex or large right coronary artery.
- Less common.
- Results in pump failure and malignant ventricular arrhythmias.

Complications of AMI

Death
- 30-50% of patients, who die from AMI, die in the first 30 minutes.
- The mortality rate is highest in the elderly, in females, in those who have a history of previous myocardial infarction, in those with extensive infarcts and in those who develop heart failure.
- The greater the degree of myocardial damage, the greater the resulting ventricular dysfunction, disability and incidence of complications.

Arrhythmias (45%)
- Electrical instability, leading to ventricular fibrillation. May be aggravated by autonomic overactivity.
- The major cause of preventable early deaths.

Pump failure (45%)
- Decreased strength of muscle contractions, leading to left ventricular failure.
- A major cause of late deaths.

Other mechanical problems (2%)
- Rupture of:
    - Myocardial wall:
        - Accounts for 10% of all hospital deaths.
        - Characterised by the sudden onset of cardiac failure (EMD), followed by sudden death due to ventricular fibrillation/asystole.
    - Interventricular septum (0.5%), leading to a ventricular septal defect (VSD).
    - Papilliary muscles, resulting in acute mitral regurgitation.
- Ventricular aneurysm.

Thromboembolism (8%):
- Late deep vein thrombosis, pulmonary embolism.
- Now rare in hospital.

Diagnosis

History

- In the Immediate Care situation, history taking should be as rapid as possible.
- There may be history of up to several days general malaise or increasingly severe angina just prior to an AMI.
- Past medical history:
  - Previous myocardial infarction.
  - Angina (20-30%).
  - Risk factors for coronary artery disease.

Symptoms/signs

Malaise
- Prodromal symptoms of pain and a lack of well-being often precede AMI.

Cardiogenic shock
- The patient may be:
  - Frightened, ill, pale, and sweating (this decreases with age).
  - Hypotensive (systolic BP <90 mmHg).
  - Peripherally shutdown.

Complaining of
- Pain (see below).
- Dyspnoea, faintness, and confusion (increases with age): pump failure.
- Nausea, vomiting, hiccoughs (inferior myocardial infarction): autonomic dysfunction.

Pain/discomfort
- Only occurs in 80-90% of patients, but is more likely to be due to an AMI in the elderly.
- May be absent, especially in the elderly.

  Nature
  - Severe, intense, heavy, crushing, "like a heavy weight", tight or frightening.

  Location
  - May be:
    - Precordial *(usual)*
    - Epigastric
    - In either shoulder, arm or in the back
    - In front of the neck or jaw
    - Any combination of these.

  Radiation
  - To neck/jaw, down either arm or through to the back.

  Time
  - More likely to occur in the late evening or early morning (the peak is between 6-11 am, possibly precipitated by the blood pressure rising on/before arousing/awakening, resulting in coronary artery plaque rupture, vessel occlusion and myocardial infarction).

  Duration
  - May last many hours.

  Course:
  - Continuous, usually without variation, but may be of increasing intensity.

Relationships
- Precipitated by:
    - Physical or emotional stress.
    - Meals, and micturition or defecation.

    But usually occurs at rest
- Not usually relieved by rest and nitrates.

Pulse
- May be low volume, rapid and irregular.

Breath sounds
- Usually normal, but there may be the signs of congestive cardiac failure, e.g. basal creps or crackles.

Heart sounds
- Often normal, but there may be a III or IV heart sound.

Low grade pyrexia
- This may take a few hours to develop

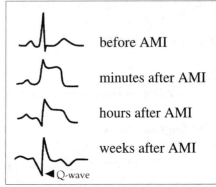

Figure 10-7 ECG changes after AMI

Investigations

Electrocardiogram: ECG in AMI
- 5-10% of those with a myocardial infarction have no ECG changes.
- 5-10% of those with myocardial infarction have doubtful ECG changes.
- 25% have probable ECG changes, and *only 50% show classical changes*.

Diagnostic criteria:
- Significant ST segment elevation "acute change" of at least 2 mm in at least two leads:
    - Anterior infarction: I, aVL, V2-6
    - Antero-lateral infarction: I, aVL, V4-6
    - Antero-septal infarction: V1-4
    - Inferior infarction: II, III, aVF
    - Postero-lateral infarction: Vl, V5-6.

- ST segment depression:
    - This may be reciprocal to ST elevation (indicates myocardial ischaemia)
        - Anterior infarction: II, III, aVF
        - Posterior infarction: V1-V4
        - Inferior infarction: I, aVL, V1-2.

- T wave:
    - Elevation: tall broad (hyperacute) in true posterior AMI.
    - Inversion (this is a late change, therefore probably indicates an old AMI).
    - Deep symmetrical T waves are found in Subendocardial infarction.

- Deep Q waves (>2 mm deep or >0.04 seconds wide):
    - This is a later sign (takes up to 24 hours to develop, and usually persists).
    - Usually indicates irreversible infarction (if present early; this indicates a previous AMI).

- R wave:
    - Progressive loss across the chest leads.

ECG examples of different types of acute myocardial infarction

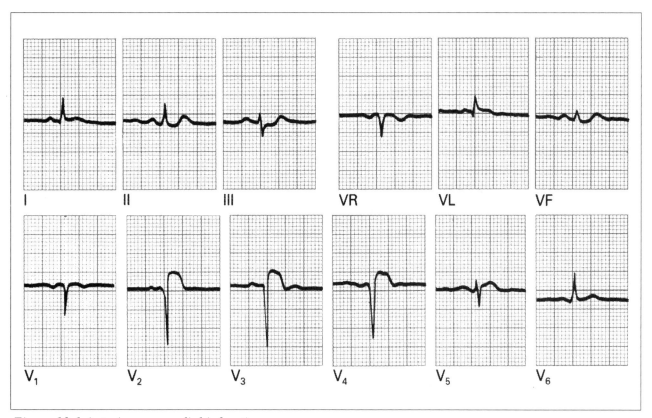

Figure 10-1 Anterior myocardial infarction

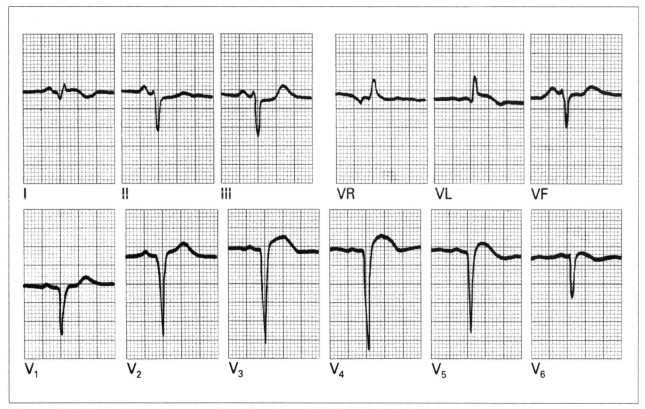

Figure 10-2 Antero-lateral myocardial infarction with left axis deviation

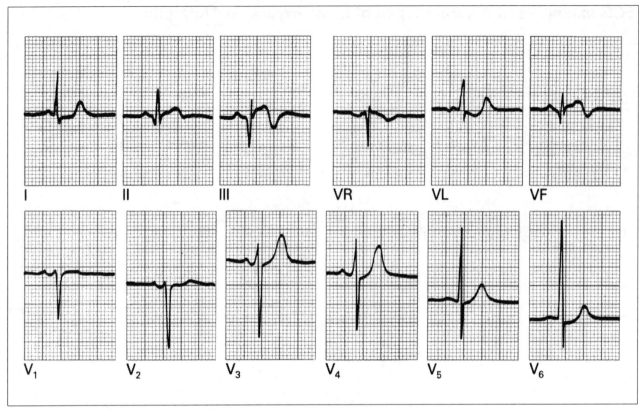

Figure 10-3 Inferior myocardial infarction

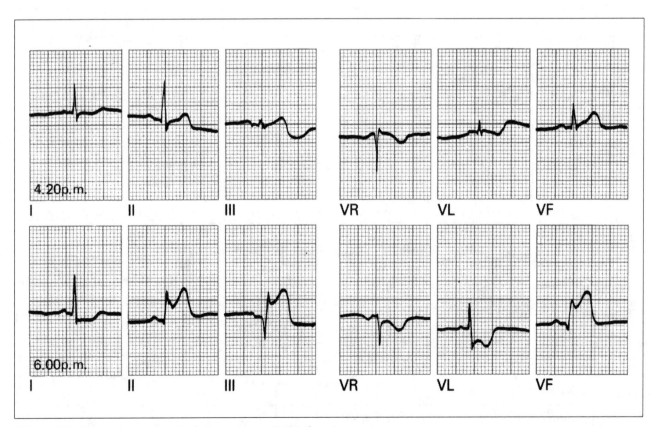

Figure 10-4 Development of inferior myocardial infarction

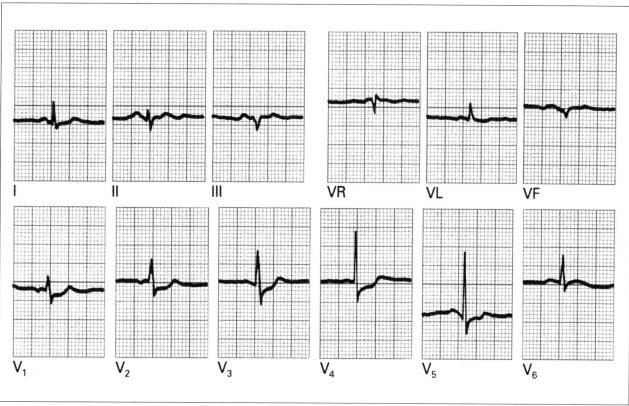

Figure 10-5 Posterior myocardial infarction

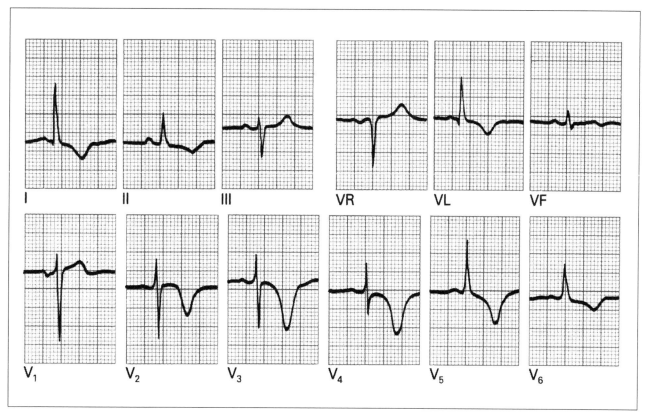

Figure 10-6 Subendocardial infarction

Differential diagnosis of chest pains

Chest wall

Herpes zoster
- There may be pain and/or hyperaesthesia up to 7 days before the appearance of the rash.

Bornholm disease
- Poorly localised acute pain with pyrexia and tender intercostal muscles.

Costal chondritis "Tietze's syndrome"/cough fracture
- Localised tenderness.

Trauma/musculoskeletal pain
- History and localised tenderness.

Diaphragmatic catch syndrome
- Negative history of trauma.
- Pain is transient and "catches the breath".
- There may be tender rib margins.

Heart

Myocardial infarction: See above

Stable angina

Aetiology
- Similar to acute myocardial infarction

Pathophysiology
- Relative impairment of myocardial muscle perfusion due to:
    - Increased myocardial oxygen demand:
        - Exercise especially after meals
        - Stress.
    - Reduced oxygen supply:
        - Spasm of coronary arteries
        - Partial occlusion of coronary arteries by plaque
        - Anaemia.

History
- Similar attacks in similar circumstances.

Symptoms/signs
- Similar to myocardial infarction, with central chest pain, but the pain is:
    - Less severe, though similar in character to AMI
    - Precipitated by and occurs during exertion, and makes the patient stop or slow down
    - Relieved by:
        - Resting or standing still for about 10 minutes
        - Glyceryl trinitrate spray or sublingual tablets within 2-3 minutes
    - The patient is not usually so shocked nor so ill
    - Dyspnoea is common and sometimes the principal feature.

ECG diagnosis
- May be normal or show:
    - Ischaemic changes
    - Evidence of an old AMI.

Management
- Rest and reassurance
- GTN: Spray or sublingual tablets
- Oxygen
- Analgesia.

Unstable angina

Pathophysiology
- Similar to angina, with progress towards infarction
- 10% progress to acute myocardial infarction (5% die)
- 35% are left with persisting angina.

Symptoms
- The pain is similar to that of stable angina but it:
    - May be more severe, more frequent, and is less predictable
    - May occur on minimal exertion or even at rest
    - Is more prolonged and may not respond immediately to rest or nitrates.
- The recent onset of increasingly severe angina.
- A change in the pattern of the patient's usual angina.

ECG diagnosis
- Associated with fluctuating ST segment (depression) or T wave changes (inversion).

Management
- Administer oxygen and buccal or sublingual nitrates.
- Give soluble aspirin: half a 300 mg tablet orally.
- Establish intravenous access.
- Give analgesia: morphine/diamorphine with an anti-emetic.
- If there is no improvement (no pain relief or resolution of ST segment changes):
    - Consider giving nifedipine (diltiziem is an alternative)
    - Then consider: atenolol 100 mg orally
    - Admit to hospital *immediately*.

Pericarditis

Incidence
- May occur in the relatively young.

History
- There may be the history and signs of systemic viral infection, and rarely neoplasm or autoimmune disease.

Symptoms
- The pain is central and may be reduced by sitting forward and aggravated by deep breathing/coughing.
- There may be a friction rub, with the signs of cardiac tamponade: raised JVP and pulsus paridoxicus.

ECG diagnosis
- There may be generalised ST elevation without Q waves.

Myocarditis

Incidence
- May be associated with chest pain especially when there is pericarditis.

Symptoms
- Usually presents with a pyrexia, malaise and a tachycardia.
- Sometimes there may be arrhythmias, cardiac failure and shock.

Aorta

Dissecting aneurysm

Symptoms
- Pre-existing hypertension.
- May be precipitated by exertion.
- Sudden onset of severe searing, tearing pain radiating to the neck, abdomen, legs or back of the chest.
- May simulate or include an AMI.

Signs
- *The blood pressure may be raised and there may be a machinery murmur on auscultation.*
- Cardiogenic shock with a raised central venous pressure, cardiac failure and ankle oedema.
- There may be absent or reduced neck or limb pulses with distended often pulsatile superficial veins.

Trachea

Tracheitis

Symptoms
- There may be a raw central pain, made worse by coughing.

Lungs

Pleurisy

Symptoms
- The pain is usually localised and lateral, and may be exacerbated by deep inspiration.

Signs
- There is usually a pleural friction rub, and evidence of pneumonia.

Pneumothorax

Incidence
- Typically seen in slim and maybe Marfanoid young males, and also the asthmatic, in whom effective management may be life saving.

History
- There may be a history of previous episodes.

Symptoms
- There is usually, but not always (especially in asthmatics) the sudden onset of acute pleuritic pain, and dyspnoea.

Signs
- There are signs of tracheal shift and reduced or absent air entry, and hyper-resonance on percussion
- If severe, it may mimic a massive pulmonary embolism (see below).

Pulmonary embolism

History
- Recent surgery, pelvic or long bone trauma, pregnancy, etc.

Symptoms/signs
- These will vary according to underlying pathophysiology:
    - *Peripheral embolus:* e.g. a small embolus blocking a peripheral branch of the pulmonary artery:
        - Haemoptysis
        - Pleuritic chest pain.
    - *Central embolus:* i.e. a massive embolus blocking a proximal part of the pulmonary artery:
        - Collapse
        - Severe dyspnoea with cyanosis
        - Pain: may be absent or severe, may mimic an acute myocardial infarction
        - Shock with a raised jugular venous pressure
        - There may also be a tachypnoea and tachycardia.

ECG diagnosis
- Often there are minimal or no ECG changes.
- May be difficult to distinguish from acute myocardial infarction, but there may be:
    - Atrial tachyarrhythmias (most common)
    - Non-specific ST segment and T wave changes
    - Right axis deviation
    - Right bundle branch block
    - Sometimes inferior Q waves and inverted T waves (S1, Q3, T3).

Gastrointestinal tract

Reflux oesophagitis/hiatus hernia

Symptoms/signs
- Epigastric/retrosternal burning pain.
- Usually related to meals and posture: lying down and bending forward.
- May be difficult to distinguish from cardiac pain, especially if unrelated to food and posture.
- Usually relieved by food, nitrates or antacids.

Oesophageal spasm

Symptoms
- Similar to oesophagitis, but even more difficult to distinguish from AMI.

Peptic ulcer, gallstones and pancreatitis

- Usually the history, the site of the pain and physical examination will distinguish these from AMI.

Guidelines for the management of AMI

Object: To resuscitate the patient and reduce myocardial damage and complications following an AMI, prior to rapid evacuation to hospital.

Basic Life Support (see chapter on Basic Life Support)

- If the patient is unconscious with no spontaneous respiration, pulse or blood pressure.

Position/posture

- The patient should be placed in the position of greatest comfort, usually sitting up, as this may reduce the venous return.

Administer oxygen

- This is essential for the patient with a suspected AMI.

Establish intravenous access

- This may be with just a cannula or an intravenous infusion may be set up.
- This will allow immediate access for intravenous drugs.
- If an intravenous infusion is started:
    - Crystalloid, e.g. Hartmann's solution or 5% dextrose, is to be preferred.
    - Intravenous fluids should be run in slowly, so as to avoid fluid overload.

Monitoring

ECG
- This is very important for the early detection of arrythmias, and confirming the diagnosis of AMI prior to the administration of an arrhythmic or thrombolytic agent.

Haemodynamic assessment
- Blood pressure.
- Pulse:
    - Rate, rhythm, and character.
- Breath sounds.
- Heart sounds.
- The patient's general condition, etc.

Pain relief/sedation

- This is also very important as pain alone causes a rise in the circulating catecholamines and may precipitate "shock", and increases the vagal tone and incidence of arrhythmias (see chapter on Pain Relief).
- In AMI, all drugs should be administered intravenously unless contraindicated as:
    - The patient may be peripherally shut down, drugs may not enter the circulation and will not be effective.
    - Haematoma formation may result if the patient receives concurrent thrombolysis.

Analgesia in AMI (for details of presentation, dosage, etc., see chapter on Pain Relief)

Opiates: morphine/diamorphine

- These are the analgesics of choice for cardiac pain because of their analgesic efficacy and anxiolytic effects.

Action
- For principal analgesic action: see chapter on Pain Relief.
- Other beneficial effects include:
    - Dilation of the resistance and capacitance vessels
    - They sometimes reduce the heart rate
    - They may also reduce cardiac work and myocardial oxygen demand (beneficial in congestive cardiac failure and AMI).

Disadvantages
- They impair the normal response to changes in posture and may precipitate hypotension.
- Care has to be taken if the patient has already taken nitrates or other vasodilators as severe hypotension may occur as a result.
- May cause nausea (which in the context of AMI may also be due to increased vagal activity).

Administration
- This should be by slow intravenous injection, diluted and titrated so as to avoid hypotension or respiratory depression, which is more likely if administration is rapid.
- They should be given together or in combination with an antiemetic to reduce nausea (see below).

Pethidine
- More rapid onset of action, shorter acting, less potent, but less likely to cause respiratory depression than morphine.
- In AMI may be considered, if the pain is not severe and in inferior infarcts.

Nalbuphine (Nubain)
- Should be considered if the patient is hypotensive or has respiratory depression.

Nitrous oxide/oxygen
- Should be considered if opiates are not available.

Antiemetics for use in AMI

- In AMI nausea and vomiting is common and may be due to the autonomic disturbance that may arise as a result of AMI itself or to the effects opiate analgesics.
- Antiemetics used in AMI include:
    - Metoclopramide (Maxolon): *probably the antiemetic of choice in AMI.*
    - Prochlorperazine (Buccastem buccal tablets, Stemetil suppositories, *not* intramuscular injection).
    - Cyclizine (Valoid), which should be used with caution and is *not recommended in AMI* as it may cause vasoconstriction.

Anxiolytics

Diazepam (see chapter on Pain Relief)
- This may also be beneficial, especially if the patient is very anxious, and can reduce the incidence of arrhythmias.
- Should be used with care when administered intravenously as may cause respiratory depression.

Administration
- Intravenously or rectally.

Nitrates

Action
- Increases the coronary blood flow by causing coronary artery vasodilation.
- Reduces the myocardial oxygen demand (workload) by causing:
  - Venodilation:
    - Reduces the left ventricular filling pressure (preload).
  - A reduction in the afterload.
- Post infarct, nitrates may help to maintain coronary artery patency during thrombolytic treatment, and improve the prognosis by limiting the infarct size and preserving left ventricular function.

Indications
- Cardiac ischaemic pain: angina.

Side effects
- Flushing, headache, dizziness, postural hypotension, tachycardia.

Presentation
- Glyceryl trinitrate:
  - Tablets: 300, 500 and 600 μg.
    - Short acting: 20-30 minutes.
    - Unstable and once opened, the tablets have a very short life of only 2 months.
  - Buccal tablets (Suscard): 1, 2, 3 mg.
    - Rapid onset, longer duration of action.
  - Sublingual spray: 400 μg metered dose.
    - Rapid onset, short duration of action, long storage life (2 years).

- Isosorbide dinitrate:
  - Tablets/sublingual spray
    - Active sublingually.
    - A more stable preparation for those patients who may use it infrequently.
    - Long duration of action.

- Isosorbide mononitrate:
  - A metabolite of isosorbide dinitrate.

Administration
- May be given:
  - Sublingually (spray, or tabs):
    - Acts rapidly to cause initial arteriolar vasodilation and subsequent venodilation.
  - Intravenously (not usually administered this way in Immediate Care).
- Act predominantly as venodilators.

Thrombolytics

Introduction
- The use of thrombolytics are now established in the early management of acute myocardial infarction. It has been shown that aspirin and thrombolytics used approprately can reduce the mortality by half, if administered early after the onset of symptoms to patients with suspected AMI; and could save up to 50 lives per 1000 patients treated. The earlier the administration, the greater the benefit, and several trials have shown an increased benefit for pre-hospital thrombolysis, especially in rural areas.

Aspirin
- An antiplatelet agent which has some thrombolytic action, when used alone, and is of additional benefit when it administered together with a specific thrombolytic. Used alone it can reduce the long term mortality rate by up to 25%, saving up to 25 lives per 1000 patients treated, but there is a a small additional increase in the incidence of stroke.

Action
- The precise mechanism of action is unknown, but a reduction in platelet aggregation undoubtedly plays a part in influencing the thrombolytic process.

Dosage
- Half of one tablet of soluble aspirin (150 mg), sucked, chewed or crushed under the tongue.

Contraindications (relative)
- Previous history of haemorrhagic shock, gastrointestinal bleed/peptic ulcer disease, recent trauma, allergy to aspirin or other NSAIDs, and recent arterial puncture.

Specific thrombolytics

Introduction
- The development of specific thrombolytics is a major advance in the management of acute myocardial infarction, and can give a 12-50% reduction in the short term mortality, and up to a 47% reduction in the long term mortality (>1 year).
- They are most effective if given immediately after the infarction, and become less beneficial as time elapses.
- They are of greatest benefit to those at greatest risk:
  - Age: >70 years
  - History of a previous myocardial infarction
  - The hypotensive
  - Females
  - Those with an anterior infarct
  - Those with a proven myocardial infarction
  - The greatest benefit occurs if they are given together with aspirin.

Action
- Thrombolytics activate the natural endogenous lytic pathways in the circulation. The precursor of this pathway is plasminogen which is converted to an active protease enzyme; plasmin. Plasmin breaks down the fibrin matrix of the thrombus, resulting in dissolution of the clot itself. It has no effect on the underlying atheromatous disease.
- Intracoronary clot lysis results in an increase in the patency of the blocked coronary artery, the restoration of blood supply to the infarcted coronary muscle and a reduction in the loss of myocardium.
- Reperfusion results in the early release of cardiac enzymes, which may be associated with cardiac arrythmias.

Disadvantages
- The overall risk of complications is low.
- Severe bleeding:
    - < 1% (0.5% have a major cerebral bleed but there is no overall increased risk of a cerebral vascular accident, although with rtPA this risk is slightly greater than with streptokinase).
    - Most bleeding is minor.
- Bradycardia, sudden severe, but transient hypotension.   } made worse by
- Life threatening ventricular arrhythmias due to reperfusion of cardiac muscle (rare) } ambulance ride
    - Allergic reactions (rare).
    - Risk of microemboli due to disintegration of pre-existing clot.
    - Expense (apart from streptokinase, which is much cheaper).
- Antigenic: no more than one dose of streptokinase or anistreplase may be given in a 1 year period, due to antibody formation.

The problem
- Myocardial infarction may be difficult to diagnose early with any certainty, when thrombolysis is most effective and beneficial.
- The major problem with diagnosis is over the exclusion of aortic aneurysm, as innappropriate thrombolysis given to a patient with an aortic aneurysm may be fatal.

Contraindications
Absolute
- Known bleeding diatheses, long term anticoagulant therapy, or chronic liver disease with portal hypertension.
- Recent bleeding from any site.
- Intracranial neoplasm, arteriovenous malformation or aneurysm.
- Surgery, major trauma, or neurosurgery in the last month.
- Gastrointestinal bleeding, or pancreatitis.
- Known potential site for pre-existing blood clot:
    - Enlarged left atrium
    - Ventricular/aortic aneurysm.
- Acute pericarditis, septic thrombophlebitis or sub-acute bacterial endocarditis.
- Cerebral vascular accident in the preceding 3 months leaving residual disability, or transient ischaemic attack within the preceeding 6 months.
- Pregnancy.
- Proliferative diabetic retinopathy.

Relative
- Recent prolonged external chest compressions.
- Severe hypertension (BP >200 mmHg systolic and/or >120 mmHg diastolic).
- Menstruation or lactation.
- Dental extraction within preceding 14 days.
- Non-compressible arterial punctures within the preceeding 14 days or required immediately.
- Allergy to streptokinase or anistreplase.
- Serious organic or psychiatric illness.
- (Administration of streptokinase or anistreplase within the preceding 5 days to 1 year is a contraindication to it being administered again.)

Indications
- Presentation within 24 hrs of the onset of chest pain of at least 30 minutes duration, unrelieved by nitrates.
- ECG changes diagnostic of AMI (see above).

Non fibrin specific plasminogen activator

Streptokinase (Streptase, Kabikinase)

Presentation
- Kabikinase: 1.5 million unit vial.
- Streptase: 7500 unit vial.

Advantages
- The original specific thrombolytic, with which most experience has been gained.
- There is a lower risk of it causing cerebral and non-cerebral haemorrhage than either anistreplase or alteplase.

Disadvantages
- It is a "foreign" (bacterial) protein and is antigenic, as a result of which patients develop antibodies to it after about 5 days. Consequently it should not be used at intervals of less than 12 months, and may not be effective in some patients if readministered within 1 year.
- Allergic reactions may occur, but rarely.

Administration
- Slowly intravenously: 1.5 million units in 100 ml normal saline over 1 hour.

Cost
- Cheapest.

CONCLUSION
- *Unsuitable for pre-hospital administration*, but is the thrombolytic of choice for hospital use.

Fibrin specific plasminogen activators

- These are fibrin specific and administration has been shown to result in better vessel patency than with streptokinase, although no clinical advantage has actually been shown.

Anistreplase: APSAC (Eminase)

Presentation
- 30 units/5 ml vial, 5 ml WFI, syringe and needle.

Advantages
- Effective and easy to administer.
- Few allergic reactions or episodes of hypotension reported so far.

Disadvantages
- Must be stored between 2-8°C.
- Antigenic: antibodies develop after 5 days and allergic reactions may occur rarely (but more frequently than with either streptokinase or alteplase).
- Should not be used within 1 year of the administration of streptokinase or anistreplase.

Administration
- 5 ml/30 units given intravenously over 4-5 minutes.

Half life
- 90-110 minutes

Cost
- Very expensive (in the UK, 7x the cost of streptokinase).

CONCLUSION
- *Thrombolytic of choice for pre-hospital administration.*

Alteplase: rtPA (Actilyse)

Presentation
- Pack of 2 x 50 mg vials, 2 x 50 ml WFI, 2 transfer devices and 2 hanging bags.

Advantages
- Non antigenic and causes less reduction in fibrinogen.
- May reduce the mortality following AMI slightly more than streptokinase.

Disadvantages
- More likely to cause cerebral vascular accidents.

Administration
- Given by slow intravenous infusion: 10 mg bolus, 50 mg over 1 hour, then 40 mg over 2 hours.

Cost
- The most expensive (in the UK, 11x the cost of streptokinase).

CONCLUSION
- *Unsuitable for pre-hospital use.* Should be reserved for patients who have had streptokinase or anistreplase within the preceding 1 year.

β-blockers

Introduction
- Judicious use of β-blockers has been shown to reduce the mortality rate following AMI by 15%, but administration is usually reserved for in-hospital use.
- Chronic administration of β-blockers after AMI has also been shown to reduce the incidence of further AMI as well as reducing the mortality, and is widely used in follow-up care.

Indications
- SVT following AMI.

Mode of action
- This is unproven, but is probably by:
    - Reducing the incidence of cardiac rupture
    - Reducing/preventing the undesirable effects of increased sympathetic activity by:
        - Reducing the cardiac workload and consequently oxygen demand
        - Reducing the pain and the size of the infarct
        - Improving the blood supply to ischaemic areas
        - Reducing the potential for developing arrhythmias: VF, VT and PVCs
        - Possibly reducing thrombus formation and platelet aggregation
        - Reduction of blood pressure and heart rate.

Contraindications
- Cardiac shock/severe heart failure: i.e. hypotension with a systolic BP <100 mmHg.
- Bradycardia: heart rate: <50 bpm.
- Second or third degree heart block.
- Current treatment with β-blockers or calcium channel blockers/calcium antagonists, e.g. verapamil.
- History of asthma or obstructive airways disease.

Atenolol (Tenormin)

Presentation
- 5 mg/10 ml ampoules, 50 mg and 100 mg tablets

Dosage
- Give 5 mg by slow intravenous infusion over 5 minutes and reassess.
- If the pulse rate <40 bpm, then give no more.
- If the pulse rate >60 bpm then give a further 5 mg after 5 minutes.
- 10-15 minutes after the intravenous dose has kept the pulse rate between 40-60 bpm, give 50 mg orally.

Metoprolol (Betaloc, Lopressor)

Presentation
- 5 mg/5 ml ampoules, 50 mg and 100 mg tablets.

Dosage
- 5 mg intravenously at a rate of 1-2 mg per minute.
  - This may be repeated at 2-5 minute intervals until a satisfactory response has been obtained, up to a maximum of 15 mg, and then 50 mg orally every 6 hours.

Note: - Intravenous thrombolytics and β-blockade may be used together in the same patient.

CONCLUSION: Not used in the Immediate Care situation at present, but recent evidence shows that they *may have a role in reducing the incidence of life threatening arrhythmias following AMI.*

Diuretics

Introduction
- Diuretics are used in the treatment of severe pump failure with acute pulmonary oedema and congestive cardiac failure.

Frusemide (Lasix)

Action
- Produces a diuresis which is maximal after about 30 minutes.

Presentation
- 10 mg/ml in 2, 5 and 25 ml ampoules.

Dosage
- By slow intravenous injection (no more than 4 mg per minute) of 20-50 mg.

Haemodynamic management of AMI

The degree of pump failure depends on the size and site of the infarct and the immediate management should therefore be directed at reducing this.

I. Normal/hyperdynamic circulation (mortality 0-5%)

Pathophysiology
- Pre-existing hypertension, sympathetic overactivity.

Management
- Thrombolysis
- Early β-blockers
- Management of hypertension.

II. Hypotension (mortality 10-20%)

Pathophysiology
- Forward pump failure, hypovolaemia, vasodilation and tamponade.

Symptoms/signs
- Dyspnoea, cyanosis, gallop rhythm and a raised jugular venous pressure (JVP).
- Bradycardia.
- Pain.

Management
- Volume adjustment:
  - Intravenous fluids.
- Inotropic support:
  - Dopamine, dobutamine.
- Atropine for bradycardia.
- Analgesia/antiemetic.
- Adequate haemodynamic monitoring.

III. Cardiac failure/left ventricular failure (mortality 35-40%)

Aetiology
- Common with large anterior infarcts, less common with inferior infarcts.

Pathophysiology
- Backward pump failure, fluid overload, acute VSD, acute muscle rupture (ventricular aneurysm).

Symptoms/signs
- Dyspnoea, acute pulmonary oedema.
- Cold, sweaty, hypotension.
- Confusion.
- Poor peripheral perfusion.

Management
- Posture: sit the patient up.
- Oxygen, analgesia.
- Diuretics intravenous, e.g. frusemide 40-80 mg intravenously.
- Opiates: morphine.
- Vasodilators, e.g. nitrates (intravenously or sublingually).
- Inotropes: dopamine/dobutamine.
- Adequate haemodynamic monitoring.

IV. Cardiogenic shock: systolic BP < 90 mmHg (mortality 85-95%)

Aetiology
- Occurs in 10% of patients with a myocardial infarction.
- Related to the size of the infarct (> 40% of ventricle).

Pathophysiology
- Left ventricular infarction leading to left ventricular failure.
- Acute pulmonary oedema.
- A reduced cardiac output, intense vasoconstriction and cyanosis.
- Results in a metabolic acidosis.

Signs
- Pallor, cyanosis, sweating, confusion, peripheral shutdown, oliguria.

Management
- Airway, oxygen.
- Analgesia.
- Position supine (if there is pulmonary oedema: half sitting).
- Establish an intravenous infusion with low volume fluid administration.
- Inotropes.
- Adequate haemodynamic monitoring.

Guidelines for the immediate management of AMI

Primary survey

Immediate assessment and management

- *Conscious, breathing, good (carotid) pulse:* - Obtain history
  - Check blood pressure and monitor heart rhythm
  - Administer buccal GTN
  - Oxygen

- *Unconscious, breathing, good (carotid) pulse:* - Maintain the airway (?put into the recovery position)
  - Administer oxygen
  - Check blood pressure and monitor heart rhythm

- *Unconscious, not breathing:*
  - *Pulse present:*   - Expired air ventilation
    - Oxygen
    - Mechanical ventilation

  - *No pulse:* - Start Advanced Life Support immediately

Secondary survey

ECG monitor: make a diagnosis if possible

Provide rapid treatment of any immediate life threatening arrhythmias or complications

Obtain intravenous access

Administer: Analgesia with an antiemetic intravenously: for relief of pain, nausea and vomiting

Aspirin, thrombolysis: to minimise myocardial damage

Treat any symptomatic arrhythmia

Admit to hospital immediately

Support and give advice to the patient and their family

11

Medical emergencies

Medical emergencies

Introduction

- All doctors should have some knowledge of the management of medical emergencies, but those active in Immediate Care may be asked to deal with the more serious problems because of their expertise.
- Their management follows the same basic guidelines: Aiway, Breahting Circulation, etc. followed by management of the cause

Acute severe asthma

- Acute potentially reversible expiratory airways obstruction, unresponsive to the patient's usual medication, resulting in a reduction in the peak flow to 40% or less of its predicted value.

Introduction

- Acute severe asthma is a life threatening condition, causing approximately 2000 deaths per year in the UK, which necessitates immediate recognition and requires rapid, aggressive and effective management.
- Most deaths occur in older people, but are more preventable in the young (80-90%) in whom the severity of the attack is often not recognised either by the patient, their parents/partner, or by their own doctor.
- The onset of an attack may be either rapid or insidious, but by the time an Immediate Care doctor or extended trained ambulanceman is involved, the patient is usually extremely ill.

Incidence

- Usually occurs in known asthmatics.
- One of the commonest medical emergencies encountered outside hospital.
- Death may occur quickly and with little warning.
- Occurs most often at night or in the early hours of the morning.
- May be precipitated by a viral or rarely a bacterial upper or lower respiratory tract infection.
- May be exacerbated by stress.
- In atopic individuals, it may be caused by sudden rise in the pollen count or airborne moulds.

Aetiology

- Over reliance on bronchodilators
- Under use of inhaled/oral steroids
- Failure to make objective measurements of severity of an attack.
- Inadequate medical supervision.

Pathophysiology

- Asthma is an acute inflammatory reaction of the airways resulting in:
    - Mucous plugging of bronchioles and alveoli (mucous gland hyperplasia).
    - Desquamation of the epithelium with thickening of the basement membrane.
    - Bronchospasm.
    - Hypoxia caused by an impairment of gaseous exchange.
    - Tachypnoea.
    - Dehydration: combination of inadequate fluid intake and increased fluid loss (increased ventilation)
    - May (rarely) be complicated by sudden development of a spontaneous pneumothorax.

History

- Previous history of asthma or atopy.

Signs/symptoms

Uncontrolled asthma

- Tracheal tug with intercostal recession and use of the accessory muscles, but normal speech.
- Pulse <110 beats per minute
- Hyperinflation with a respiratory rate <25 breaths/minute.
- Peak expiratory flow rate (PEFR) >50% of best or predicted.

Acute severe asthma

- Increasing wheeze and breathlessness, so that the patient has difficulty with speaking (unable to complete a sentence in one breath), get up from a chair or bed, or feed.
- A persistently increased respiratory rate: >25 breaths per minute (>50 breaths per minute for children).
- Tachycardia: >110 bpm (>140 bpm for children).
- Reduced peak expiratory flow rate: <50% of the predicted value or if this is not known <120 l/m.
- Pulsus paradoxus with an inspiratory fall in systolic blood pressure of >10 mmHg.
- Reduced SaO_2.

Life threatening asthma

- "Silent Chest" or severe wheezing.
- Cyanosis.
- Bradycardia.
- Exhaustion, restlessness, confusion and unconsciousness.
- Reduced peak expiratory flow rate: <33% of predicted.

Note:- **Spontaneous pneumothorax**:
- An uncommon, potentially fatal complication of asthma characterised by sudden circulatory collapse, and sometimes by pain.
- **In young children**:
    - Asthma can be very difficult to diagnose.
    - The differential diagnosis includes:
        - Croup
        - Inhaled foreign body
        - Acute viral pneumonitis
        - Cystic fibrosis.

Management

- The management of acute severe asthma needs to be rapid and aggressive, if lives are going to be saved.
- The patient's response to treatment should be constantly monitored, observing changes in the patient's appearance and vital signs.
- Serial peak flow meter readings should be obtained initially and after treatment.
- The management of acute asthma can be especially difficult in children under the age of 18 months as they may respond poorly to treatment.

Breathing/ventilation: hypoxia

Oxygen
- Oxygen *is mandatory*.
- Use a high concentration oxygen mask with as high a flow rate as possible, as most patients who die, do so as a result of hypoxia.
- Retention of carbon dioxide is not aggravated by oxygen therapy in patients with acute severe asthma.

Bronchospasm/mucous plugging

β_2 adrenergic agonists (salbutamol, terbutaline)

- These are best administered via a nebuliser (preferably oxygen driven).
- Great care should be exerted as a transient fall in PaO_2 may occur, resulting in a respiratory arrest in the severely hypoxaemic patient. This is thought to be due to a direct vascular effect, and is caused by a reversal of the compensatory pulmonary vasoconstriction in poorly ventilated areas of the lung, which leads to an increase in the ventilation/perfusion mismatch. The fall in PaO_2 is usually transient and ends once the bronchi dilate and ventilation becomes more homogeneous, but in the severely hypoxaemic patient the additional reduction in PaO_2 may lead to a respiratory arrest. Oxygen, should therefore always be administered before giving β-agonists, if the nebuliser is not oxygen driven.
- If a nebuliser is not available:
  - Consider using an inhaler fitted with a large spacer (a plastic cup may suffice for children) filled with the inhalant from 2 puffs from the inhaler; repeated 10-20 times.
- If there is minimal response to the nebulised preparation (possibly due to mucous plugging), then administration by slow intravenous and/or subcutaneous injection, may be tried.
- In severe refractory cases an intravenous infusion may be considered and the infusion rate titrated against the patient's response (the value of parenteral administration has not yet been proven and may only increase the incidence of side effects).

Salbutamol (Ventolin)

Presentation
- Nebules: 2.5 mg, 5.0 mg.
- Respirator solution: 0.5 % or 5 mg/ml.
- Intravenous injection: 0.5 mg in 1 ml, 0.25 mg in 1 ml.
- Intravenous infusion: 5 mg in 5 ml.

Dosage
- By nebuliser: 2.5-5 mg (recommended maximum: 15 mg).
- Intravenously: 200 μg over 10 minutes.

Terbutaline (Bricanyl)

Presentation
- Respules: 5 mg in 2 ml.
- Respirator solution: 100 mg in 10 ml.
- Intravenous injection: 1 ml ampoule: 0.5 mg.
- Intravenous infusion: 5 ml ampoules: 0.5 mg/ml.

Dosage
- By nebuliser: 5-10 mg (recommended maximum 10 mg).
- Intravenously: 250 μg over 10 minutes.

Anticholinergics

Ipratropium bromide (Atrovent)

- May be particularly useful in young children under 1 year, who may not have fully developed β-receptors, and in whom β-agonists may be relatively ineffective.
- Can also be useful in the treatment of residual bronchoconstriction after using an inhaled β-agonist, without causing the side effects of β-agonists.

Presentation
- Nebuliser solution 0.025% (0.25 mg/ml).

Dosage
- Adults: 0.4-2.0 ml solution (0.1-0.5 mg).
- Children (3-14 years): 0.4-2.0 ml solution (0.1-0.5 mg).

Administration
- Usually administered by nebuliser.
- May either be administered together with a β-agonist in the same nebuliser, or given separately afterwards.
- May take longer to be effective than β-agonists (30-60 minutes), but has a longer duration of action.

Note:- Patients with severe asthma benefit more from combination therapy than those with less severe asthma.

Steroids

Hydrocortisone (sodium succinate/phosphate)

Presentation: See under anaphylactic shock.

Dosage
- Adults: 200 mg   Children: 100 mg.

Administration
- By intravenous injection.

Side effects
  - Paraesthesiae, which may be painful and unpleasant, most often experienced in the genital area, and occasionally generalised, but is usually short lived.

Prednisolone

- Considered by many to be a better alternative to hydrocortisone (unless the patient is unable to take oral medication), and may be given alone or in combination with hydrocortisone 200 mg intravenously.

Presentation
  - Tablets 5 mg (enteric coated are probably best).

Dosage
  - Adults: 30-60 mg orally.
  - Children: 2 mg/kg initially (maximum 40 mg).

Note: - Steroids are slow to take effect and have a short duration of action. They should therefore be administered as soon as possible. Some consider that they have a limited role in the Immediate Care of acute severe asthma.

Adrenaline

- This may have a role in the management of acute severe asthma, where there is a major atopic element.
- For further details see the chapter on (Anaphylactic) Shock.

Methylxanthenes (aminophylline)

- The use of these are well established, but they have a narrow therapeutic range, and serious toxic side effects, such as arrhythmias and convulsions may occur before other less serious symptoms of toxicity: nausea, vomiting and tachycardia.

Presentation
  - Ampoules of 250 mg/10 ml.

Dosage
  - Adults: 250-500 mg (5 mg/kg).
  - Children: 5 mg/kg initially.

Administration
  - Should be administered by slow intravenous injection over 20 minutes.

Note: - Aminophylline should *never* be administered to the patient already receiving a methylxanthene (aminophylline, theophylline) as fatal overdosage may occur.

Assisted ventilation

- Intermittent positive pressure ventilation may be needed in a small number (0.5-1%) of patients, but can be difficult to achieve due to the high inflation pressures which may be necessary, and the need to suppress the patient's spontaneous ventilatory effort, which may necessitate heavy sedation.
- In the past the mortality rate has been between 9 and 38%, but this has been reduced recently by using "Controlled hypoventilation", a technique which uses high inspired oxygen concentrations and low flow rates and inflation pressures.

Pneumothorax

- Insertion of a chest drain (see under Management of Chest Injuries).
- Ventilation.

Dehydration

- This is caused by a combination of inadequate fluid intake and increased fluid loss due to increased ventilation.

Intravenous fluids: crystalloid

Hartmann's/Ringer-lactate solution: Sodium lactate intravenous compound (see chapter on Shock)

- An intravenous infusion may be started in all patients with prolonged acute severe asthma as significant dehydration may occur.

Monitoring

- Serial peak expiratory flow rates.
- Oxygen saturation:
    - Try to maintain SaO_2 >92% (chronic asthmatics may manage on lower levels).
    - A sudden fall in SaO_2 may indicate a pneumothorax.

Guidelines for the management of acute severe asthma

In unstable asthma

- Administer:
  - Nebulised β₂ agonist:
    - Salbutamol 5 mg or terbutaline 10 mg (half doses in very young children), using an oxygen driven nebuliser if available (if not available, use an aerosol inhaler with a spacer).
- Observe and if there is *minimal response after 15-20 minutes*, i.e PEF >50-70 predicted or best, manage as acute severe asthma.

In acute severe asthma

- Add:
  - Oxygen (in as high a concentration as possible).
  - Steroids:
    - Oral prednisolone 30-60 mg or intravenous hydrocortisone 200 mg (both if the patient is very ill). For children administer prednisolone 1-2 mg/kg body weight (maximum 40 mg) initially.
  - Observe and if there is *minimal response after 15-20 minutes*, manage as life threatening asthma.

In life threatening asthma

- Add:
  - Nebulised ipratropium bromide 0.5 mg (0.25 mg for children or 0.125 mg for very young children) to the nebulised β₂ agonist.
  - Intravenous aminophylline 250 mg (5mg/kg for children) slowly over 20 minutes (if the patient is not already taking a methylxanthene), or subcutaneous/intravenous terbutaline 250 μg over 10 minutes.
  - Intravenous hydrocortisone 100 mg (children only).
- If there is *little or no improvement*, consider intubation and ventilation.

Note:- Consider use of intravenous adrenaline if there is a major atopic element of the patient's asthma.

Hospital admission

- Admit to hospital *without delay* if:
  - Any immediately life threatening features are present.
  - Any potentially life threatening features persist inspite of treatment.
  - The PEFR 15-30 minutes after treatment is still 40% below the predicted/best.
- Consider hospital admission if:
  - Attack is in the afternoon or evening.
  - Recent onset of nocturnal or worsening symptoms.
  - There have been previous severe attacks, especially if they have been of rapid onset.
  - The patient or their relatives are unlikely to respond appropriately to any deterioration in the patient's condition.
  - There is concern over the patient's social circumstances.

Acute epiglottitis

Introduction

This is an acute life threatening condition, and rapid effective treatment can save lives.

Incidence

- Occurs much less often than croup.
- Usually occurs in children between 18 months and 7 years old (peak incidence 2-3 years).
- Much less common in adults.
- Boys are more often affected than girls.

Aetiology

- Usual causative pathogen:
    - Children: *Haemophilus influenzae* type B.
    - Adults: *Haemophilus influenzae, Streptococcus pyogenes.*

Pathophysiology

- Infection results in acute inflammation of the supraglottic structures of the larynx, resulting in the rapid development of severe pharyngeal oedema and consequent airway obstruction.

Symptoms/signs

- *History:*
    - Sore throat with the rapid (usually less than 6 hours) development of respiratory distress and severe dysphagia.

- *General appearance:*
    - Very unwell, anxious, toxic with a temperature often >40 °C.

- *Tripod position:*
    - Chin forward, extended neck, with mouth open, protruding tongue and often drooling saliva (as swallowing is so painful).
    - The child resists attempts to make him lie down.

- *Airway:*
    - *Stridor:*
        - Soft low pitched, with the rapid onset of inspiratory wheeze *only*.
    - There is *no* cough, and the voice is muffled (in croup the voice is abnormal or absent).
    - Severe dysphagia with saliva tending to pool in the pharynx.

- *Breathing:*
    - Intercostal, subcostal, costal and sternal recession, with reduced air entry.
    - Tachypnoea, tachycardia, cyanosis, use of the accessory muscles:
        - Ala nasae
        - Sternomastoids.
    - Respiratory arrest may occur suddenly and without warning.

- *Circulation:*
    - Poor peripheral perfusion, proceeding to shock.

CAUTION:
    - If acute epiglottitis is suspected do *not* attempt to examine the child's throat by depressing the tongue with a spatula or other instrument, as this may push the epiglottis down onto the larynx and provoke total airway obstruction.

Management

- Strong reassurance to keep the child as calm as possible
- Oxygen:
    - Administer 100% oxygen if possible.
- If acute respiratory distress develops:
    - Cricothyrotomy or tracheotomy.
- Do *not* delay transportation to hospital:
    - *Always accompany the child to hospital* (he may develop severe respiratory distress proceeding to respiratory arrest *very* rapidly).
- Antibiotics:
    - Amoxycillin
    - Co-amoxyclav
    - Erythromycin.

Note: - Endotracheal intubation should only be attempted by the very experienced if the child is moribund, as it can exacerbate an already critical situation, and is probably *not appropriate* in Immediate Care. If it is attempted:
    - The endotracheal tube should be non cuffed, and two sizes smaller than that normally used in children of that age, to prevent later pressure necrosis of the subglottic region.
    - It is advisable to pass an introducer, e.g. a gum elastic bougie, first.

Croup: acute viral laryngotracheobronchitis

Incidence

- Usually (6%) occurs in children aged between 2 months and 9 years old (peak 18 months).
- The peak incidence is between October and December in temperate climates.

Aetiology

- Viral infection:
    - Most commonly:
        - *Para-influenzae* (commonest)
        - *Influenza A+B*.
    - Less commonly:
        - *Respiratory syncitial* virus
        - *Echo* virus
        - *Coxsackie A* virus.

Pathophysiology

- Acute inflammation of the larynx, trachea and bronchi with subglottic oedema resulting in airway narrowing.

Symptoms/signs

- History of prodromal (usually 48-72 hrs) viral upper respiratory tract illness.
- The child is not usually toxic and the temperature is usually <39 °C.
- The child is usually restless, but not acutely ill.
- Harsh inspiratory or biphasic stridor, of gradual onset.
- Sore throat, with a barking "seal like" cough and an abnormal hoarse voice.
- The chest is clear, and there is no intercostal recession.

Management

- Reassurance.
- Nebulised water/steam.
- Rehydration with frequent small volumes of clear fluid.
- Admit to hospital if the child develops signs of increasing airways obstruction:
    - Severe stridor or stridor at rest.
    - Evidence of respiratory distress:
        - A steadily increasing respiratory rate.
        - Intercostal recession.
        - Exhaustion.
        - Cyanosis.
    - Increasing pulse rate.
- Consider:
    - Adrenaline: 3-5 ml of 1:1000 administered by nebuliser.
    - Cricothyrotomy or tracheotomy in very severe cases.

Bacterial laryngotracheobronchitis (LTB)

- This is a rare, but life threatening illness.

Incidence

- Uncommon.
- Occurs mostly in children >5 years old.

Aetiology

- Often caused by *Staph. aureus* secondary to a viral infection.
- May also be caused by Streptococci or *Haemophilus influenzae*.

Pathophysiology

- Inflammation and ulceration of the glottis.
- Necrosis of the tracheal mucosa.
- Production of copious purulent secretions and a thick, crusting exudate (pseudomembrane).

Symptoms/signs

- Similar to acute viral LTB, but the systemic disturbance is much greater.

Management

- Initially similar to acute viral LTB.
- Antibiotics:
    - Flucloxacillin
    - Co-amoxiclav.

Differential diagnosis of acute epiglottitis

Croup (viral larygotracheobronchitis): see above

Bacterial laryngotracheobronchitis: LTB

Asthma
Signs:
- Expiratory stridor/wheeze.

Inhalation of foreign body

Rarely:
- Angio-oedema
- Retropharyngeal abscess
- Diptheria
- Steam inhalation burn.

Angio-oedema

Incidence

- This a relatively uncommon problem, which can present as an acute medical emergency.

Aetiology

- Occurs in individuals who are allergic to a variety of stimulants including:
    - Food
    - Medication
    - Toxins, e.g. β-haemolytic streptococcal infection.
- Occurs in hereditary angio-oedema (HANE), where individuals have a deficiency of complement C-1 enterase inhibitor.

Pathophysiology

- Localised allergic type I reaction affecting parts of the face and upper airway, with severe oedema and swelling, which may result in upper airway obstruction.

Symptoms/signs

- There is usually a personal or family history of allergy/atopy and sometimes of previous attacks.
- There may be swelling of the face, lips, tongue and sometimes the tissues surrounding the airway.

Management

- If any airway obstruction is present or looks as if it might develop:
    - Treat as anaphylactic shock:
        - Adrenaline *(treatment of choice)*:
            - 0.5-1.0 ml of 1:1000 administered subcutaneously slowly over 5 minutes.
        - Antihistamines:
            - Chlorpheniramine (Piriton): 2-5 mg administered intravenously.
        - Steroids:
            - Prednisolone 30-60 mg orally.
            - Hydrocortisone: 100-200 mg administered intravenously.
    - Consider:
        - Endotracheal intubation.
        - Cricothyrotomy.
- In hereditary angio-oedema, the patient may carry a preparation of the missing complement which should be administered to them immediately during an attack.
- Patients with known angio-oedema may carry adrenaline for self-administration.

Diabetic emergencies

- Diabetic coma is a very serious complication of diabetes with a high mortality.

Hypoglycaemia

- Mortality rate is 2-4%.

Incidence
- This is a relatively common occurrence in insulin dependent diabetics, whose diabetic control is poor, especially the newly diagnosed, the young, the solo, the long term diabetic and the elderly:
    - Severe hypoglycaemia affects about 20-30% of patients annually with an incidence of 1.1-1.6 episodes per patient per year.
- Only rarely occurs in non-insulin dependent diabetics (tends to be at night).

Aetiology

- A relative excess of insulin caused by either:
    - An overdose of injected insulin (commonest), or natural over production of insulin, e.g. the rare insulin secreting tumour of islets of Langerhans.
    - A relative overdose of oral hypoglycaemics, especially sulphonylureas.
    - Excessive excercise resulting in rapid sugar metabolism without extra carbohydrate intake.
    - Starving, i.e. missing carbohydrate intake.
- May be precipitated by prior alcohol consumption.

Pathophysiology

- Very low blood sugar levels result in:
    - Sympathetic overactivity (may be masked in those taking β-blockers).
    - Altered cerebral function.

Symptoms/signs

- These may develop very quickly with little or no warning, especially in insulin dependent diabetics who may lose those warning signs of hypoglycaemia due to sympathetic overactivity. Those particularly at risk are those whose diabetes is well controlled and those on human insulin (in whom there may also be a reduced catecholamine response).

Initially
- Confusion, drowsiness, irritability, aggression.
- Headache, tremor, dizziness, diplopia, weakness, emptiness, hunger and palpitations.
- Pale, sweaty countenance, with a tachycardia, a full pulse and normo- or hypertension.
- Appearance of intoxication, and sometimes hypothermia.

Later
- May become unconscious, unrousable and lapse into fits, coma, and death.

Investigation

- Blood sugar level testing with test strips (Dextrostix, BM Stix) and glucometer confirm low blood sugar.

Management

- If the patient is *conscious:*
    - Glucose: 10-20 gm orally in a solution *or*
    - Carbohydrate in a readily absorbable form.

Note:- Hypostop:
    - This is a convenient glucose preparation carried by many diabetics.
    - It is a gel, which can be smeared on the gums or inside of the mouth allowing absorption of glucose. Honey or non-diabetic jam are alternatives.
  - All diabetics should have some carbohydrate available.

- If the patient is *unconscious:*
    - Care of the airway, oxygen.
    - Administer either:
        - *Glucose* (may cause thrombophlebitis or localised tissue necrosis if extraversation occurs):
            - Adults: 50 mls of 50% glucose administered intravenously.
            - Children: 0.5-1.0 mg *or*
        - *Glucagon* (acts more slowly than dextrose):
            - 1 mg/ml administered intramuscularly, intravenously or subcutaneously (particularly useful if the patient's veins are difficult to inject or the patient is restless).
            - May cause nausea, vomiting and headache

- Blood sugar levels should be monitored during treatment.

Note:- If the patient has been unconscious for some time, the response to treatment may be slow (probably due to cerebral oedema or irreversible cerebral damage).

Hyperglycaemia: diabetic keto-acidosis

- Mortality rate is 5-10%: due to cerebral oedema and irreversible damage.

Incidence

- More common in women than men.
- Occurs about once per 100 diabetics per year (recurrence rate is 10%).

Aetiology

- May be the presenting feature of diabetes mellitus (insidious onset).
- Reduction in, failure to increase or accidental omission of insulin dose.
- May be precipitated by stress or illness:
    - Upper respiratory tract infection
    - Lower respiratory tract infection: 65%
    - Abscess
    - Urinary tract infection
    - Mental stress
    - Menstruation
    - (Cerebral vascular accident)
    - Trauma.

Pathophysiology

- Hyperglycaemia may be ketoacidotic, lactic acidotic or non ketoacidotic hyperglycaemia.
- The relative deficiency of insulin, results in an extracellular increase in osmolarity and cellular dehydration.
- Ketoacidosis: A fall in blood pH (acidaemia), and compensatory hyperventilation, results in still further fluid loss.
- Potassium enters the extracellular and intravascular compartments from the cells and is excreted in the urine causing potassium loss. This may result in cardiac arrhythmias and death.
- There may be gastric stasis and vomiting.

Symptoms/signs

- The gradual onset of polydypsia, polyuria, malaise, thirst, polyphagia and weight loss.
- Often associated with infection, nausea and vomiting (and a failure to increase the dosage of hypoglycaemic agents in known diabetics).
- Ketoacidosis: smell of acetone on breath.
- Warm, dry skin and mucous membranes.
- Hyperventilation, or deep sighing "Kussmaul" respiration.
- Dehydration and salt depletion: rapid, weak and irregular pulse, and hypotension.
- Constipation, abdominal pain/cramps (often severe enough to mimic an acute abdomen) and diplopia are common.

Diagnosis

Urine: Glycosuria, ketonuria.
Blood sugar: Levels raised on testing with glucometer and test strips.

Management

Airway
- Intubation, ventilation and gastric emptying may be indicated to protect the airway in the unconscious patient, as vomiting is a common complication and cause of death.

Hypoxia
- All unconscious patients may suffer from hypoxia, and should therefore be given oxygen.

Dehydration
- An intravenous infusion of normal saline should be administered, as a buffered solution, e.g. Hartmann's solution, may exacerbate the lactic acidosis.
- Infuse 1 litre of fluid immediately, followed by a further 1 litre administerd over 2 hours and a further 2 litres each administered over 4 hours:
    - This should be reduced in the young, the elderly, or if there is renal or cardiac impairement.

Hyperglycaemia
- Although insulin is needed, administration is not appropriate in the Immediate Care situation.

Infection
- Broad spectrum antibiotics if a precipitating infection is suspected.

Epilepsy

Incidence

- This is a relatively common cause of collapse, and is one of the situations with which all those involved in Immediate Care should be familiar.
- The overall mortality for people with epilepsy is 2-3 times that of the general population and is even higher in the younger age groups.
- Common causes of death in epileptics include:
    - Accidents, e.g. drowning, head injury, amd road traffic accidents
    - Status epilepticus
    - Neoplasia
    - Cerbrovascular disease
    - Chest infections
    - Sudden Unexpected Death.

Aetiology

- The likely cause of fitting varies according to age:

    - *All ages*
        - Infection:
            - Meningitis
            - Encephalitis
        - Trauma
        - Congenital cerebral lesions

    - *Neonatal*
        - Birth trauma
        - Metabolic:
            - Hypoglycaemia
            - Hypocalcaemia
        - Congenital cerebral lesions

    - *6 months to 5 years*
        - Febrile convulsions

    - *Young adult*
        - Alcoholism
        - Drug abuse
        - Cerebral tumour

    - *Elderly*
        - Cerebrovascular disease
        - Cerebral tumour
        - Subdural haematoma

Grand mal epilepsy: "major epilepsy"

Aetiology

- Usually, but not always occurs in known epileptics.
- May be precipitated by:
    - Illness
    - Stress
    - Poor management of medication: deliberate or accidental
    - Reduced efficacy of medication; due to altered hepatic metabolism, e.g. as a result of:
        - Other drugs
        - Alcohol
        - Hepatic disease.

Pathophysiology

- A spontaneous cortical discharge which may be generalised or localised.
- The focal point may be scar tissue, tumour, etc.

Symptoms/signs

- Previous history of epilepsy.
- May be preceded by aura/visual disturbance.
- Sudden collapse with generalised or localised (focal Jacksonian) tonic/clonic fitting.
- May bite tongue, and/or be incontinent of urine and/or stools.
- After fitting may be drowsy and disorientated, complaining of a headache and will usually go to sleep.

Differential diagnosis

- Hypoglycaemia:
    - Test with Dextrostix/BM Stix.
- Poisoning.
- Tetany with carpopedal spasm.
- Head injury:
    - Always examine the head carefully, as head injury may be either the cause of fitting or occur as a result of fitting.
- Hysteria.
- Cerebral space occupying lesion:
    - Tumour
    - Cerebral abscess.
- Collapse:
    - Think of all possibilities.

Management

- Most fits are self limiting and do not require medical treatment.

Safety
- Move the patient away from hard objects and other hazards, e.g. fires.
- Loosen the patient's clothing.

Airway
- Make sure that the airway is not obstructed by false teeth, etc.
- There is very little danger of the tongue causing airway obstruction, and attempts to prevent this or tongue biting, often only damage the patient's teeth.

Convulsions
- Administer diazepam (Valium, Diazemuls, Stesolid), midazolam (Hypnovel) or clobazam (Rivotril) by:
    - Slow intravenous injection.
    - Rectally (Stesolid): The route of choice in children.
- Titrate the dose against ptosis, and beware of apnoea, which may be delayed.

Clobazam (Rivotril)

- May be used as an alternative to diazepam, and is apparently equally effective, but there has been little experience in its use in Immediate Care.

Presentation: 1 mg in solvent/1 ml dilutent ampoules.

Administration: By slow intravenous injection.

Dosage: Children: 0.5 mg.
          Adults: 1 mg.

- If fitting continues; sedate heavily and be prepared to intubate and ventilate.
- After fitting has ceased, put the patient into a safe position:
    - The recovery position.
    - In small children, across their mother's knees.

Status epilepticus

Introduction

- This is a life threatening condition; the longer fitting continues, the more difficult it is to control, and the higher the morbidity and mortality.

Definition: Prolonged fitting lasting more than 10 minutes, or consisting of several distinct concurrent episodes of fitting without regaining consciousness.

Aetiology

Known epileptic

- Poor anti-convulsant compliance.
- Recent change in medication.
- Alcohol withdrawal/pseudostatus.

New presentation

- Acute cerebrovascular accident
- Acute head injury
- Meningo encephalitis
- Cerebral neoplasm
- Metabolic disorders:
    - Renal failure, hypoglycaemia, hypercalcaemia
- Drug overdose:
    - Tricyclics, phenothiazines, theophylline
- Inflammatory arteritides:
    - Systemic lupus erythematosis.

Pathophysiology

- Tonic/clonic status.
- Permanent neuronal damage may occur if fitting is very prolonged.

Management

Airway care
- Airway maintenance.
- Oxygen.
- Recovery position.

Breathing
- Ventilate.

Fitting
- Control fitting with diazepam (Stesolid or Diazemuls)/midazolam.

Note: Check the patient's blood sugar if they are unknown, and administer 50% glucose if appropriate.

Febrile convulsions

- A convulsion or fit occuring in a child aged from 6 months to 5 years, precipitated by fever arising outside the nervous system in a child who is otherwise neurologically normal.

Incidence

- In the United kingdom, nearly 3% of all children will have at least one febrile convulsion without evidence of intracranial infection or defined cause (other than infection outside the central nervous system), and of these, just over one third will have one further convulsion.
- Febrile convulsions are the most common cause of fitting in children. The parents usually think that the child is dying.
- Age: usually 6 months to 5 years. The patient can be older, but there is nearly always a previous history.

Aetiology

- Cause of pyrexia:
    - Usually a virus infection.
- Family history:
    - There is sometimes a family history of febrile convulsions.

Pathophysiology

- This is not fully understood as the fits are not clearly associated with either the level or the duration of the pyrexia, but may be associated with a rapid rise in temperature. The immature brain responds with a generalised cortical discharge.
- With increasing age, this tendency is outgrown, although some children take longer than others.
- Very few (2.4% of those previously normal) go on to develop epilepsy.

Symptoms/signs

- Prior to a fit the child may appear jittery.
- Tonic-clonic type of fitting, usually lasting <20 minutes, with complete recovery within 1 hour.
- The tonic phase may be characterised by a frightened cry followed by abrupt loss of consciousness with muscular rigidity. During this phase, which may last up to 30 seconds, breathing may cease and the child be incontinent of urine and faeces.
- The clonic phase which follows consists of repetitive jerking movements of the limbs or face.

Management

- The object of treatment is to prevent a prolonged fit (lasting more than 15 minutes), which may result in permanent brain damage, epilepsy, and developmental delay.

Airway
- Make sure that the child has a clear airway, by lying them on their side or prone with their head on one side, so as to avoid aspiration following vomiting.

Cooling
- Remove clothing, put in cool room with window open.
- Consider:
    - Tepid sponging.
    - Putting in a cool, but not cold, bath.
- If appropriate administer copious oral fluids.
- Administer oral paracetamol elixir in the maximum recommended dose for the child's age.

Convulsions
- Rectal diazepam (Stesolid) 1 mg + 1 mg for each year of age.

Differential diagnosis of febrile convulsions

Meningitis
- See below.

Hypoglycaemia
- Test blood with Dextrostix/BM stix.

Breath holding
- Benign apnoeic attacks in toddlers.

Incidence:
- Usually begins at 9-18 months, ceases by 5 years.

Aetiology:
- Usually after a painful or frustrating experience.

Pathophysiology:
- The infant cries vigorously, and suddenly holds his breath.
- He may then become cyanosed, and in severe cases lose consciousness.
- The limbs may become rigid (rarely), with a few clonic movements, lasting a few seconds.
- The infant then begins breathing and regains consciousness.

Management:
- Exclude other conditions.
- Reassure the mother.

Meningitis

Bacterial meningitis/septicaemia

- This is a significant cause of childhood morbidity and mortality.

Incidence

- More prevalent in winter.
- Increasing over the last 5 years (in 1989, there were 1142 notified cases of meningococcal meningitis in the UK with 203 deaths).
- This is the commonest cause of death from infectious disease; meningococcal meningitis was responsible for 95 childhood deaths in 1987.
- All age groups may be affected, but children <1 yr old are the most susceptible.
- More common among poor families, who live in over-crowded conditions.

Aetiology

- Commonly caused by:
    - *Neiseria meningitides:* meningococcus (usually type B in the UK, types A and C in Africa, Saudi Arabia and India).
    - Pneumococcus.
    - *Haemophilus influenzae* (type B is the most common infecting organism in pre-school children).
- Rarely caused by:
    - *E. coli,* Streptococci Gp B, *Listeria monocytogenes, Mycobacteria tuberculosis* or Leptospira.
- Mortality:
    - Meningococcal: 7% (20% in pure septicaemia)
    - *Haemophilus influenzae*: 5%
    - Pneumococcal: 20%.

Symptoms/signs

- These may be of sudden onset, with rapid deterioration in the patient's general condition
- Only a small number of patients exhibit the typical features of bacterial meningitis, which tend to vary depending on the causative organism.
- In the early stages of the illness, there are *no* features which can reliably distinguish between bacterial and viral meningitis.

Infants:
- Non specific:
    - Drowsiness, irritability, off feeds, distress on being handled.
    - Vomiting and/or diarrhoea.
    - Pyrexia.
- More specific:
    - Neck stiffness with a positive Kernig's sign (see below) and a positive Bradzinski's sign.
    - Tense or bulging fontanelles.
    - Purpuric or petechial rash:
        - Does not blanch on applied pressure
        - Initially the rash is localised, but later may become generalised.

- Late:
    - High pitched or moaning cry
    - Coma
    - Neck retraction
    - Shock
    - Widespread haemorrhagic rash.

Older children/adults:
- Non specific:
    - Vomiting
    - Pyrexia
    - Headache
    - Back or joint aches/pains.
- More specific:
    - Neck stiffness with evidence of meningeal irritation, i.e. a positive:
        - **Kernig's sign**: Pain on passive extension of the flexed knee, with the hip flexed.
        - **Brudzinski's sign**: Lower limb flexion on flexing the neck.
    - Photophobia
    - Confusion
    - Purpuric or petechial rash that does not blanch under pressure.
- Late:
    - Coma
    - Shock
    - Widespread haemorrhagic rash.

Note:- Meningism may *not* always be present.
- The combination of *pyrexia,* with *shock* and a *petechial* or *purpuric rash* constitutes an *acute medical emergency* and treatment must be started *immediately.*

Management

- Administer by slow intravenous *(best)* or intramuscular injection:
    - **Benzyl-penicillin (penicillin G)** immediately.

    Presentation: 600 mg powder for reconstitution.

    Dosage: 2.5-5 mg/kg.
    - Infants under 1 year: 300 mg.
    - Children 1-10 years old: 600 mg.
    - Adults/children over 10 years old: 1200 mg.

- If there is a history of *penicillin anaphylaxis*, administer:
    - **Chloramphenicol**

    Presentation: 300 mg, 1 g and 1.2 g vials of powder for reconstitution.

Dosage: 25 mg/kg :				
	Infants	<3 months	(approximately 5 kg)	0.125 g
		3 months-1year	(approximately 10 kg)	0.25 g
	Children	1-5 years	(up to 15 kg)	0.50 g
		5-10 years	(up to 30 kg)	0.75 g
		10-15 years	(up to 55 kg)	1.0 g

- Oxygen and an intravenous infusion of crystalloid, if the patient is unconscious or shocked.
- Admit *immediately* (accompany the very sick child to hospital, as very rapid deterioration may occur).

Prophylaxis of meningococcal infection

- Only required for those who have had intimate contact with a patient with menigococcal meningitis or septicaemia.
- If resuscitation of the patient has been necessary, this may include medical, ambulance and nursing staff.

Rifampicin

Dosage:
- Infants (3 months-1 year): 5 mg/kg every 12 hours for 2 days.
- Children: 10 mg/kg every 12 hours for 2 days.
- Adults: 600 mg every 12 hours for 2 days.

Sulphadimidine (if the strain is known to be sensitive)

Dosage:
- Infants (3 months-1 year): 250 mg/kg every 12 hours for 2 days.
- Children: 500 mg/kg every 12 hours for 2 days.
- Adults: 1 g every 12 hours for 2 days.

Viral meningitis

Incidence

- More common than bacterial meningitis.
- With the exception of mumps meningitis, the maximum incidence is in children < 5 years.

Aetiology

- May be caused by the following viruses:
    - Mumps
    - Enteroviruses
    - Echo coxsackie
    - Poliomyelitis
    - Herpes simplex.

Symptoms/signs

- Usually slower onset than bacterial meningitis (prodromal period is 3-4 days).
- The patient is not so ill.
- There is no rash.
- Consciousness is not usually impaired.

Management

- Admit to hospital for confirmation of diagnosis.
- Symptomatic relief of symptoms.

Rectal bleeding

Incidence

- Nearly always only found in the elderly.

Aetiology

- The source of the bleeding is usually from colonic diverticulae.
- Rarely from carcinoma or polyps of the rectum/sigmoid colon.

Symptoms/signs

- There may be profuse fresh blood loss.

Management

- Treatment of hypovolaemic shock.

Haematemesis

Incidence

- Usually occurs in the over sixties.
- Mortality is 10%.
- An important cause of emergency admission to hospital.

Aetiology

- Commonly occurs as a result of :
    - Peptic ulceration
    - Erosive gastritis
    - Mallory Weiss syndrome.
- Less commonly:
    - Gastric carcinoma
    - Oesophageal varices
    - Oesophageal ulceration
    - Cardiovascular malformation
    - Bleeding dyscrasias
    - Systemic disease: renal failure, connective tissue disease
    - Rupture of the aorta or other artery into the gastrointestinal tract.

Symptoms/signs

History
- Alcohol abuse.
- Melaena stools.

Forceful vomiting:
- With history of alcohol abuse in males: Mallory Weiss syndrome.
- Other causes of protracted vomiting:
    - Migraine.
    - Alcoholic gastritis.
    - Medication, e.g. NSAIDs.
    - Intestinal obstruction.

Hypovolaemoc shock:
- Pale, sweaty.
- Rapid, weak, irregular pulse, hypotension.

Liver disease:
- Liver palms, spider naevi, jaundice.
- Blood vessel malformation in skin and mucosa.

Anaemia:
- Skin pallor with pale sclera.

Malignancy:
- Emaciated, cachectic.

Management

- Oxygen
- Intravenous infusion:
    - Set up two intravenous lines with large bore cannulae.
    - If shocked:
        - Colloid followed by crystalloid.
    - If not shocked:
        - Crystalloid.
- Careful monitoring of obvious blood loss and haemodynamic state.

Massive haemoptysis

Definition: The expectoration of 200-1000 ml of blood in 24 hours.

Incidence

- Relatively rare.

Aetiology

- Usually occurs due to erosion of blood vessels secondary to neoplasia of lungs or mediastinum and associated structures.
- May rarely be secondary to severe thoracic trauma.

Pathophysiology

- The usual cause of death is asphyxia rather than hypovolaemic shock.

Management

- *Aim:* To prevent asphyxiation and treat hypovolaemia.

- Oxygen.
- Position:
    - If the side of the bleeding can be lateralised: the patient should lie head down on the side of the haemorrhage to prevent aspiration of blood into the unaffected lung.
- Do not suppress any cough:
    - Patients should be encouraged to clear their airway with gentle coughing.
- If the patient is unconscious or in danger of asphyxiation:
    - Consider intubation
    - Ventilation
    - Suction.
- Intravenous infusion with colloid.

Hyperventilation

Incidence

- Relatively common especially in the young and female.

Aetiology

- Hysteria: mostly occurs in younger women.
- May be precipitated by:
    - Pain.
    - Metabolic acidosis:
        - Diabetic ketoacidosis
        - Aspirin overdose
        - Uraemia
        - Hepatic cirrhosis/coma
        - Hypoxaemia
        - Gram negative septicaemia.
    - Organic central nervous system disturbance.

Pathophysiology

- Anxiety results in hyperventilation, which in turn results in an increase in anxiety and so a vicious cycle develops.
- There is a resulting acute respiratory alkalosis, with a fall in the arterial PCO_2, and elevation of PO_2 and blood pH. The plasma HCO_3^- is reduced by renal excretion and tetany may occur due to a fall in the ionised plasma calcium levels.

Symptoms/signs

- The patient will be:
    - Anxious, possibly with a history of emotional problems.
- She may be complaining of:
    - A funny feeling/parasthesiae/coldness in the hands and face, especially around the mouth, hands and feet (this may be bilateral or unilateral).
    - Dyspnoea, palpitations, atypical chest pains, chest tightness, faintness or dizziness.
    - Poor memory/concentration, and/or a feeling of unreality.
- Rapid deep sighing breathing, tachycardia.
- Carpopedal spasm, tetany.

Management

- Massive reassurance.
- Treatment of the cause (if appropriate).
- Rebreathing using a paper or plastic bag:
    - This results in a rise in the inspired CO_2 and corrects the respiratory alkalosis.
- Nitrous oxide/oxygen via an Entonox or Nitronox apparatus.

Differential diagnosis of collapse

Aetiology

Airway/breathing
- Upper airway obstruction:
    - Foreign body
    - Laryngeal oedema
    - Epiglottitis.
- Lower airways:
    - Asthma
    - Anaphylactic shock
- Pneumothorax.

Circulatory
- Cardiac:
    - Acute myocardial infarction
    - Arrhythmias: ventricular fibrillation, ventricular tachycardia, complete heart block.
    - Electrocution.
- Vascular:
    - Neurogenic shock (syncope): vasovagal, micturition, cough, carotid sinus
    - Pulmonary embolism
    - Hypovolaemic shock.
    - Bacteriological shock (peritonitis, pelvic infection).

Disability (CNS)
- Epilepsy
- Infections: meningitis, encephalitis.
- Stroke: cerebral vascular accidents, transient ischaemic attacks, sub-arachnoid haemorrhage.
- Cerebral tumours and abscess.
- Head injury
- Poisoning and drug overdosage: accidental/deliberate, including alcohol.
- Hysteria.

Endocrine/metabolic
- Diabetes:
    - Hypoglycaemia
    - Hyperglycaemia.
- Thyroid disease
- Renal failure
- Liver failure
- Adrenal failure
- Hypercalcaemia
- Hypothermia and hyperthermia.

12

Poisoning and overdosage

Poisoning and overdosage

Introduction

- Although this topic may not be an obvious part of Immediate Care, it is part of emergency medicine and the management of poisoning and overdosage is a subject with which the Immediate Care doctor should be familiar.

Definitions:
- **Poisoning:** Exposure to substances that are intrinsically harmful.
- **Overdosage:** Exposure to substances that are only harmful when taken in excess.

Incidence

- Very common in children under the age of 5 years (50%):
    - Usually accidental, although non-accidental poisoning may occur.
    - Deaths are very rare (under 10 per year)
- Self poisoning/non accidental overdosage:
    - Accounts for about 5% of all emergency medical admissions.
    - 60% are female.
    - Most common in the 15-19 year old age group.
    - Analgesics, especially paracetamol are involved in over 50% of cases.
    - Hypnotics and tranquillisers (usually benzodiazepines) are the next most commonly involved.
    - 50% have taken alcohol in addition to their primary poison.
    - Carbon monoxide is a major cause of death (motor vehicle exhaust fumes: 1000 deaths per year).

Aetiology

- Usually involves ordinary household chemicals:
    - Detergents, bleaches, etc.
- May be accidental:
    - Children, the elderly.
- May be deliberate:
    - Suicide, parasuicide: drugs, carbon monoxide.
- In self poisoning more than one substance may be involved, especially alcohol and drugs.

Pathophysiology

- The substances involved may produce both systemic and local effects depending on the route of absorption.

Through the dermis

- Absorbed: chemicals.
- Bite: insect, snake.
- Injected: plants, intravenous drug abuse.

Effects
- *Local:*
    - Erythema, blistering, etc.
- *Systemic:*
    - Bee stings: anaphylactic shock.
    - Organophosphates.

Inhaled

- Noxious gases, etc.

Effects
- *Local:*
    - Respiratory tract: laryngeal and bronchial oedema.
    - Lungs: pulmonary oedema.
- *Systemic:*
    - Specific to the poison.

Ingested

Effects:
- *Local:*
    - Burning of lips, mouth, oesophagus, vomiting, and abdominal pain.
- *Systemic:*
    - Specific to the poison.

Systemic effects

- **Blood**
    - Reduce available oxygen in the circulation:
        - Carbon monoxide
        - Cyanide.

- **Brain**
    - Produce generalised cerebral depression
        - Narcotics
        - Tricyclic antidepressants.
        - Alcohol.
    - Produce specific effects
        - Respiratory depressants.

- **Heart**
  - Arrhythmogenic:
    - Tricyclic antidepressants.
    - β-blockers
    - Calcium antagonists.

- **Lungs**
  - Respiratory muscle paralysis:
    - Snake bite
    - Organophosphates
    - Botulinus toxin.
  - ARDS:
    - Paraquat.

- **Liver**
  - Hepatic damage:
    - Paracetamol.
    - Amanita mushrooms.

- **Kidneys**
  - Renal damage:
    - Paracetamol.

- **Tissues**
  - Cyanides.

- **Multisystem**
  - Anaphylactic shock:
    - Insect bites.
  - Infective shock:
    - Bacterial endotoxins and toxins.

Guidelines for the management of poisoning/overdosage

Assess the scene

Rapidly assess what has happened

Protect yourself from any obvious danger

Move the casualty away from direct contact with the poison and remove to a place of safety
- Remove contaminated clothing and wash/hose down the skin with water.

Primary survey

Assess the patient's vital signs, including pupil size

Perform basic/advanced life support:
- Airway.
- Breathing.
- Circulation.

Secondary survey

Identify the cause of the poisoning from:
- Medicines:
    - Shape, colour of pills/capsules
    - Labels of container/bottle.
- Chemicals;
    - Container labels
    - HAZCHEM code.
- Dead snake/insect.
- Uneaten food, leaves, fruit, berries, etc.

Consider inducing emesis: ipecacuanha, or gastric emptying
- This is of *doubtful value* after more than 4 hours except for:
    - Salicylates (24 hrs)
    - Tricyclics (8 hrs).
- It is *dangerous* in drowsy/comatose patients unless there is:
    - A good cough reflex
    - Airway protection with a cuffed endotracheal tube.
- *Not advised* for:
    - Petroleum products:
        - These are more dangerous in the lungs than the stomach: aspiration pneumonitis.
    - Corrosive compounds
    - Pregnant patients.
- Generally seldom practicable until the patient has reached hospital.

Method
- Administration of Paediatric Ipecacuanha Emetic Mixture BP (*not* tincture).

Dosage
- Children: 6-18 months: 10 ml.
                18 months-14 years: 15 ml.
- Adults: 30 ml.
- The dose should be followed by a glass of water or orange juice and may be repeated once after 20 minutes as necessary.

Adsorbants: activated charcoal
- Activated charcoal given orally can bind and reduce the absorbtion of many poisons, including;
    - Tricyclic antidepressants
    - Opioids
    - Organophosphates
    - Aspirin
    - Mefenamic acid
    - Phenothiazines.
- Usually only effective if given within 1-2 hours of ingestion of the poison.
- Ineffective against:
    - Lithium
    - Cyanide
    - Corrosive agents
    - Iron salts
    - Organic solvents.

- Activated charcoal adsorbs ipecacuanha, rendering it ineffective.
- Activated charcoal should be considered if induction of emeses is unsuccessful or not advisable.

Dosage
- Optimal dose is 5-10 times the amount of drug ingested: often up to 50 g.

Specific treatment
- Use specific antidotes if applicable/available.
- Information should be obtained from the local Poisons Information Centre (see list at the end of this chapter).

Inform receiving hospital of
- The cause, effects, and treatment of poisoning
- The time of:
  - Ingestion
  - Onset of symptoms
  - Treatment carried out.

If possible send to hospital
- The chemical/pill container/syringe
- The chemical code number
- Dead snake/insect
- Uneaten fruit/mushrooms, etc.
- Any suicide note
- A sample of vomit.

Specific problems

Bites

Insect bite

- These are usually only dangerous if anaphylactic shock occurs, or if a bite in the mouth or on the tongue causes upper airway obstruction and respiratory distress.

Incidence
- Life threatening problems are rare.

Aetiology
- Stings from: ants, bees, wasps, and hornets.

Symptoms/signs
- Local pain and tenderness.
- A circle of erythema and swelling sometimes with a haemorrhagic centre (especially if it has been sucked!).
- Development of an anaphylactic reaction.

Management
- Respiratory obstruction:
    - Consider cricothyrotomy.
- Anaphylactic shock:
    - Basic/advanced life support, adrenaline, etc. (see under Management of Anaphylactic Shock).
- Cleanse area, apply cooling lotion or topical antihistamine.
- Oral antihistamine, eg. chlorpheniramine (Piriton).
- If the mouth is affected:
    - Sucking ice may be helpful.
- Bee sting:
    - Remove by scraping off with knife.
    - Do *not* try to remove sting with fingers or tweezers as this may result in further injection of venom.

Snake bite

Incidence
- Rare in the UK; the only indigenous poisonous snake is the Adder.
- Usually only occurs in warm weather.
- Rarely fatal, except in the very debilitated patient who receives a large amount of venom.

Symptoms/signs
- Local:
    - Swelling (which may spread to involve the whole limb)
    - Erythema
    - Ecchymosis
    - Pain.
- Systemic:
    - Nausea, vomiting, colicky abdominal pain and diarrhoea.
    - Tachycardia, bradycardia and hypotension.
    - Dizziness, restlessness, agitation, confusion, fits and coma.

Management
- Remove all rings, etc. from the affected limb so as to avoid impairment of the peripheral circulation, if swelling occurs.
- Clean and cover the bite with a dressing and firmly (but not occlusively) bandage the affected limb:
    - This increases the systemic vascular resistance, and reduces the venous return, thus reducing local spread and the possibility of the venom causing systemic side effects.
- Immobilise the limb in a sling or splint, and keep it below heart level, but not dependent (to reduce the venous return).
- Consider using antihistamines.
- Get a good description of the snake.
- Do *not*:
    - Allow the patient to walk on the affected limb, as this will increase the blood supply (ideally the patient should not be allowed to walk at all).
    - Allow the patient to drink alcohol as this may exacerbate any CNS depression.
    - Apply a tourniquet.
    - Lance, squeeze or suck the bite.
    - Remove the bandage once it has been applied.

Dangerous chemicals

Acids

Aetiology
- Found in rust removers, car batteries, toilet cleaners, descalers, etc.

Pathophysiology
- Skin:
    - Produces localised burns.
- Ingestion:
    - Burning/pain around the mouth and oesophagus, with dysphagia.
    - Abdominal pain, nausea and vomiting.
- Inhalation:
    - Dyspnoea.

Symptoms/signs
- As for burns.

Management
- Ingestion:
    - Do *not* induce vomiting
    - Give copious water immediately.
- Burns:
    - See under burns/eye injuries.

Alkalis

Aetiology
- Found in bleach, washing soda, drain cleaner, ammonia and oven cleaner.

Pathophysiology
- Skin:
    - Produces localised burns.
- Ingestion:
    - Burning/pain around the mouth and oesophagus, with dysphagia.
    - Abdominal pain, nausea and vomiting.
- Inhalation:
    - Dyspnoea.

Symptoms/signs
- Burning/pain around mouth and oesophagus.
- Pain/difficulty in swallowing.

Management
- Do *not* induce vomiting.
- Administer milk or water orally.

Petrol and petrol distillates

Incidence
- Petrol ingestion is a rare problem in the UK.
- Ingestion of petrol distillates is very common.

Aetiology
- Petrol ingestion is usually caused by siphoning petrol.
- Petrol distillates are a common constituent of many household products, e.g. lighter fuel, furniture polish, white spirit and turpentine.

Pathophysiology
- Only toxic when ingested or inhaled in high concentrations.
- Highly irritant to the respiratory mucosa, and may cause pulmonary oedema.
- May result in vomiting and an aspiration pneumonia.
- Absorption may result in cerebral and cardiac toxicity.

Symptoms/signs
- Respiratory distress with cough, choking, cyanosis and pulmonary oedema.
- Severe abdominal pain.
- Cerebral irritability, convulsions and coma.
- Hypoglycaemia may occur.
- Cardiac arrhythmias may occur.

Management
- Do *not* induce vomiting, as this may result in aspiration pneumonia.
- Oxygen, and airway care with intubation to protect the lungs from aspiration.
- Suction of any secretions (which may be copious).
- Circulatory support:
    - Intravenous infusion.
- Cardiac monitoring.
- All patients should go to hospital, even if they appear well initially (a chest X-ray is advisable for most patients).

Note: - Petrol sniffing can result in lead poisoning.

Methyl alcohol: methanol, wood alcohol

Incidence
- Accidental poisoning is relatively common in the desperate and poor alcoholic, who uses it as a substitute for ethyl alcohol, resulting in chronic poisoning.

Aetiology
- Found in paints, paint thinners, paint removers, varnishes and antifreeze.
- Usually only toxic when ingested.

Pathophysiology
- Can cause a profound metabolic acidosis.
- Methanol is metabolised to formic acid, which cannot be further metabolised by the body and commonly results in blindness.

Symptoms/signs
- Alcoholic odour.
- Tachypnoea with deep respirations.
- Hypotension and shock.

Management
- Induce emesis.
- Oxygen.
- Circulatory support:
    - Intravenous infusion of crystalloid.
    - If the patient shows signs of a metabolic acidosis:
        - Consider administration of 50 ml 8.4% bicarbonate intravenously.
- Cardiac monitoring.
- Give one measure of whiskey every hour (ethanol selectively impairs the metabolism of methanol to formic acid and thus promotes its excretion unaltered).

Cyanide

- May cause cardiac arrest and death very rapidly and poisoning is therefore an acute medical emergency.

Incidence
- Relatively rare, usually occurs as a result of deliberate ingestion.

Aetiology
- May occur by ingestion, absorption or inhalation.

Pathophysiology
- Cyanide interferes with oxygen metabolism at the tissue level, resulting in cellular hypoxia.

Symptoms/signs
- History of exposure.
- Skin contact:
    - Irritation, erythema and local pain.
    - Burns can also occur.
- Ingestion:
    - Burning sensation in the throat, with nausea and vomiting.
- Inhalation:
    - Odour of almonds on the patient's breath.
    - Chest pain.
- Systemic:
    - Absence of pallor.
    - Chest tightness and respiratory distress with dyspnoea, and a tachypnoea leading to bradypnoea.
    - A rapid, weak pulse.
    - Red discolouration of the venous blood (on fundoscopy; arteries and veins look the same colour).
    - Dizziness, confusion, coma, convulsions and death.

Management
- 100% oxygen and airway maintenance.
- If the casualty is not breathing after cyanide ingestion:
    - Ventilate with a bag and mask.
- If the casualty is breathing:
    - Break two amyl nitrite capsules beneath his nose, so that he inhales the vapour.
- If the patient is unconscious or is losing consciousness:
    - Administer dicobalt edetate (Kelocyanor) 300 mg intravenously immediately, followed by 50 ml 50% dextrose. This can be repeated up to 900 mg maximum.
- Provide circulatory support: Intravenous infusion.
- Monitor the cardiac rhythm.

Note:- Dicobalt edetate can cause flushing, collapse and convulsions if the patient *does not* have cyanide poisoning and should therefore be used with caution.
- As an alternative, sodium nitrite may be given intravenously, followed by sodium thiosulphate.

Pesticides

Organophosphates
- Poisoning may be fatal.

Incidence
- Found in many insecticides, herbicides and fungicides, as powders or dissolved in organic solvents and in chemical warfare "nerve" agents.

Aetiology
- May be absorbed accidentally through intact skin, accidentally or deliberately ingested or accidentally inhaled (rarely).

Pathophysiology:
- Causes parasympathetic stimulation; by inhibition of cholinesterase activity, leading to a build up of acetylcholine at muscarinic and nicotinic receptors.
- May be absorbed through the skin, with symptoms similar to inhalation or ingestion.
- May cause pulmonary oedema and general muscular paralysis.

Symptoms/signs
- Skin contact:
    - Mild local erythema and irritation, followed by systemic effects.
    - Muscarinic effects:
        - Nausea, excessive sweating, and profuse salivation *(early)*.
        - Epigastric and retrosternal discomfort, with abdominal cramps, vomiting and diarrhoea.
        - Rhinorrhoea, bronchoconstriction with profuse bronchial secretion, dyspnoea, respiratory distress, pulmonary oedema and hypoxia, leading to respiratory arrest.
        - Bradycardia, arrhythmias.
        - Urinary and faecal incontinence.
    - Nicotinic effects:
        - Muscle twitching, followed by weakness, convulsions and flaccid paralysis, including ocular and respiratory muscle paralysis (in approximately 6 hours).

- Central nervous system effects:
    - Anxiety, restlessness, dizziness, confusion and headache *(early)*
    - Pupil constriction *(early)*
    - Convulsions.
- Metabolic problems:
    - Hyperglycaemia and glycosuria (without ketonuria).

Management
- Oxygen (100%) with frequent removal of bronchial secretions.
- Consider ventilation.
- Remove clothing and decontaminate the skin with water and possibly use soap.
- Consider induction of emesis.
- Start an intravenous infusion.
- Give:
    - Atropine:
        - Give 2 mg intravenously immediately.
        - Repeat the intravenous dose every 5-10 minutes, until there are signs of atropinisation, i.e. dilated pupils, dry mouth, pulse rate >80 bpm.
    - Pralidoxime 1 g every 4 hours: if available, administer intravenously (slowly).
    - Diazepam: 2-15 mg intravenously, if fitting.

Note:- *Never* administer morphine or aminophylline as these exacerbate the effects of organophosphates.

Paraquat

Incidence
- Used to be responsible for a considerable, but now rapidly decreasing number of deaths.

Aetiology
- Used to be a commonly used chemical in farming and market gardening.
- Only toxic when ingested, but highly irritant to the eyes and skin.

Pathophysiology
- Local cytotoxic effect.
- Causes pulmonary fibrosis due to proliferative alveolitis and bronchiolitis.
- Renal failure.

Symptoms/signs
- Eyes:
    - Corneal and conjunctival ulceration.
- Skin:
    - Irritation, blistering, and ulceration.
- Inhalation of spray mist or dust:
    - Epistaxis, sore throat.
- Ingestion:
    - Nausea, vomiting, diarrhoea.
    - Ulceration of the lips, tongue and fauces within 36-48 hr.
- Large overdose:
    - Multiple organ failure within 6-48 hr.
- Milder overdose:
    - Dyspnoea and hypoxia after initial recovery.

Management
- Eyes:
    - Copious washing, antibiotic eyedrops.
- Ingestion:
    - Activated charcoal, Fuller's earth or bentonite to adsorb the poison and reduce absorption.
    - Careful gastric lavage/emptying (not emesis), and then further Fuller's earth/magnesium sulphate.
    - Intravenous fluids.
    - Analgesia.

Noxious gases

Carbon monoxide: Colourless, odourless and tasteless gas.

Incidence
- Commonest inhaled agent involved in causing death: up to 1000 deaths every year, up to 200 occurring during the winter months and at home.
- Often used in successful suicide: motor vehicle exhaust, etc. (over 800 deaths per year).

Aetiology
- Produced by incomplete combustion of fossil fuels, e.g. gas, petrol.
- Accidental poisoning:
    - Inhalation of smoke, car exhaust or fumes caused by blocked flues from fires and boilers or the incomplete combustion of gases in confined spaces.

Pathophysiology
- Carbon monoxide has a very high affinity for haemoglobin, with which it combines to form carboxyhaemoglobin, displacing oxygen and causing tissue hypoxia.
- Levels of carbon monoxide do not need to be high to cause poisoning.

Symptoms/signs (may be difficult to recognise initially)
- Lethargy, muscular weakness, a throbbing headache, nausea and vomiting.
- Dizziness, confusion and disorientation, followed by convulsions and coma.
- A bounding pulse, dilated pupils, cyanosis and pallor (the cherry red colour of the lips, so often described is in fact rarely seen during life).
- Pulmonary oedema, with respiratory depression.
- (Investigation: Take blood and put into EDTA or lithium heparin bottle for carboxyhaemoglobin estimation. Do *not* get it spun down, or take blood for blood gas analysis, as many blood gas analysers will also give carboxyhaemoglobin levels).
- ECG: ischaemic changes.

Management
- Oxygen (100%), using a tight fitting mask and a circuit which minimises rebreathing.
- Hyperbaric oxygen (if available) is most important if the patient:
    - Has been unconscious
    - Has neurological symptoms or signs
    - Is pregnant
    - Has carboxyhaemoglobin levels >20%.
- Respiratory support.

Freons

Incidence
- Rarely encountered except in solvent abuse which is an increasing problem in some parts of the UK and is usually found in children and young adolescents.

Aetiology
- Used as refrigerants and propellants in aerosols.
- The mortality rate is high with significant exposure, usually in solvent abusers.

Pathophysiology
- Usually only toxic when inhaled.
- Cardiotoxic.

Symptoms/signs
- Dyspnoea.
- Headache, nausea, drowsiness, and unconsciousness.
- Hyperactivity.
- Cardiac arrest.

Management
- Basic Life Support.
- Oxygen.
- Cardiac monitoring.
- Intravenous infusion.
- Consider using lignocaine for tachycardias.

Toluene

Incidence
- This is the major substance involved in child solvent abuse (glue sniffing), resulting in the deaths of up to two children per week in the UK. May also be ingested.

Aetiology
- Used as a solvent in: glue, paint, cleaning fluids, nail varnish remover.
- Poisoning usually occurs as a result of accidental overexposure.

Pathophysiology
- Hallucinogenic, can cause intoxication.
- Nervous system depressant: may cause respiratory and cardiac arrest.

Symptoms/signs
- Dry throat with cough, and chest tightness.
- Dyspnoea and pulmonary oedema.
- Drowsiness, confusion and unconsciousness, fits, coma and death.

Management
- Oxygen/fresh air.
- Airway care, with monitoring of the vital signs.
- Reassurance.
  (Recovery is usually fairly rapid and may be full within 20 minutes.)

Sulphur dioxide, chlorine, phosgene

Incidence
- Relatively rare, but poisoning may be fatal.
- Chlorine poisoning is the most common.

Aetiology
- Inhalation is the usual mode of poisoning.
- Usually only found in accidental industrial poisoning.
- Chlorine poisoning may occur:
    - In the home when lavatory cleaner and bleach are mixed.
    - In public swimming baths.

Pathophysiology
- Acidic gases causing:
    - Lung tissue damage resulting in pulmonary oedema, etc.

Symptoms/signs
- Coughing, choking (except phosgene).
- Breathlessness and cyanosis (this may develop suddenly up to 36 hr following exposure).

Management
- Observation for more than 36 hr.
- If symptomatic:
    - Oxygen
    - Steroids.

Note:- For poisoning with other dangerous chemicals please refer to:
- "Dangerous Chemicals: Emergency First Aid Guide" *and/or*
- Contact the nearest Poisons Information Centre (see end of this chapter).

Medicines

Narcotic analgesics: opiates: morphine, heroin, methadone, codeine, and dextropropoxyphene.

Incidence
- Overdosage is relatively rare in the UK, except amongst drug addicts, due to the difficulty in obtaining these drugs, legally and in any quantity, except for dextropopoxyphene, which is widely prescribed in combination with paracetamol (co-proxamol).

Pathophysiology
- Cause respiratory and central nervous system depression (exacerbated by alcohol).
- Death may result very rapidly.

Symptoms/signs
- Bradypnoea leading to apnoea.
- Hypotension.
- Constricted pupils, drowsiness, unconsciousness and coma.
- Needle marks, thrombosed veins in drug addicts.

Management
- Basic Life Support.
- Oxygen.
- Naloxone (400 µg/ml: 1/2 ml amps):
    - *Dosage:-* 0.8-2.0 mg given as an intravenous bolus.
        - This has a short half-life so administration may be repeated as required, according to the patient's response.
        - Reversal of symptoms should begin within about 1 minute, but beware of "recovery" followed by further collapse (for more information: see chapter on Pain Relief)
- Circulatory support with an intravenous infusion.
- Consider use of activated charcoal if the opioid has been ingested.

Non steroidal anti-inflammatory drugs (NSAIDs)

Aspirin

Incidence
- Accidental poisoning is commonly encountered in young children.
- Used to be a very popular method of overdosage in adults, but is declining.

Pathophysiology
- Absorption and hence onset of symptoms may be delayed for up to 24 hours or more.
- Produces an initial respiratory alkalosis caused by hyperventilation, followed by a metabolic acidosis.
- Pulmonary oedema.
- Renal failure.

Symptoms/signs
- Nausea, vomiting, haematemesis.
- Vasodilation, pyrexia, sweating, hyperventilation.
- Dehydration.
- Tinnitus, deafness, vertigo, headache.
- Confusion, coma and fits (very severe poisoning only).

Management
- Induce emesis.
    - Rehydration:
        - Intravenous infusion
        - Consider bicarbonate: forced alkaline diuresis.
- Fits: treat with diazepam.

Mefenamic acid (Ponstan)

Incidence
- Relatively uncommon.

Symptoms/signs
- Fits, usually very brief.

Management
- Induction of emesis/gastric emptying.
- Fitting: intravenous diazepam/midazolam.

Ibuprofen

Incidence
- Serious overdosage is relatively uncommon.

Symptoms/signs
- Nausea, vomiting, tinnitus.

Management
- Gastric emptying or induction of emesesis, if more than 10 tablets have been ingested.

Paracetamol

Incidence
- Very commonly used in deliberate overdosage, and in accidental overdosage in children.

Pathophysiology
- As few as 20-30 tabs may cause delayed hepatic (hepatocellular) necrosis, and less commonly renal tubular necrosis.

Symptoms/signs
- Often the patient does not appear ill.
- Nausea, vomiting (usually settles within 24 hours).
- Persistence of vomiting is usually associated with right subcostal pain/tenderness and indicates hepatocellular necrosis.

Management
- All cases should go to hospital, even if they appear well, so that appropriate treatment may be started.
- Gastric emptying within 4 hours of ingestion.
- Hepatic protection may be provided within 10-12 hours of ingestion by:
    - *N-Acetylcysteine* in 5% dextrose as an intravenous infusion.
        Dosage: 150 mg/kg in 200 ml over 15 minutes then 50 mg/kg in 500 ml over 4 hours, followed by 100 mg/kg over 16 hours.
    - *Methionine*: administered orally (do *not* administer activated charcoal as well).
        Dosage: 2.5 g initially followed by a further 2.5 g every 4 hours, up to a total of 4 times (10 g).

Note: - Paracetamol concentrations should be obtained if available.

Co-proxamol: Dextropropoxyphene and paracetamol

Incidence
- Commonly used in overdosage.

Pathophysiology
- Initial effects are those of opiate overdosage.
- Respiratory arrest is very common.
- Cardiovascular collapse may also occur.

Management
- Basic and Advanced Life Support in extreme cases as indicated.
- Induction of emesis/gastric emptying.
- As opiate and paracetamol overdosage.
- Use naloxone (see under opiates).

Hypnotics and anxiolytics

Barbiturates

Incidence
- Used to be commonly used in overdosage, but now uncommon in the UK as their prescribing has almost ceased, except for epileptics.

Pathophysiology
- Depressants of nervous tissue especially the central nervous system, resulting in depression of the level of consciousness.
- May also cause severe respiratory depression.

Symptoms/signs
- Drowsiness, confusion, unconsciousness, coma.
- Pupil size may vary.
- Respiratory depression, bradypnoea, with shallow respirations, or Cheyne Stokes respiration.
- Vomiting and aspiration, resulting in pneumonia.
- Signs of shock, hypotension, etc.
- Erythema, skin blisters (barbiturate blisters).
- Hypothermia.
- Metabolic acidosis.

Management
- If unconscious:
    - Airway support, i.e. oxygen, ventilation, etc.
- If conscious:
    - Activated charcoal orally immediately.
- Cardiac monitoring.

Benzodiazepines: temazepam, nitrazepam, lorazepam, diazepam, chlordiazepoxide

Incidence
- Still a relatively popular drug of overdosage in the UK, often combined with alcohol.

Pathophysiology
- General CNS depressants but causes less severe respiratory depression, which is rarely by itself fatal.
- May potentiate effects of other CNS depressants taken at the same time, especially alcohol.

Symptoms/signs
- Ataxia, dysarthria.
- Drowsiness, unconsciousness and coma.
- Hyporeflexia, hypotension.

Management
- Induction of emesis/gastric emptying is not indicated.
- Care of the unconscious patient.
- Flumazenil:
    - Not usually necessary, but indicated if there is respiratory depression (may be of diagnostic use in patients with a mixed overdosage, in whom diagnosis is difficult).
    - Should be administered with care and titrated against the patient's response (for details of administration see chapter on Pain Relief).

Note:- Flumazenil may be associated with convulsions in mixed tricyclic and benzodiazepine overdosage.

Antidepressants

Tricyclics

Incidence
- Often used in deliberate overdosage.

Pathophysiology
- May cause CNS depression and cardiac dysrhythmias.

Symptoms/signs
- Dry mouth.
- Respiratory failure, metabolic acidosis.
- Sinus tachycardia, hypotension, cardiac conduction defects/arrhythmias.
- Hypothermia.
- Hyperreflexia, extensor plantar response, dilated pupils, urinary retention, and convulsions.
- Drowsiness/unconsciousness, and coma.

Management
- Care of the unconscious patient.
- Activated charcoal immediately (orally: only if the patient is conscious).
- Gastric lavage, even after 6 hours post ingestion.
- Cardiac monitoring.
- If there is hypotension or arrhythmia administer:
    - Sodium bicarbonate (0.5-1 mmol/kg) intravenously.
- If there is a serious arrhythmia: consider administration of amiodarone (lignocaine is contraindicated).
- If the patient is fitting:
    - Administer intravenous diazepam/midazolam.

Lithium salts

Incidence
- Uncommon.

Aetiology
- Poisoning may be deliberate or accidental.

Symptoms/signs
- May be delayed more than 12 hours after ingestion.
- Non specific apathy, restlessness.
- Vomiting, diarrhoea
- Ataxia, weakness, dysarthria, muscle twitching/tremor.
- Severe poisoning:
    - Convulsions, coma, hypotension, renal failure and electrolyte imbalance.

Management
- Induction of emesis/gastric emtying.
- Supportive.
- Intravenous infusion:
    - Buffered solution of crystalloid, e.g. Hartmann's solution.
- Convulsions:
    - Intravenous diazepam/midazolam.

Phenothiazines

Incidence
- Fairly commonly used in self poisoning.

Pathophysiology
- Centrally acting dopamine antagonists.

Symptoms/signs
- Hypotension.
- Hypothermia.
- Sinus tachycardia, cardiac arrhythmias.
- Dystonic reactions (these can also occur with therapeutic doses).
- Convulsions (severe cases only).

Management
- Arrhythmia control.
- Hypotension:
    - Intravenous fluids.
- Convulsions:
    - Intravenous diazepam/midazolam.
- Dystonic reactions:
    - Orphenadrine.
    - Procyclidine.

Iron compounds

Ferrous sulphate, ferrous gluconate, etc.

Incidence
- Common in accidental poisoning of children.
- Has an appreciable mortality.

Pathophysiology
- Hepatocellular necrosis.

Symptoms/signs
- Nausea, vomiting, abdominal pain, diarrhoea, haematemesis and rectal bleeding.
- Hypotension, shock with apparent recovery between 8-24 hours.
- Later:
    - Hypotension, coma, and hepatocellular necrosis.

Management
- Gastric emptying:
    - Emesis/gastric lavage.
- X-ray stomach to show tablets.
- Catharsis/whole gut lavage.
- Desferrioxamine (chelating agent).

    Dosage: By mouth: 5-10 g in 50-100 ml of water.
    By intravenous infusion: Up to 15 mg/kg/hour (maximum: 80 mg/kg).

Note: - Intravenous desferrioxamine may cause hypotension and an anaphylactic reaction.

Alcohol

Acute intoxication

Incidence
- Common in adults, but may also occur in children.
- Involved in 10% of all road traffic accidents: resulting in 800 deaths and 22,000 casualties annually in the UK.
- Drunken drivers account for 1/3 of all fatal RTAs (2/3 of all fatal RTAs between 10 pm and 4 am).
- 1/3 of drivers in injury accidents fail the breath test.

Aetiology
- Acute alcohol poisoning itself carries a significant risk of death.
- Alcohol ingestion may predispose the patient to other life threatening conditions especially trauma.
- Every year people die because their condition is presumed to be due to alcohol, rather than the real cause, e.g. head injury.
- The patient may have taken other drugs as well as alcohol.

Pathophysiology
- Alcohol is a CNS depressant, which depresses the inhibitory centres first resulting initially in inebriation.
- Vomiting whilst unconscious can be a problem.
- Causes vasodilation especially of cutaneous vessels, resulting in increased heat loss and may precipitate hypothermia.

Symptoms/signs
- History of alcohol ingestion.
- Smell of alcohol on breath (Unreliable as a guide of the blood alcohol level).
- Nausea, vomiting.
- Impaired level of consciousness:
    - Drowsiness, slurred speech, nystagmus, unsteady gait, irrational behaviour, aggression, stupor, coma and death.
- Flushed, warm skin, hypothermia.
- Hypotension, tachycardia.
- Metabolic acidosis.
- Hypoglycaemia, convulsions (especially in children).

Note: - Even if the patient's breath smells strongly of alcohol; other causes of impaired consciousness should be positively looked for:
- Head injury
- Hypoglycaemia
- Physical illness, etc.

Management
- Induce emesis/gastric emptying.
- Care of the unconscious patient, especially the airway as vomiting may occur and the patient may have a reduced gag reflex and respiratory drive.
- Full examination to exclude other cause for the patient's condition.
- If the patient is confused and violent, sedation should be considered, e.g. with chlorpromazine.
- Respiratory depression, cardiac dysrhythmias and shock should be treated as detailed in the appropriate chapter.
- Blood glucose monitoring and intravenous/oral glucose if indicated.

Acute alcohol withdrawal (delirium tremens: DTs)

Aetiology
- Only found in alcoholics.
- Usually comes on within 24-72 hours of the last drink, but may be delayed for up to 10 days.
- Has a high mortality.

Symptoms/signs
- History and signs of alcoholism.
- Confusion, tremor, restlessness, agitation.
- Hallucinations of spiders, snakes, etc.
- Convulsions.

Management
- Reassurance and sedation:
    - Intravenous chlormethiazole (Heminevrin) may help sedate patients with acute withdrawal symptoms.
- Intravenous infusion of crystalloid.
- Treatment of fits:
    - Intravenous diazepam/midazolam.

Note: - Alcoholics are also at risk from other acute problems, e.g. haematemesis.

Poisonous plants and fungi

Incidence

- This is the third most common cause of poisoning after ingestion of drugs and household chemicals.
- Fungi: accidental ingestion is a relatively uncommon cause of poisoning in the UK.
- Abuse of hallucinogenic fungi "magic mushrooms",e.g. Amanita Psylocybus, is fairy common.

Aetiology

- Young children are most at risk from ingesting poisonous plants accidentally.
- Adults may accidentally ingest poisonous fungi in the mistaken belief that they are edible.
- Young adults may ingest hallucinogenic fungi.

Symptoms/signs

- Can be almost anything depending on the plant/fungi.
- Symptoms of poisoning with Amanita mushrooms may be very delayed (main effect is hepatic failure).

Management

- Resuscitate as necessary.
- Reassure and obtain history:
    - Botanical or common name of plant if known.
    - If possible sample of plant, or if not possible obtain a good description.
    - Type and severity of exposure: skin contact, ingestion, etc.
    - If ingested, how much and which parts of the plant were eaten.
    - Time of exposure/ ingestion, onset of symptoms and any treatment carried out.
    - Age of patient.
    - Symptoms.
- Decide whether or not plant is toxic.
- Contact your local poisons centre.
- Induce emesis if advised.
- Activated charcoal (5-10 g) will bind most plant toxins, and reduces the severity of poisoning.

Dangerous chemicals/medicines and their specific antidotes

Drug	Antidote
Cyanide	Dicobalt edetate
Organophosphates	Atropine Pralidoxime
Opioids	Naloxone
Paracetamol	N-Acetylcysteine Methionine
Benzodiazepines	Flumazenil
Phenothiazines	Orphenadrine Procyclidine
Iron compounds	Desferrioxamine
Disinfectants	Milk, liberal fluids

Poisons information centres

Centre	24 hour telephone number		
Belfast	0232	240 503	ext 2140
Birmingham	021	554 3801	ext 4109
Cardiff	0222	709 901	
Dublin	010	379 966 *or* 964	
Edinburgh	031	229 2477 228 2441	ext 4786 (viewdata)
Leeds	0532	430 715 432 799	ext 3547
London	071	635 9191 *or* 955 5095	
Newcastle	091	232 1525 5131	(9am-5pm) (after 5pm)

13

Heat related injury, drowning and dysbarism

Heat related injury

Introduction

- Heat related injury is being encountered more and more due to the increased leisure time that many people enjoy, spending it on outdoor persuits, when with inadequate experience and wearing innappropriate clothing, they may be unexpectedly exposed to the extremes of our climate.

Sunburn

Incidence

- Common in the summer months.
- More likely to occur in those who are unaccustomed to exposure to the sun.

Aetiology

- Caused by excessive exposure to ultraviolet light.
- Gradual exposure can lessen the effect due to tanning.
- People with a fair complexion are the most at risk.

Pathophysiology

- Similar to burns.
- If large areas are involved, sunburn may result in heat hyperpyrexia.

Symptoms/signs

- **Initially**
  - Erythema and itching.

- **Later**
  - Pain, oedema and bullae.
  - Malaise, headache and nausea.

Management

Shock
- Rehydration: usually oral fluids are sufficient.

Pain
- Sedation and antihistamines, e.g. chlorpheniramine.

Dermal injury
- Prick large blisters.
- Calamine lotion.

Hyperthermia

Heat cramps

Incidence
- Uncommon in the UK except in very hot weather and with prolonged vigorous exercise, e.g. marathon running, troops in training.

Aetiology
- Occurs with vigorous exercise in hot climates.

Pathophysiology
- Profuse sweating results in salt and water depletion.
- This results in muscle cramps.

Symptoms/signs
- The sudden onset of pain and cramps in the extremities.
- There may be nausea and hypotension.
- Hyperventilation.

Management
- Move the patient to a cool environment.
- Give copious oral fluids with added glucose, if nausea is not present.
- If there is nausea or hypotension, establish an intravenous infusion with normal saline or dextrose 5%.
- Treatment of hyperventilation (see under Medical Emergencies).

Heat exhaustion

Incidence
- See above.

Aetiology
- Progression from heat cramps, i.e. it is a more severe condition.
- This condition is more likely in the dehydrated, the unfit, the elderly and the hypertensive.

Pathophysiology
- Salt and water loss, with additional peripheral pooling.

Symptoms/signs
- Headache, fatigue, dizziness, confusion, nausea and abdominal cramping.
- Syncope, collapse.
- Profuse sweating, pale, with clammy skin.
- A rapid, weak pulse, with hypotension and tachypnoea.
- Normal or slightly elevated (<39°C) body temperature.

Management
- Move the patient to a cool environment.
- Cooling:
    - Fan
    - Tepid sponging
    - Immersion in luke warm water.
- Administer copious fluids (water) unless nausea is present.
- Establish an intravenous infusion:
    - Crystalloid: Hartmann's solution or normal saline.

Heat hyperpyrexia/heat stroke

- This is an *acute medical emergency* with a mortality rate of 25-50%.

Incidence
- Rarely encountered in temperate climates, except for those taking part in physical activities requiring extreme exertion, carried out in very hot weather.
- Most commonly occurs in men over the age of 40.

Aetiology
- The same as heat exhaustion.

Pathophysiology
- Begins as heat exhaustion.
- As the body's attempts to lose heat fail, the core temperature rises rapidly, and irreversible tissue damage occurs principally affecting the brain, kidneys and liver.
- Circulatory collapse.

Symptoms/signs
- Headache, dizziness, dry mouth.
- Hot, flushed, dry skin.
- Hyperpyrexia (typically >40°C):
    - It is very important to take the rectal temperature, preferably with an electronic thermometer.
- Strong, bounding pulse initially, followed by collapse.
- Convulsions, coma and death.

Management
- Rapid cooling:

  Method 1
    - Put the patient in a cool environment, e.g. a tepid bath (do *not* use ice).
    - If the periphery is cooled too rapidly, however, peripheral cutaneous vasoconstriction may occur and this may prevent further core cooling.

Method 2 (method of choice)
- Evaporative cooling in which the skin is kept moist while it is fanned strongly. This may be achieved with the patient lying on their side or supported in the hands and knees position, whilst the skin is wet with a spray of atomised water under pressure at 15 °C and fanned with warm air.
- This maintains a high water pressure gradient from skin to air, facilitating rapid heat loss, without causing peripheral vasoconstriction.

- Fluids:
  - Oral fluids (water or special glucose and electrolyte solution), if possible (may cause vomiting).
  - Intravenous infusion:
    - Rapid infusion of large volumes of crystalloid, plus colloid if there is any haemorrhage.
- Cardiac monitoring.
- Treatment of fits.

Hypothermia
- Exists when the body core temperature is <35°C

Incidence
- Immersion is a major cause in the UK.
- Dry hypothermia:
  - Incidence and mortality are doubled with each 5°C fall in ambient outside temperature
  - Males are more likely to die than females.

Aetiology
- Occurs when the rate of heat produced by metabolism is less than the rate of heat loss from the body.
- Water immersion.
- Dry hypothermia usually occurs in the elderly:
  - Following a fall, they may be unable to get up.
  - May be due to poor heating and impaired cold perception.
  - May occur due to diabetes mellitus.
- May be due to cold exposure:
  - Accidents in bad weather/hostile environments.
  - Alcoholic intoxication.
  - Sporting events: mountaineering, climbing, marathons in cold wet weather.

Pathophysiology
- The elderly (less efficient metabolism, myocardium and circulation) and the young (greater relative surface area and small subcutaneous fat and energy stores) are particularly susceptible.
- A fall in the body temperature results:
  - *Initially:*
    - In increased heat production: shivering
    - In reduced heat loss: peripheral vasoconstriction.
  - *Later* (at body temperatures below 35°C):
    - Shivering stops.
    - A reduction in ventilation and later ventilatory arrest.
    - Slowing of body metabolism: reduction in oxygen requirement carbon dioxide production.
    - Cardiovascular:
      - Hypotension
      - The myocardium becomes electrically unstable: cardiac arrhythmias (usually VF)
      - Sludging of the blood
      - Cardiac arrest.
    - A metabolic acidosis.

Symptoms/signs

Moderate hypothermia (body temperature between 35 and 32°C)
- Behavioural/personality changes, slurred speech, incoordination, confusion, drowsiness, apathy/lethargy.
- Shivering, pallor, cold skin.
- Stumbling and slowing of physical activity.
- Low rectal/oral temperature (use a low reading thermometer).

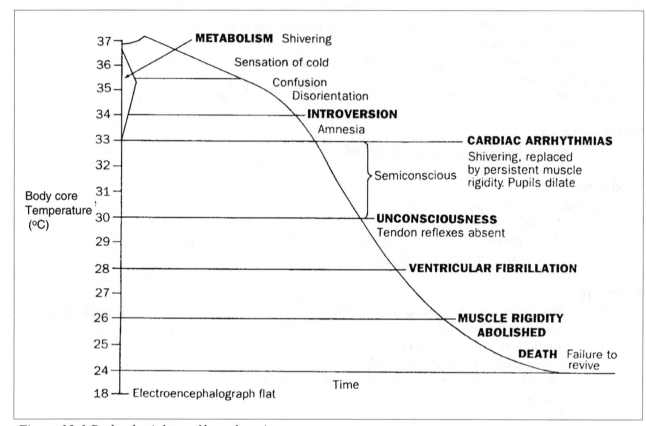

Figure 13-1 Pathophysiology of hypothermia

Severe hypothermia (body temperature below 32 °C).
- The patient may be: unconscious or stuporose, with non reacting pupils.
- The skin may be ice cold.
- Bradypnoea.
- No detectable pulse or blood pressure, with inaudible heart sounds.

Management
- Protect yourself: do not expose yourself to the risk of becoming a cold casualty:
    - Do not become exhausted
    - Do not donate your protective clothing to others, including the casualty you are trying to help.

All cold casualties
- Lay the casualty flat, treat any significant injuries and resuscitate if indicated.
- Prevent further heat loss by enclosing the casualty (including the head, but allowing for ventilation) in:
    - Heavy gauge plastic bags (if available)
    - Sleeping bag
    - Space blankets (not so robust and may be ineffective in a hostile environment).
- Insulate the casualty from the ground and provide overall wind and waterproof protection, as necessary.

- Provide further protection from the elements by finding/creating a shelter if possible.
- Remove the casualty, lying flat, to a warmer environment, so as to reduce any further heat loss.
- Gently rewarm the casualty, without removing their insulation (so as to avoid rapid surface rewarming).
    - Consider "airway insulation" with a heat and moisture exchanger. If this is not available. a scarf over the mouth and nose will help.
    - Oxygen may be beneficial, but should not be used if the cylinder is very cold.
- Consider body surface rewarming with hot water bottles or hot packs (beware of direct contact as this may cause burns), and be careful as rapid rewarming of the surface may result in severe hypotension.
- Carefully monitor the patient's respiration and pulse

Cold, conscious or confused casualties
- Once under shelter:
    - If their clothing is wet, replace it with dry clothing.
    - If their clothing is dry, keep them wrapped up and allow them to rewarm slowly.
- Give the casualty a warm sweet drink (but no alcohol), but only if they are able to swalllow easily (may have little effect on body temperature, but can be comforting).
- Obtain any significant medical history, e.g. dibetes mellitus, epilepsy.
- If immediate evacuation to a hospital is not possible:
    - Immerse the casualty up to the neck in warm water (maintained at approximately 40°C, which is comfortable both for your elbow and the casualty).
    - Remove any heavy outer clothing before immersion and any remaining clothing later after the casualty has been put into the bath.
    - Cessation of shivering should occur shortly after immersion, but this is *not* an indication for removal from the hot water.
    - When the casualty is comfortably warm, remove them from the bath, encourage them to lie flat, dry them and cover them with blankets (if they complain of feeling hot or dizzy, make them get out of the bath).
    - Keep the casualty lying flat until they feel warm, and have a near normal body temperature.

Unscious or semiconscious casualties
- Remove the casualty from the cold to a warm environment, wrapped up in blankets or a sleeping bag.
- Gently remove any wet clothing (be very careful, as rough handling may precipitate ventricular fibrillation).
- Carefully place the casualty in the recovery position, until they regain consciousness, and then keep them lying down until they are warm.

Cardiopulmonary resuscitation of cold casualties
- In spite of appearing to be dead, patients with severe hypothermia can survive, and every effort should be made to continue the attempt to resuscitate them, until they have been rewarmed to normal body temperature. The patient should not be confirmed deceased until the body temperature has been brought up to near normal or attempts to raise core temperature have failed.
- Full neurological recovery is possible even after prolonged arrest, as hypothermia reduces the cerebral oxygen requirements.

Basic Life Support
- Maintain the airway.
- If breating is absent, is less than 5 breaths per minute, becomes obstructed or stops, perform expired air ventilation at a rate of 8-12 cycles per minute.
- Administer oxygen.
- Only start chest compressions if:
    - There is no carotid pulse detectable after palpating for at least one minute (the pulse is often slow and weak in severe hypothermia).

- Cardiac arrest is observed, i.e. a pulse was present, but has subsequently disappeared.
- There is a reasonable possibility that the cardiac arrest occurred within the previous 2 hours.
- There is a reasonable expectation that effective CPR can be provided continuously (or with only brief interruptions to allow for movement of the casualty), until they can be removed to a location where full ALS can be provided.
  - If at any time a pulse is detectable, chest compressions should be stopped.
  - Hypothermia may cause stiffness of the chest wall, which can result in increased resistance to chest compression.

Advanced Life Support
- Monitor the cardiac rhythm:
  - If the patient is in asystole or ventricular fibrillation, start Basic/Advanced Life Support.
- Defibrillation may not be effective at temperatures below 30ºC.
- Drugs should be administered in a reduced dosage during rewarming, so as to reduce the amount of peripheral pooling.
- Use bretylium (5 mg/kg) instead of lignocaine, which is not effective at low temperatures.
- Arrhythmias other than VF tend to revert to normal sinus rhythm spontaneously as the core temperature rises, and do not require treatment.
- Continue ALS until the patient is fully rewarmed, or until effective respiration and circulation return.
- Administer an intravenous infusion of warmed fluid at 40ºC, preferably via a central vein:
  - Use a buffered solution of crystalloid, with sodium bicarbonate if cardiac arrest is prolonged.
- Insert a nasogastric tube.
- Monitor the patient's rectal temperature, using a low reading thermometer or thermocouple.
- Convey to hospital in the head down position.

Frost bite

Incidence
- Rarely encountered in the UK, except in extreme weather conditions.

Aetiology
- Exposure of the extremities to subzero temperatures may occur in cold climates, or may be due to exposure to very cold liquids/gases.

Pathophysiology
- The heat injury is very similar to burns as the mechanism is similar.
- Usually affects the fingers, toes and exposed extremities (may also very rarely affect the male genitalia).

Symptoms/signs
- Pricking pain, loss of sensation, followed by severe pain as the affected part warms up.
- Skin discolouration: waxy white, mottled blue.
- Blistering.
- Hardness.
- Impaired movement.

Management
- Removal of the patient from the cold.
- Management of hypothermia.
- Gentle removal of clothing, avoiding damage to the skin, or bursting of blisters, etc.
- Rewarm in warm water at about 40ºC (checked with a thermometer) until completely rewarmed.
- Analgesia, as required, from aspirin up to and including morphine.
- Do *not* allow the patient to smoke as nicotine may cause peripheral vasoconstriction.

Near drowning

Introduction

- The problems associated with swimming is a relatively specialised part of Immediate Care and only something that those who live on or near the coast, or near large inland waterways, will experience with any regularity. However, all of us go on holiday, often near the sea, and so should have some idea as to the problems involved.

Drowning

- Children often survive after near drowning in the British Isles, especially if they have been hypothermic (30% of children with fixed dilated pupils may survive fully neurologically intact).

Incidence

- Usually occurs in summer, particularly in children and teenage males.
- Drowning is the third most common cause of accidental death in the UK, responsible for about 1000 deaths and over 5,000 near drownings per annum in the UK (most occurring inland).
- 50% occur within 5m of land, 75% occur in an unsupervised area.

Aetiology

- In young adults alcohol plays a major part.

Pathophysiology

- Unlike other situations respiratory arrest occurs before cardiac arrest.
- Often associated with hypothermia (see previous section).

Cold challenge
- The colder the temperature; the longer the heart can remain stopped without major problems. The main limiting factor is the development of ventricular fibrillation.

Lung injury
- Water inhalation: 10% have no water in the lungs, and there is rarely more than 1.5 litres in the lungs.

Brain injury
- Hypoxia, resulting in cerebral oedema.
- The lower the temperature, the less the injury.
- Cerebral oedema may increase as the patient warms up.

Electrolyte changes
- Relatively unimportant.
- Hypokalaemia: salt and fresh water.
- Hypernatraemia: salt water.
- Hyponatraemia: infants in fresh water.

Cold water drowning (temp <10 °C or below)
- Initial response:
    - The patient gives an inspiratory gasp followed by hyperventilation.
    - This can precipitate death by inhalation of water and wet drowning.
    - May also precipitate sudden hypertension and severe cardiac arrhythmias and arrest.
- Short term (up to 15-20 minutes):
    - Inability to cope with cold shock:
        - Hyperventilation continues and swimming/breathing becomes uncoordinated, leading to water inhalation and wet drowning.
- Long term:
    - Hypothermia:
        - Wet drowning
        - Ventricular fibrillation.
- Post rescue:
    - During immersion, the hydrostatic pressure of the water supports an otherwise compromised circulation.
    - When the body is removed from the water, this support is suddenly removed, and may cause catastrophic circulatory collapse (similar to suddenly deflating a PASG).
    - This effect may be exacerbated by rapid rewarming.

Management

Respiratory problems

No apparent water inhalation

- If some water is aspirated:
    - Adult respiratory distress syndrome (ARDS) may develop 0-72 hours later.
        - *Signs:*
            - Cough, rising respiratory rate, crackles on chest auscultation.
        - *Management:*
            - Observation for 24 hours:
                - If they develop signs of ARDS: early aggressive ARDS management (O_2, PEEP).

Note:- 12-20% of patients with no apparent water inhalation die for no known reason --"dry drowning":
    - This may possibly be due to a primitive diving reflex:
        - Results in laryngeal spasm and bradycardia.
    - In children, spontaneous respiratory effort is associated with a full recovery.

Some water inhalation, but adequate ventilation

Incidence:
- Commonest group.

Signs:
- Respiratory distress, cyanosis and painful wheezy breathing.

Management:
- Oxygen.
- Admit for observation.

Water inhalation and inadequate ventilation

Management:
- Clear the airway: if it is blocked by water consider:
  - Inversion.
- Mouth to mouth/mask, expired air resuscitation.
- Oxygen (100%) using an oxygen reservoir (because of the severe hypoxia resulting from drowning).
- Ventilation: high pressures may be needed due to increased pulmonary compliance.
- Frequent suctioning (or turn the patient onto their side to allow drainage of fluid from the mouth).
- If the patient is unconscious consider:
  - Intubation
  - Insertion of a nasogastric tube.

Note: - Most water is usually in the stomach; getting it out by any method other than by a nasogastric tube risks causing pulmonary aspiration of the gastric contents.

No ventilation or cardiac output

Management
- Basic Life Support (this should be started in the water if possible).
- Advanced airway and cardiac management.

Cardiovascular problems

Cardiac arrest
- This may often be delayed.
- Ventricular fibrillation is the usual mode of death.

Symptoms/signs
- Pulse: feel for the carotid pulse for at least 10 seconds
- The skin colour is often misleading.

Management
- Basic life support:
  - If the heart restarts, the survival rate increases from 8% to 70%.
  - This should be continued for at least 1 hour or until the body temperature is greater than 32 °C (34 °C core temperature).
- ECG and temperature monitoring should be carried out continuously.
- Advanced Cardiac Life Support:
  - Defibrillation should be performed for ventricular fibrillation, but not until the patient's temperature >32 °C (the myocardium is not responsive to defibrillation at very low temperatures).
- If the patient has poor peripheral perfusion, with signs suggestive of hypovolaemia, then administer an intravenous infusion of colloid (with sodium bicarbonate 8.4%, if resuscitation is prolonged).

Circulatory collapse

Management
- The body should be held as horizontally as possible before removal from the water.
- If there are signs of circulatory collapse, a PASG may be applied and the BP and pulse monitored.
- Rewarming should be carefully controlled.

Cold injury

Management
- If the patient is conscious:
    - Rapid rewarming is indicated, if immersion has been brief
    - Gradual rewarming, if immersion has been prolonged.
- If the patient is unconscious:
    - Rewarm slowly in clothing with insulation (plastic bag, etc.). This reduces the risk of increasing any cerebral oedema, or circulatory collapse.
- Monitor the patient's temperature continuously with a rectal thermometer or thermocouple.

Brain injury

Management
- Basic and Advanced Life Support (to improve/maintain cerebral oxygenation).

Associated problems

- Head/Neck injuries:
    - Immobilise the cervical spine in a rigid cervical collar, if there is *any* possibility of a cervical spine injury.
- Myocardial infarction
- Cerebral vascular accidents
- Epilepsy
- Hypoglycaemia
- Alcoholic intoxication
- Drug abuse
- Diving dysbarism.

Guidelines for the management of near drowning

Basic Life Support (this should be started in the water if possible)
- Airway management: with stabilisation of the cervical spine if injury is suspected (cervical collar).
- Breathing: expired air ventilation.
- Circulation: external chest compressions.

Remove from the water: without allowing the casualty to pull you in!

Advanced airway management

Hypothermia: Dry and start rewarming

Monitor temperature continuously

Advanced Cardiac Life Support: as the temperature rises and it is likely to be effective.

Treat any associated problems

Resuscitation should be continued for at least 45 minutes and/or until the body temperature is near normal.

Dysbarism

Introduction

- This is a condition caused by rapid changes in the environmental pressures to which the patient is subjected.
- Many patients suffering from dysbarism may also be suffering from other associated problems, e.g. near drowning, hypothermia, injury accidents.
- Dysbarism is a relatively rare problem and is only something that military doctors and those who have an interest in diving, climbing or flying will come across in normal circumstances.

High altitude: low pressure dysbarism

Incidence

- Virtually unknown in the UK, as there are no mountains over 1500 m high, but may occur due to sudden depressurisation in aircraft.

Aetiology

- A significant reduction in atmospheric pressure may occur during flying/climbing at altitudes greater than 3500 m (aircraft cabin pressures go up to 2750 m).

Pathophysiology

- At high altitudes, there is less oxygen due to the reduced atmospheric pressure, and hypoxia develops.
- Too rapid an ascent does not allow physiological compensation to occur.
- Mountain sickness, due to mild cerebral oedema, may occur at heights >2500 m, affecting 70% of people at heights between 3500-4000 m.
- At heights above 4000 m, about 2% of people develop high altitude pulmonary oedema (HAPO), resulting in cardio-respiratory failure and cardiac arrest.
- At heights above 4500 m, about 1% of people will develop high altitude cerebral oedema (HACO), usually resulting in death.
- Above 5000 m, 50% of people will suffer from flame shaped retinal haemorrhages, which may result in blindness.

Symptoms/signs

Mountain sickness
- Dyspnoea, tachycardia and insomnia.
- Headache, nausea, anorexia, vomiting and diarrhoea.

High altitude pulmonary oedema (HAPO)
- Rapid onset of severe breathlessness, nocturnal dyspnoea, chest pain and cough with haemoptysis

High altitude cerebral oedema (HACO)
- Headache, drowsiness, ataxia, nystagmus and papilloedema.
- Irrationality, hallucinations, unconsciousness, coma and death.

Management

- Removal to a low altitude.
- Oxygen.
- Mountain sickness:
    - Antiemetics: prochlorperazine buccal preparation (Buccastem), metoclopramide.
    - Oral electrolyle replacement: Dioralyte, Rehidrat, Electrolade.
- High altitude pulmonary oedema:
    - Diuretics.
    - Intubation and ventilation (possibly with PEEP).
    - Nifedipine 20 mg S/R 6 hourly.
- High altitude cerebral oedema:
    - Dexamethasone: 8 mg initially followed by 4 mg 6 hourly, or betamethasone.

Diving diseases: low altitude: high pressure dysbarism

- Diving is a very popular sport with over 50000 participants in the UK.
- Some 150-200 cases of serious dysbarism occur annually in the civilian population.
- Although most patients present to coastal centres, a significant number present to their GP or local Accident and Emergency department as the onset of symptoms is often delayed and not recognised as being diving related.
- Diving to deeper than 50 metres is usually done only by professional divers, who have their own specialist occupational health and medical backup offshore. Any problems that they may encounter are beyond the scope of this book.

Compression barotrauma (compression dysbarism)

Aetiology
- Only found in divers or fliers.

Pathophysiology
- As a diver descends in the water the pressure around him increases by 1 atmosphere for every 10 metres (33 ft) descended.
- As the pressure increases, gas becomes compressed.
- Human tissues are incompressible, but hollow spaces, e.g sinuses, the lungs, etc. are not.
- Unless extra gas enters these spaces:
    - The space will either collapse (lungs, chest or abdomen)   *or*
    - Extra fluid or tissue will be drawn into the space (sinuses).

Ear compression barotrauma

Incidence
- This is a relatively common problem, especially in inexperienced divers.

Pathophysiology
- If the pressure on one side of the tympanic membrane is very much greater than that on the other side, injury to the membrane will result.
- This may be:
    - Haemorrhage
    - Rupture, sometimes with obliteration of the middle ear space by a serosanguinous exudate.

Symptoms/signs
- Pain in the ear: usually very severe.

Management
- Prevention:
    - Clearing the ears (Valsalva manoeuvre): this allows pressure equalisation on both sides of the tympanic membrane.
- Analgesia:
    - Oral analgesics are usually adequate.
    - Do *not* use nitrous oxide when there is any indication of decompression sickness.

Round window rupture

Incidence
- Rare.

Symptoms (similar to those from inner ear decompression sickness)
- Tinnitus
- Disorientation
- Giddiness.

Management
- Urgent assessment by an ear, nose and throat consultant or specialist.

Sinus compression barotrauma

Pathophysiology
- If the openings to the sinuses become blocked due to catarrhal swelling, polypi or a deviated nasal septum, pressure equalisation between the sinuses and the upper respiratory tract cannot take place.
- On descent, the volume of air in the sinus decreases and because the bone of the sinus is rigid, a negative pressure develops inside the sinus, which then becomes filled with transudate.
- During ascent, the air in the sinus re-expands, and aggravates the injury to the previously traumatised mucosa (lining) of the sinus.
- If large vessels are involved there may be severe haemorrhage.
- May (rarely) result in facial nerve neuropraxia.

Symptoms/signs
- There may be severe pain.
- Haemorrhage from nose.
- Facial weakness (may be difficult to distinguish from weakness caused by gas embolism, or cranial nerve involvement in decompression sickness).

Management
  - Pain relief.
  - Treatment of shock, if the haemorrhage is severe.

Pulmonary compression barotrauma

Incidence
  - Only occurs in breath holding divers and is very rare.

Pathophysiology
  - As the diver descends, the volume of gas (air) in the lungs decreases and it becomes more dense, due to the increase in pressure:
    - At 30 metres (99 ft) depth the pressure increases to 4 atmospheres (atmospheric pressure + 3 atmospheres).
  - In the breath holding diver, the lung volume gets smaller until it approaches the residual volume, resulting in a change in the chest configuration from one of inspiration to one of expiration. Further descent and resulting pressure increase will result in haemorrhage into the alveoli (*chest squeeze*).
  - In order to overcome these problems, the diver needs to be supplied with air, which is at the same pressure as the surrounding water. This is done either by:
    - Supplying air at the appropriate pressure via an air line *or*
    - A self-contained underwater breathing apparatus (SCUBA), which supplies air at the appropriate pressure via a demand valve.

Symptoms/signs
  - Dyspnoea, with respiratory distress and cyanosis.
  - Ventilatory insufficiency, and pulmonary oedema.

Management
  - Careful evacuation to the surface.
  - Oxygen.
  - Artificial ventilation, using PEEP, if there is low arterial oxygen tension.

Decompression illness/decompression barotrauma

Aetiology

  - Occurs on return to atmospheric pressure following significant exposure to increased pressure (depth and time) as a consequence of inert gas bubble formation (see below):
    - Too rapid an ascent from depth without due regard to the Diving Tables. These dictate the speed of ascent and the number of stops necessary, depending on the depth dived and the time spent at that depth:
      - Poor diving discipline.
      - Following equipment failure.
      - Accident and panic.
      - Submarine escape.
      - May occur from *any* dive in which air is breathed from a SCUBA.
  - May even (rarely) occur if standard decompression procedures (Diving Tables/Computers) are followed rigorously.
  - Sudden decompression in an aircraft.

Pathophysiology

- As pressure is reduced, gases expand.
- If the reduction in pressure is too rapid, it may cause problems for the human body in two ways:

Systemic decompression barotrauma: the "bends"
- Gases which are usually dissolved in the blood and tissues, form bubbles.
    - These bubbles may be intravascular and/or extravascular, and they cause problems in two ways:
        - Have a mechanical effect: blocking arterioles, etc.
        - There is a reaction at the bubble/tissue interface resulting in:
            - Protein denaturation
            - Lipid emboli
            - Red cell sludging
            - Platelet aggregation
            - Activation of clotting mechanisms
            - Histamine release.

Pulmonary decompresssion barotrauma: air embolism
- As the diver ascends, the air in the lungs expands. He should breathe out, but if he does not, or if a mucous plug obstructs an alveolus, pressure builds up in the alveoli and alveolar rupture may occur.
    - The rupture may extend:
        - Through the visceral pleura to cause a pneumothorax.
        - Anteriorly to cause a pneumopericardium, mediastinal emphysema and subcutaneous emphysema.
        - Into the pulmonary veins to cause a pulmonary air embolism, resulting in an arterial air embolism usually in the brain or limbs, but it may affect any part of the body.

Note:- In practice the disease has a wide spectrum of symptomatology, and it is frequently not possible to distinguish between the two types of illness.

Symptoms/signs

- These may vary very considerably depending on the individual patient's physiology, the rate of ascent, and the duration and depth of the dive.

Mild decompression illness

- Symptoms usually begin within the first hour of surfacing, but may be delayed for up to and occasionally more than 24 hours.
- Unexplained fatigue, malaise and anorexia.
- Transient pruritis especially of ears, hands and wrists (common).
- Musculoskeletal pain around synovial joints (*Limb or joint bends*):
    - This usually begins as an ache, and initially is often attributed to physical exertion, lifting heavy equipment, etc.
    - Initially it may flit from joint to joint, before becoming localised and more severe.
        - Most common sites:
            - Shoulder
            - Knee.
    - It is rare for there to be associated tenderness; if this is present, consider another cause.

- Skin rashes:
    - Trunk/abdomen:
        - Patches of cutaneous venous stasis and cyanosis.
    - Limbs:
        - Cutaneous and subcutaneous oedema, occasionally with swelling and tenderness of the regional lymph nodes.
    - Any part of the body:
        - Local oedema due to bubble formation in lymphatics (rare).

More severe decompression illness

- Usually appears within a few minutes of surfacing, but may be delayed for several hours.

Neurological effects (the most common)
- Usually affects the brain or spinal cord, and very rarely the peripheral nerves.
- Any neurological deficit or combination of lesions may occur (often from more than one site)
    - Cerebral decompression illness:
        - Unconsciousness
        - Visual disturbance, particularly of peripheral vision
        - Migraine-like headaches
        - Behavioural alteration: cognitive dysfunction, personality and mood changes
        - Symptoms/signs of a cerebral vascular accident.
    - Spinal decompression illness:
        - Paralysis or paresis of limbs (commonly)
        - Paraesthesiae
        - Girdle pains of the trunk
        - Bladder, sphincter or sexual dysfunction.
    - Inner ear decompression illness:
        - Vertigo with nausea and vomiting (*Staggers*).
        - Tinnitus (this may be difficult to distinguish from barotrauma to the middle ear).

Pulmonary effects (*Chokes*)
- May develop slowly, and are rarely associated with neurological damage:
    - Chest pain due to:
        - Pneumothorax.
    - Retrosternal pain on inspiration.
    - Dyspnoea.
    - Signs of hypoxia in severe cases.

Circulatory effects (occurs due to the rise in capillary permeability)
- Hypovolaemia.
- Haemoconcentration.
- Hypotension.
- Peripheral circulatory failure.

Dermatological effects
- Subcutaneous emphysema (additional symptoms include change of voice quality).

Management

- Recompresssion (treatment of choice):
    - This should be done as soon as possible; the patient will be taken down to the depth of his dive, and then very slowly decompressed.
    - Any delay may lead to deterioration in the patient's condition.
- Prior to and during transport:
    - Oxygen:
        - 100% which may displace the less soluble nitrogen from the air bubbles.
    - Intubation:
        - If the patient requires intubation, the cuff should be filled with water rather than air (volume change during recompression).
    - Ventilation:
        - Should be done with great care, and chest drains inserted immediately if there is any evidence of a pneumothorax.
    - Intravenous infusion:
        - In every severe case.
        - If there is evidence of hypovolaemia.
        - Crystalloid is generally preferred to colloid, although some think that Dextran 40 may have specific advantages due to its low molecular size, in spite of the risk of it causing renal tubular necrosis.
    - Steroids:
        - Dexamethasone: 16 mg administered intravenously immediately followed by 10-12 mg 6 hourly may be considered for patients with cerebral problems.
    - Analgesia:
        - Not often used.
        - Paracetamol is preferred (aspirin make aggravate capillary bleeding within the nervous system).
        - Nitrous oxide/oxygen mixture (Entonox/Nitronox) is *absolutely contraindicated*.
    - Sedation/fits
        - Intravenous midazolam or diazepam.
    - Catheterisation
        - It is prudent to assess whether or not the patient can empty his bladder. If not, he should be catheterised, and the catheter balloon filled with water and *not* air.

Note:- Any symptoms presenting within 36 hours of a dive should be considered to be due to dysbarism until proven otherwise.

Transportation of the patient with high pressure dysbarism

- If air transport is used, e.g. helicopter:
    - The pilot should fly at as low an altitude as possible, as any significant reduction in pressure will aggravate the patient's condition.
- With road transport:
    - In mountainous areas the lower altitude route is to be preferred.
- In order to assist the doctor receiving the patient for recompression, the following information should be supplied:
    - Depth and duration of last two dives.
    - Any problems with ascent or descent.
    - Did the patient get unduly cold or work particularly hard during his dive.
    - Was his diving discipline good or did he omit any decompression procedures (stops).
    - All the diving equipment used and the patient's diving partner "buddy" should always accompany the patient.

Other diving problems

- Diving dysbarism in particular may be associated with other problems, which may considerably complicate management:
    - Near drowning.
    - Hypothermia.
    - Breathing bad air: carbon monoxide is the commonest.

Advice on medical diving problems

- The Royal Navy provides a **24 hour emergency advice service**, which will give information on:
    - The location of the nearest medical diving problem treatment facility (recompression chamber).
    - The emergency management of diving related illness.

- The **emergency telephone number** is: **0831 151523** (cellular telephone)
    - If there is difficulty in obtaining a reply, use:
      Portsmouth (0705) - 822351 ext. 41769 during the working day (0800 - 1600)
                        - 818888 out of hours.

- Please state that you have a medical diving problem.

14

Head injuries

Head injuries

Introduction

- Head injury is probably the most significant single injury encountered in Immediate Care, as either in isolation or in combination with other injuries, its severity affects the eventual outcome more than any other injury.
- Half of all those patients who die as a result of head injury, do so before they reach hospital. The skilful and aggressive pre-hospital management of these injuries is the only way that this appalling waste of (mostly young) life may be reduced.

Incidence

- Head injury is common in the UK:
    - Nearly 2000 patients per 100000 attend an Accident and Emergency department annually of whom approximately 250 per 100000 population require admission as a result.
    - Occurs in 60-70% of all road traffic accidents.
- Approximately 9 per 100000 population die as a result, the majority of these die within the first 24 hours following injury.
- 25% of all multiply injured patients who die, do so as a result of their head injury.
- Head injury is the commonest cause of death in the 15-24 age group.
- Children:
    - Head injury is the commonest single cause of death in children aged over 1 year accounting for:
        - 25% of deaths in children aged 5-15 years
        - 15% of deaths in children age 1-15 years.
    - Half of all those admitted with a head injury are under 20 years old.

Aetiology

- The commonest causes are:
    - Road traffic accidents
    - Assaults
    - Falls.
- Other significant causes are:
    - Sporting accidents, especially golf (in children), riding.
    - Industrial accidents.
- Alcohol related head injury is very common.

- Commonest cause of head injury in:
    - Males: Road traffic accidents.
    - Females: Domestic accidents.
    - Children:
        - Road traffic accidents: 76% (most as pedestrians)
        - Falls: 13%
        - Aspiration of vomit (10% died before reaching hospital).

Pathophysiology

- Head injury is a dynamic situation, involving both acceleration and deceleration.
- Injury often involves all three tissues: scalp, skull and brain.
- Head injuries may be subdivided according to their cause:

Penetrating (or open) head injuries

Aetiology
- The head is usually static or moving at a low velocity, and is struck by a small relatively high velocity, often sharp, object.

Pathophysiology
- The outer coverings of the brain are penetrated, resulting in exposure of the intracranial compartment to the exterior.
- Fragments of bone, scalp, hair, clothing, the vehicle and road may be carried into the brain substance:
    - This may be both epileptogenic and act a focus of infection resulting in meningitis, brain abscess and osteomyelitis.
- There is often no history of unconsciousness.
- If the injury is in a neurologically "eloquent" area of the brain, focal neurological deficits may occur.

Blunt (closed or concussional) head injuries

Aetiology
- The head is subjected to sudden acceleration and deceleration often associated with rotation.
- There is usually a period of unconsciousness.

Pathophysiology
- These injuries may be classified according to the duration of unconsciousness or coma into:

Major head injury
- There may be prolonged or profound loss of consciousness:
    - Coma lasting >6 hours.
    - Post traumatic amnesia >24 hours.

Minor head injury
- Accounts for the majority of head injuries.
- The injury is frequently trivial.
- Short initial period of unconsciousness (<6 hours).
- Post traumatic amnesia is short (<24 hours).
- The majority recover fully.

Scalp injury

Pathophysiology

- There may be:
    - Contusion:
        - Bruising may indicate the site of impact and thus of underlying injury.
    - Laceration:
        - Caused by impact with sharp objects.
    - Avulsion:
        - Caused by a tangential force.
- The scalp has an extremely good blood supply, and often haemorrhage may be profuse, and if left untreated, may result in hypovolaemic shock, especially in children and the elderly.
- The absence of scalp injury does not preclude brain injury.

Management

- Haemorrhage:
    - Application of direct pressure:
        - Pressure dressing (skin flaps should be restored to their anatomical position before applying any dressings, so as to avoid causing ischaemia in a creased flap).
    - Clips/artery forceps:
        - If used, these should be applied to the cut edge of the galea, which should then be pulled up so as to compress the blood vessels between the galea and the skin (usually, just hanging the forceps over the edge of the skin flap, will produce sufficient control, by virtue of their weight alone).
        - *No* attempt should be made to grasp the bleeding vessel itself.
    - Undersewing with a quick tacking stitch (not usually possible in the pre-hospital situation)
    - Intravenous infusion with colloid to prevent/treat any hypovolaemic shock (see below).

Skull injury

Pathophysiology

- A deforming force such as a deceleration impact applied to the skull will tend to produce a fracture.
- Fractures are usually linear and extend from the impact site.
- The length and shape of fracture lines depend on the degree of force, the area that the force is applied to, and the structure and thickness of the skull.
- The severity of any fracture is an indication of the degree of force involved/used.
- Fracture usually involves the vault or less often the base of skull, or occasionally both.
- Skull fractures are not usually significant in themselves, but their presence indicates a greatly increased risk of:
    - Cerebrospinal fluid leakage.
    - Cranial nerve damage.
    - Intracranial haematoma.

Symptoms/signs

- Mastoid bruising (Battle's sign):
    - Indicates a probable fractured base of skull (middle cranial fossa).

- Periorbital haematoma:
  - In the absence of an injury to the eye itself, this may be indicative of:
    - Blow-out fracture of the orbital floor
    - Anterior (middle third) skull fracture.

Management

- Airway care with stabilisation of the cervical spine if indicated:
  - Maintenance of adequate oxygenation.
- Breathing: maintenance of adequate ventilation.

Complications of head injury

CSF leak

Aetiology/pathophysiology
- Indicates a compound skull fracture with an associated dural tear:
  - Rhinorhoea (most common cause of CSF leak) indicates:
    - Anterior fossa fractures (25%), including the frontal ethmoid or sphenoid sinuses, especially the cribriform plate (50% of patients will have anosmia).
    - Fracture of the petrous temporal bone (rarely).
  - Otorrhoea indicates:
    - Fracture of base of skull (7%)
    - Laceration or perforation of the eardrum.

Sign
- CSF may be a clear or bloodstained fluid, which if put on a slide will separate out so that the red cells concentrate in the centre of a drop of fluid the "Ring Test" for CSF.

Aerocoele

Cranial nerve palsy

Incidence
- Occurs in about 30% of patients with severe head injuries
- Commonest:
  - I: Anosmia: may occur in association with fractures of the cribriform plate, followed by:
  - VII: Facial nerve palsy.
  - VIII: Deafness.
- Less common:
  - III: Traumatic midriasis: pupil dilation (may indicate uncal herniation associated with cerebral oedema).
- Others are rare.

Aetiology
- May occur as a result of a fracture of:
  - Cribriform plate: I (may also occur in mild head injury without skull fracture).
  - Orbit (apex) or cavernous sinus: II, III, IV and VI.
  - Base of skull: VI (diplopia)
  - Petrous temporal bone: VII, VIII.

Management
- Very little in the Immediate Care situation, other than recording any obvious deficit and drawing the attention of the receiving doctor to it.

Intracranial haemorrhage

- This is the major cause of preventable early death following head injury.

Pathophysiology

- Occurs as a result of laceration of blood vessels:
    - Within the skull, e.g. middle meningeal artery.
    - Adjacent to bone, e.g. the major dural sinuses.

Extradural (epidural) haemorrhage

Incidence:
- <2% of all head injury admissions.

Aetiology:
- Usually associated with skull fracture.

Pathophysiology:
- Middle meningeal: temporal or parietal haematoma.
- Dural sinuses: frontal or occipital haematoma.

Subdural haemorrhage

Aetiology:
- Occurs as a result of rupture of the bridging veins from the cortex to the dural sinuses.

Brain injury

Pathophysiology

- Sudden deceleration results in distortion of brain tissue; the actual amount of brain damage being related to the degree of stretching.

Mechanism of injury

- Contusion *coup* and *contra coup* (often worse).
- Laceration:
    - On sharp bits of skull, e.g. sphenoidal ridge.
- Shearing injury:
    - If rotational forces are involved.
- "Brain stem" injury:
    - This is the cause of unconsciousness (reticular activating system).

Natural history
- Brain is a:
    - Fluid, and is therefore incompressible.
    - Biological tissue and its response to injury is swelling.
        - Intracranial swelling leads to elevation of intracranial pressure.
        - An elevated intracranial pressure threatens cerebral perfusion, and reduces venous outflow, thus further increasing cerebral oedema and pressure (worse if there is CO_2 retention).
        - Cerebral perfusion is all important, and depends on adequate blood pressure and oxygenation:
            - Perfusion pressure = mean arterial blood pressure - intracranial pressure.

Compensation mechanisms
- Cerebral spinal fluid:
    - Increased absorption.
    - Displacement with compression of the ventricles.
- Venous:
    - Venous compression.
- Arterial:
    - Cushing's reflex:
        - This results in a rise in blood pressure, an early reduction and later elevation in the pulse rate and widening of the pulse pressure.
        - Rising intracerebral pressure eventually results in herniation of brain tissue through the tentorial opening and/or foramen magnum.

Decompensation mechanisms
- Brain shift:
    - Compartmental herniation.
- Loss of compensation results in an exponential deterioration in the patient's condition.
- Secondary brain stem compression "secondary head injury":
    - Reduction in the level of consciousness.
    - Deterioration of respiratory and cardiac function.
    - Untreated (untreatable) herniation results in secondary brain stem infarction.

Causes of death following head injury

First injury -------------------- Severe brain injury

Second injury --------

Intracranial complications
- Haemorrhage or oedema resulting in:

Increased intracranial pressure
- Shown by:
  - Deterioration in the level of consciousness
  - Reduction in pulse rate
  - Rise in blood pressure
  - Increase in respiratory rate
  - Vomiting and/or fitting

Chest complications
- Reduced ventilation: inhalation, pneumothorax

Multiple injuries
- Hypovolaemia

Assessment

History

- Obtaining and providing an accurate history is probably more important in the head injured patient than in any other type of injury, as the patient's hospital management depends on exactly what has happened to him. It is up to those at the scene of the accident to obtain and provide it.
- The history should include:
  - The time of injury.
  - The type of injury.
  - The estimated speed of impact/amount of deceleration.
  - The mechanism of injury, especially if there is any indication of associated injury to the cervical spine, e.g. hyperextension of the neck.
  - Whether or not the head injury was secondary to some other event: syncope, AMI or fit.
  - Whether or not a crash helmet, seat belt, etc. was worn.
  - Whether or not alcohol was involved.
  - The patient's condition immediately afterwards and any changes in that condition.
  - Any periods of altered consciousness: If so when ? how long ?
  - Amnesia:
    - Retrograde amnesia.
    - Post-traumatic amnesia.

Practical point: If the casualty was wearing a crash helmet of any type, it should be sent with him to hospital, as careful examination of it may give a very good idea as to the mechanism of injury/impact and the amount of force involved.

Symptoms/signs

- It is extremely important in head injured patients to record the patients's symptoms, and obtain and record serial observations of their vital signs.

Primary assessment

Airway
- Impaired consciousness may result in airway obstruction by the tongue, dentures, vomit.

Breathing
- Increased respiratory rate, irregularity of respiration.
- Oxygen saturation:
    - A reduced saturation indicates reduced ventilatory efficiency, and the cause should be looked for and treated.

Circulation
- Blood pressure.
- Pulse: rate, volume, regularity.
- Never assume that hypotension is caused by head injury.

Disability (neurological state)
- State of higher functions:
    - Confusion, unconsciousness.
    - Irritability (indicates hypoxia).
- "Vegetative" disorders: vomiting.
- Hypersecretion: bronchus, saliva.
- Motor dysfunction: decerebration.
- Fits
- Pupil abnormalities:
    - Pupil size changes are usually a late and serious sign, and are unlikely in the alert patient.
    - Unilateral pupil dilation:
        - Indicates an uncal herniation with occulomotor lobe dysfunction.
        - Associated brain stem compression may indicate a developing space occupying lesion, e.g. haematoma.
    - Bilateral dilation and loss of reactivity indicates secondary brain stem compression, with a risk of brain stem infarction, an increasing amount of brain stem injury and eventually an irreversible situation.
- Temperature elevation.

Initial neurological assessment
- This is especially important in head injuries, and is useful both as a prognostic indicator, and as a guide to further management.
- Measure/establish the base lines (including temperature if possible/practicable).
- Compare these with the history.
- Record them for future reference.

AVPU scale

A: Alert
V: Responds to verbal stimuli
P: Responds to painful stimuli
U: Unresponsive

Management

- The first priority is to reduce any cerebral hypoxia and hypercapnia and to preserve the vital functions.

Airway care

- Airway protection
    - From obstruction: position, airway.
    - From aspiration, especially if there is a history of alcohol ingestion: intubation.
- Oxygen (vital)
    - In as high a concentration as possible, as even slight hypoxia results in an increase in brain swelling and intracranial pressure.
- Cervical spine protection

Note:- It must be assumed that the unconscious head injured patient has a cervical spine injury until proven otherwise, and they must be handled accordingly, and the neck immobilised in a rigid cervical collar.

Breathing: ventilation care

- Ventilation
    - This should be considered especially if the patient has an associated chest injury, depressed respiration or a compromised airway necessitating intubation.
    - If there is evidence of inadequate ventilation, consideration should be given to hyperventilating the patient so as to reduce brain swelling and increase oxygenation.
    - In children intubation should be considered due to the high risk of gastric aspiration.

Note: - Chest injury is often (in up to 40% of patients) associated with serious head injury, and exacerbates any hypoxia (the prognosis is much worse).
    - Head injured patients tolerate hypoxia badly, so it is very important to treat any chest injury impairing efficient respiration, e.g. pneumothorax, flail chest, early.

- Sedation
    - The commonest cause of cerebral irritability is hypoxia, which requires immediate treatment.
    - Cerebral irritability results in inappropriate muscular action, and exacerbates hypoxia, by diverting the circulation to the skeletal muscles, which metabolise the already scarce oxygen.
    - Sedation may be appropriate in the confused hypoxic and violent patient in whom airway and respiratory care to correct their hypoxia is not possible because of the difficulty experienced in restraining them and preventing them from removing airway devices, e.g. oxygen mask, airway.
    - The drug of choice is midazolam or diazepam, titrated to the patient response (for dosage, see chapter on Pain Relief).

- Fitting
    - This usually indicates severe cerebral injury with focal injury or increased intracranial pressure.
    - It may result in impairment of oxygenation and ventilation, making efficient management of the patient difficult, and will exacerbate hypoxia.
    - The treatment is administration of midazolam or diazepam (see above).

Cardiovascular care

- Hypotension
    - This is *not* caused by head injury (patients with a head injury do not regulate their blood pressure when there is coexistant blood loss).
    - If hypotension is present, it *must* be due to hypovolaemia, which if not treated will exacerbate any hypoxia.

Management
    - Establish an intravenous infusion which will reduce hypoxia if the patient is hypovolaemic.
    - Colloids are preferred to crystalloids, as they are less likely to cause cerebral oedema.
    - Treatment of the cause of the hypovolaemia, e.g. splinting of fractures.
    - Analgesia:
        - This is important especially if the patient is restless and in pain, as pain itself may result in a rise in intracranial pressure
        - It is mandatory to record the patient's neurological status before and after administration of analgesics, especially opiates, which may cause a change in the patient's pupil size, level of consciousness and respiratory state, together with the time the drug was administered.
    - The patient's response to treatment should be carefully monitored (see below).

General care

- Treat other injuries:
    - Dress lacerations/abrasions
    - Splint fractures.

Associated problems affecting management

- Alcohol:
    - Coma will be present with alcohol levels >400 mg/100 ml.
    - Intoxication is usually evident at 100 mg/100 ml.
- Drugs:
    - If the patient has pinpoint pupils: administration of naloxone 4 mg intravenously may be beneficial.
- Hypoglycaemia:
    - If hypoglycaemia is a possibility, intravenous glucose or glucagon may be administerd (it can do no harm and may be beneficial).

Evacuation

- If the patient has a significant head injury, he should be evacuated to a Neurosurgical Unit, if circumstances and local geography permit.

Monitoring

Secondary neurological assessment

- It is very important to carry out serial observations of all the vital signs, at regular intervals so as to detect any changes or "trends" in the patient's condition.
- Should be performed in the pre-hospital situation *only* if it will not cause unnecessary delay in evacuation of the patient.

Glasgow coma scale

- This is based on eye opening, best verbal and motor reponses and is a practical method of monitoring changes in the patient's condition and level of consciousness.

Eye opening	Spontaneously	4
	To verbal command	3
	To pain	2
	No response	1
Best motor response	To verbal command: Obeys	6
	To painful stimulus: Localises pain	5
	Flexion/withdrawal	4
	Flexion decorticate	3
	Extension decerebrate	2
	None	1
Best verbal response	Orientated/converses	5
	Disorientated/confused	4
	Inappropriate words	3
	Incomprehensible sounds	2
	Nil	1
	Total	**(3-15)**

PRACTICAL POINT:- *The coma scale may be expressed as: E1, M1, V1, etc. (This may be useful when communicating by radio.)*

Head/skull

- Examination of the patient's head for:
    - Abrasion or laceration to the scalp
    - Scalp haematoma formation
    - Depressed fracture
    - CSF rhinorrhoea or otorrhoea
    - Bleeding from the ear
    - Mastoid bruising.

Sensation

- A brief examination, including the perianal area.

Reflexes

- Deep tendon reflexes (including plantar responses).

Prognosis

Factors associated with poor prognosis:
- Increasing age.
- Abnormal motor signs.
- Pupil abnormalities.
- Massive lesions.
- Diffuse bilateral CT lesions.
- Multiple injuries.
- Increasing intracerebral pressure.

Guidelines for the management of patients with a recent head injury

Criteria for skull X-ray after recent head injury

- Skull X-rays can be helpful, but clinical judgement is necessary and the following criteria will be refined by further experience.
- The presence of one or more of the following indicates a need for X-ray in patients with a history of recent head injury:
    - Loss of consciousness or amnesia at any time.
    - Neurological symptoms or signs.
    - Cerebrospinal fluid or blood from the mouth or ears.
    - Suspected penetrating injury or scalp bruising or swelling.
    - Alcohol intoxication.
    - Difficulty in assessing the patient, e.g. in the young, epileptic, intoxicated.

Note: - Simple scalp laceration does not meet these criteria.

Criteria for admission after a recent head injury

- The presence of one or more of the following:
    - Confusion or any other depression in the level of consciousness at the time of admission.
    - Open skull fracture.
    - Neurological signs or severe headache or persistent vomiting.
    - Difficulty in assessing the patient, e.g. due to alcohol, in the young, in epilepsy.
    - Other medical conditions, e.g. haemophilia, epilepsy (due to the risk of a secondary injury during a fit).
    - The patient's social conditions or lack of a responsible adult or relative.

Note: - Post-traumatic amnesia with full recovery is not an indication for admission.

Criteria for consultation with a neurosurgical unit

- The presence of one or more of the following:
    - A fractured skull in combination with:
        - *Either:* Confusion or other depression of the level of consciousness.
            - *or:* Focal neurological signs.
            - *or:* Fits.
    - Confusion or other neurological disturbance persisting for more than 12 hours, even if there is no skull fracture.
    - Coma continuing after resuscitation.
    - Suspected open fracture of the vault or the base of skull.
    - Depressed fracture of the skull.
    - Deterioration in the patient's condition.

15

Facial injuries

Facial injuries

Introduction

- Severe facial injuries are often associated with other severe injuries especially of the head, neck and chest and can result in life threatening conditions and require effective Immediate Care if these complications are to be prevented.

Incidence

- Severe facial injuries are relatively uncommon.

Aetiology

- Isolated injury: this usually occurs as a result of blows to the face.
- Commonly caused by road traffic accidents (less so since the introduction of compulsory seat belt wearing).
- Usually associated with head and often chest and abdominal injury.
- Facial fractures are relatively uncommon and are usually the result of very considerable force, e.g. high velocity ejection.
- Fractured mandibles and the zygomatic complex are usually the result of assault and road traffic accidents.

Pathophysiology

- The airway:
    - This may become blocked by vomit, blood, local oedema, fractured teeth, or dentures, displaced bones or debris.

- Circulation:
    - The facial soft tissues have a good blood supply and tend to swell easily and bleed profusely.

Symptoms/signs

- Facial deformity: swelling, oedema.
- Epistaxis.
- Haemorrhage from the mouth.
- There is usually surprisingly little associated pain, except on movements involving the fracture site.
- Inability to close/clench the teeth properly:
    - Anterior open bite indicates a middle 1/3 fracture.

Management

Airway care
- This is especially important in the unconscious patient.
- Airway aids:
    - Oropharyngeal airway.
    - Nasopharyngeal airway (*not* if there is an associated fractured base of skull).
    - Intubation.
- Rarely, there may be difficulty with intubation if this is necessary, due to the distorted anatomy/ swelling, in which case consider cricothyrotomy.
- Put in the lateral position, this:
    - Prevents the tongue causing obstruction of the airway.
    - Allows blood, etc. to drain out of the mouth.
- Remove debris from the mouth: fractured teeth, dentures.

Note:- Always beware of the possibility of an associated cervical spine injury, and take appropriate care when moving the patient.

Circulation care:
- Consider putting up an intravenous infusion.

Soft tissue injury of the face

Pharynx

Pathophysiology
- The pharynx may become swollen from retropharyngeal haemorrhage and oedema.

Symptoms/signs
- Blood in the mouth.
- Difficulty with breathing and swallowing.
- Associated injury: fractured teeth or dentures.

Management
- Gently clear away any debris with suction, under direct vision, if possible (this may not be easy with a conscious patient).

Tongue

Aetiology
- Lacerations:
    - These are usually caused by the teeth, typically by a blow to the underside of the jaw.
    - May also be caused by the patient's dentures, which may be intact or fractured.

Pathophysiology
- The tongue:
    - Has a good vascular supply and tends to bleed profusely.
    - May swell considerably if traumatised.
- Injury may cause major problems with airway maintenance, especially if there is a transverse laceration or a fractured mandible involving the lingual blood vessels.
- Bilateral fracture of the mandible may result in an unstable anterior segment, which may be displaced backwards with the tongue and compromise the airway further.

Symptoms/signs
- Bleeding from the mouth.

Management
- Insert a suture in the tongue to pull it forward.

Method
- Using a curved needle, insert the needle transversely into the dorsum of the middle third of the tongue.
- Tie the suture and pull the tongue forward.

PRACTICAL POINT:- *If a suture is not available, a safety pin and tape or string may be utilised to do the same thing.*
- *If this is not possible, e.g. in severe transverse laceration of the tongue and intubation is not possible, consider a cricothyrotomy.*

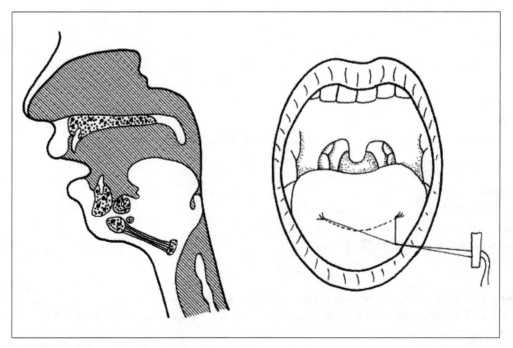

Figure 15-1 Securing the displaced tongue

Larynx/hyoid

Aetiology
- This is a very uncommon injury.
- May be caused by incorrectly adjusted seat belt, or by hanging.

Pathophysiology
- May result in airway obstruction.

Symptoms/signs
- Local swelling and tenderness.
- Dyspnoea.

Management
- Cricothyrotomy if intubation is not possible due to laryngeal disruption.

Eye

Incidence
- Eye injury is now relatively uncommon in road traffic accidents, as a result of the law making the wearing of seat belts compulsory.
- Ocular trauma is responsible for 5% of blind eyes in pre-school and school children.
- More common in males due to sporting, shooting, industrial and DIY activities, drunkenness and subsequent assault and RTAs.
- One third of domestic eye injuries occur in children under 16.

Aetiology
- Usually caused by a direct blow, or penetration by a sharp object, e.g. windscreen and spectacle glass.
- In industry, corneal foreign bodies are the commonest form of occular injury (25-80%), with 60% caused by hammer/chisel fragments.
- Chemical splash injury is also fairly common, especially in the manufacturing and building industries.

Pathophysiology

Penetrating injury of the eye
- Where there is a perforation of the eye, any rise in extraocular pressure may result in extrusion of part of the intraocular contents, especially the iris.

Bruising of the eye and lids
- This often occurs as a result of assault, or sometimes in sporting activities, especially ball games, e.g. squash, badminton, cricket and football:
    - Squash balls are hard, travel very fast (over 100 mph) and fit the eye socket exactly.
    - Badminton quoits may also cause a surprisingly severe degree of injury.
    - Accidental blows from the edge of sports raquets, and elbows can also cause severe injury.

Chemical burns of the eye
- The severity of the injury is related to the duration of contact, and the concentration and pH of the chemical involved.
- Alkalis, including cement and building lime react to form soluble compounds which penetrate the cornea almost immediately.
- Weak acids have much more limited tissue penetration.

Symptoms/signs

Penetrating injury
- Usually there is obvious damage to the cornea, with accompanying lacerations of the face and eyelids and with deformity of the pupil and sometimes prolapse of the iris or vitreous, the presence of uveal tissue in the wound, and sub-conjunctival haemorrhage.

High velocity penetration
- Penetration by small metallic foreign bodies may not be obvious in the Immediate Care situation.
- *Any patient who has felt something go into the eye whilst striking one piece of metal with another, especially a hammer and cold chisel, must be assumed to have sustained a penetrating eye injury until this has been excluded by a full ophthalmological examination including suitable X-rays of the globe.*
- Penetrating injuries of this type are frequently absolutely pain free, seldom cause infection, and visual loss may not occur for days, weeks or even months after the original injury. Failure to recognise them may result in permanent visual loss for the patient and medico-legal proceedings against the doctor concerned.
- *If a penetrating eye injury is suspected urgent ophthalmological follow up is mandatory.*
- May result in brain injury (the commonest cause of death from airgun pellets, in which penetration is through the eye).

Blunt injury
- Lid swelling and bruising.
- Subconjunctival haemorrhage (classical sign of zygomatic complex fracture).
- Unilateral dilated pupil --"traumatic mydriasis".
- Distortion of the pupil:
    - This is due to splits in the iris or to the root of the iris being torn away in one area (iridodonesis).
- Hyphaema:
    - Blood in the anterior chamber, with blurred vision.
- Vitreous haemorrhage:
    - The patient complains of floaters and blurred vision.
- Retinal tears:
    - The patient may complain initially of flashing lights (photopsia), new floaters or visual impairment, including dense shadows in the vision or visual field loss.

Chemical injury
- Severe conjunctival injection with profuse lacrimation and pain.

Management

- Pad the eye.

Prevent complications
- Avoidance of coughing, sneezing, straining, struggling or anything else which might raise either the intraoccular or extraocular pressure.

Chemical burn
- Immediate prolonged copious irrigation with tap water or a buffered solution, if available, is vital.
- The patient's eye may need to be held open by an assistant during irrigation.
- All solid matter, such as particles of cement should be removed with cotton wool buds, if conditions permit, however painful this may be for the patient (consider using amethocaine as a local anaesthetic).
- In severe cases irrigation should be continued for at least 30 minutes.

PRACTICAL POINT: *In the pre-hospital situation an infusion solution of saline or Hartmann's solution attached to a giving set may be used to irrigate the eye.*

Injuries of the facial bones

General

Diagnosis
- Facial fractures are not always obvious.
- If suspected, they should be looked for by careful assessment of the facial contours and teeth, and palpation for surgical emphysema, which may be present when the para-nasal sinuses have been fractured.

Management
- Airway care.
- Treatment of haemorrhage from any cancellous bone exposed at the fracture sites (rare if the fragments are adequately stabilised).

Maxilla

Incidence
- Relatively uncommon injury (although fractures of the zygomatic complex alone is relatively common).

Aetiology
- Usually caused by a direct blow.

Pathophysiology
- If fractured, the maxilla may be displaced backwards and downwards causing/aggravating obstruction of the airway.

Symptoms/signs
- Severe swelling and deformity of the face around the mouth, nose and eyes: "dish or long face".
- There may be obvious mobility of the maxilla and associated fractures of the teeth, which may be ascertained by gripping the upper teeth and adjoining gums and trying to move them. Any movement of the teeth and adjoining gum suggests a Le Fort fracture.
- Cerebrospinal rhinorrhoea.
- Anaesthesia in the area of the infraorbital nerve is often present.
- Irregularities of the dentition may suggest a maxillary or Le Fort fracture.

Management
- If the maxilla is mobile, stabilise it:

Method
- Place a thumb in the arch of the palate and grasping the maxilla by the alveolar margin, lift it upwards and forwards, to try to stabilise it.
- If there is gross displacement and the back of the soft palate is causing airway obstruction (this usually occurs only if there is an associated mandibular fracture), and manual disimpaction is unsuccessful, and intubation is not possible:
  - Perform a cricothyrotomy.
- Management of haemorrhage (which may be profuse):
  - Intravenous infusion.

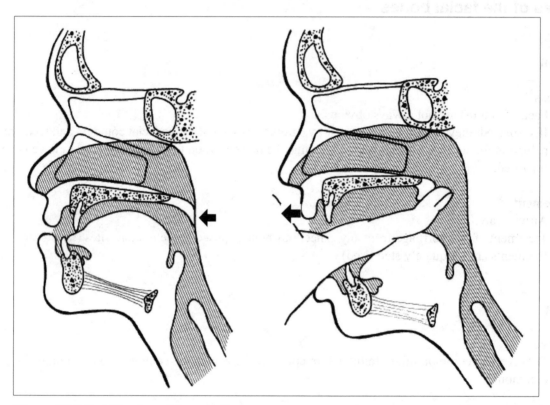

Figure 15-2 Stabilisation of the maxilla

Nasal bones

Incidence
- This is a relatively common injury.

Aetiology
- Usually arises from a direct blow.
- Sometimes associated with significant head injury.

Pathophysiology
- Buckling of the nasal septum or depressed fractures may cause nasal obstruction.
- Associated haemorrhage (which may be severe) and local oedema of the nasal passages may also result in their occlusion.
- If there is any associated obstruction of the oropharyngeal airway, the patient will rapidly asphyxiate.

Symptoms/signs
- Nasal deformity.
- Nasal obstruction: on one or both sides.
- Epistaxis.

Management

Airway
- Position the patient in the lateral position so that blood can drain out of the nose.
- Airway management in the unconscious patient, with care of the cervical spine:
    - Oropharyngeal airway.
    - Intubation.
- If in any doubt, hold the teeth apart with your hands.

Note:- Do *not* hold the jaw forward as this may occlude the oropharyngeal airway.

Haemorrhage
- Apply local pressure (with a cold pack or ice if available).
- Institute an intravenous infusion if the haemorrhage is profuse.
- If haemorrhage is uncontrollable and intubation impossible, consider cricothyrotomy.

Orbit and zygoma

Orbital fracture

Incidence
- This is a relatively common injury.
- Fractures of the inferior orbital floor, "blow-out fracture", are the most common, followed by fractures of the medial orbital wall.

Aetiology
- It is usually caused by a direct blow to the orbit or cheek, by a fist or squash ball.
- There is usually, but by no means always, an associated injury to the eye.

Pathophysiology
- The contents of the orbit may herniate through the inferior orbital floor, "blow-out fracture".
- In particular, the inferior rectus muscle may be trapped and anchored producing total inability to elevate the eye on the injured side.

Symptoms/signs
- Conjunctival/subconjunctival injection or haematoma.
- Periorbital swelling and tenderness.
- Restricted eye movement, especially on attempted upgaze, with double vision.
- Parasthesiae or anaesthesia over the area supplied by the inferior orbital nerve.
- Fractures of the zygoma will often result in a triangular shaped lateral sub-conjunctival haemorrhage and numbness over the cheek.
- If surgical emphysema is present, there must be paranasal sinus involvement, whether or not the patient is symptomatic.

Management
- Pad the affected eye.

Mandible

Incidence
- A relatively common injury.

Aetiology
- Usually caused by a direct blow to the mandible.
- The commonest fracture is through the extracapsular part of the condylar neck, and is usually caused by a blow to the chin. It may be unilateral or bilateral.
- A fracture through the angle of the mandible is also common.

Pathophysiology
- Fractures through both sides of the jaw may result in posterior displacement of the tongue and result in airway obstruction.
- If the blow to the mandible is forceful enough, it may be sufficient to drive the head of the mandible backwards, resulting in fracture of the squamous temporal bone and result in cerebral spinal fluid leak and haemorrhage from the external auditory meatus.

Symptoms/signs
- Deformity of the jaw.
- Associated fractures of the teeth.
- Loss of bite, malocclusion of teeth, often producing a lateral crossbite.
- Bleeding and lacerated gum margins with ecchymosis on the lingual gingivae.
- Anaesthesia of half of the lower lips and chin supplied by the mental nerve on that side (caused by trauma to the inferior dental nerve).
- Absence of forward movement of the condylar head on opening the mouth.

Management
- Maintaining the airway: pull the tongue forward as described above.
- Control/treat any haemorrhage.

Tempromandibular joint subluxation

Incidence
- This is relatively rarely encountered in Immediate Care.

Aetiology
- May occur spontaneously (usually by yawning) or as a result of a blow to the open mouth.

Management
- Immediate reduction may be possible, if necessary using nitrous oxide/oxygen anaesthesia.

Method
- Standing in front of the patient, insert the thumb of both hands into the mouth and apply pressure to the lower molar teeth angle of the jaw pushing the jaw downwards and backwards, and at the same time tilting the chin upwards.

Teeth

Teeth

Aetiology
- The teeth are often damaged in facial injuries.

Pathophysiology
- Teeth may be displaced, fractured or dislodged from their sockets.

Management
- Any loose whole teeth displaced from the mouth should be collected, wrapped carefully in moist tissue or plastic foil, or (better) put in milk and sent with the patient to hospital for later possible replantation.
- If the patient is fully conscious the teeth may be held in the buccal cavity between the cheeks and jaw.
- If a tooth is only partially avulsed or if only one tooth is avulsed, it should be pushed back into its socket.

Notes

16

Chest injuries

Chest injuries

Introduction

- Chest injuries either by themselves or in conjunction with other major injuries are a major cause of death following road traffic accidents.
- Their correct immediate management has a major beneficial effect on the mortality and morbidity following major trauma.

Incidence

- Common in high speed road traffic accidents, especially those:
    - Unrestrained by seatbelts.
    - Ejected from vehicles.
    - Injured when there is significant side intrusion into the vehicle of which they are an occupant.
    - Motorcyclists who part with their bicycles at high speed.

Aetiology

- Often associated with head and abdominal injury.
- May be caused in road traffic accidents by:
    - The steering wheel (sternum).
    - Seatbelt, especially if there is high speed deceleration.
    - Side door intrusion.
    - Collision with other vehicle occupants.
    - Massive decceleration.

Pathophysiology

- Any structure in the chest may be involved:
    - Skin.
    - Ribs, sternum.
    - Pleura.
    - Lungs.
    - Heart and mediastinum.
- Liver and spleen within the bony thorax.

Assessment

- Chest injuries may be difficult to assess especially if the patient is unconscious due to an associated head injury.
- Chest injury should always be positively looked for in these circumstances.

- **Pain**
    - Especially on inspiration or coughing.

- **Dyspnoea**
    - Difficulty with breathing, feeling of chest tightness.

- **Inspection**
    - This should be carried out with good lighting if possible:
        - Obvious bruising, external wounds.
        - Paradoxical chest movement.
        - Increased/reduced respiratory rate.
        - Raised jugular venous pressure on examination of the neck veins.
        - Respiratory distress.
        - Surgical emphysema.

- **Palpation**
    - The crackling sensation of surgical emphysema.
    - Springing of ribs produces pain over fracture site.
    - Clunking sensation over fractured ribs/sternum.
    - Tracheal deviation.

- **Percussion**
    - This is usually difficult due to the high ambient noise levels, usually encountered in Immediate Care.
    - Hyper-resonance over a pneumothorax.
    - Dull over a haemothorax.

- **Auscultation**
    - Reduced air entry over a pneumothorax or haemothorax.

- **ECG**
    - Damage to coronary vessels may produce ECG changes suggestive of AMI.

- **Pulse oximetry**
    - Hypoxia is indicated by a reduced oxygen saturation (SaO_2).

Management

Priorities
- Care of the:
    - **A**irway with cervical spine stabilisation:
        - Upper airway obstruction:
            - Maintain the correct neck position
            - Use an oro- or nasopharyngeal airway
            - Consider endotracheal intubation.
    - **B**reathing:
        - Tension pneumothorax:
            - Insert a chest drain.
        - Seal any open wound.
        - Flail chest:
            - Stabilise
            - Support respiration.
    - **C**irculation with control of haemorrhage:
        - Monitor the pulse and blood pressure, and if these are normal, infuse sparingly.
        - Pulmonary oedema may be aggravated by use of crystalloids, and so colloids are the infusion fluid of choice.
    - **D**isability.
    - **E**xposure.
    - Relieve pain which may be impairing respiration.

Open chest wounds

Incidence

- These are relatively rare in the UK.

Aetiology

- A stab wound is one cause.

Pathophysiology

- The depth of penetration/damage may be deeper than may be immediately apparent.
- There is nearly always some degree of lung damage and a risk of developing a pneumothorax/tension pneumothorax.

Management

- Closure of the wound with airtight/waterproof occlusive dressing, leaving one edge of the dressing free, so as to form a one way valve, and prevent the development of a tension pneumothorax.
- Consider insertion of a chest drain.
- If there is a knife in the chest, do *not* remove it.

Rib fractures

Incidence

- This is a relatively common injury in road traffic accidents especially in those patients who are not restrained by seat belts.

Aetiology

- In road traffic accidents, rib fractures may often be caused by:
    - Impact of the chest with the steering wheel (uncommon in the belted driver).
    - Seat belt injury, when there is massive deceleration.
    - Side intrusion.
- A flail chest is often associated with major underlying lung injury, i.e. pulmonary contusion.

Pathophysiology

- Blunt trauma of the chest may result in:
    - An isolated rib fracture.
    - Multiple unilateral fractures.
    - A flail chest:
        - This occurs when the integrity of the thoracic cage is breached in two places, and one part is able to move independently of the rest.
        - Expansion of the underlying lung does not occur and respiration is impaired.
        - The extent to which the flail segment compromises effective respiration depends on its size, and the severity of the underlying lung injury.
        - May be complicated by a developing pneumothorax.
        - There may be:
            - A unilateral flail segment affecting only one side of the chest.
            - Bilateral flail segments affecting both sides of the chest (this is a very serious injury, as respiration is severely impaired).
            - A flail sternum which occurs when the ribs on both sides of the sternum are fractured.
            - A posterior flail segment in which the thoracic cage is often relatively stable and this injury rarely causes problems.
            - A lateral or anterior flail segment, which often results in severe respiratory distress.

Symptoms/signs

- Pain.
- Dyspnoea, respiratory distress, cyanosis when breathing air only.
- Loss of chest movement on the affected side, paradoxical movement, e.g. in flail chest.
- Reduced oxygen saturation (SaO_2).

Management

- Oxygen:
    - This should be administered in as high a concentration as possible.
- Ventilation:
    - Intubation and ventilation should be considered if there is any respiratory distress due to ineffective chest expansion, but beware of a pneumothorax as this may become a tension pneumothorax with intermittent positive pressure ventilation.
- Stabilisation:
    - With a firm pad and bandage (flail chest only).
    - Consider lying the patient with the injured side over a sandbag (unilateral flail chest only).
    - Position/turn onto the affected side during transport.
- Pain relief:
    - This is very important and is often overlooked, as the degree of chest expansion may be very considerably reduced due to pain.
    - Be cautious with:
        - Respiratory depressants.
        - Nitrous oxide/oxygen (may aggravate/exacerbate, *but not cause,* a tension pneumothorax).
    - Consider an intercostal nerve block.

Pneumothorax

Aetiology

- This is nearly always associated with an overlying rib fracture, but can also occur spontaneously due to the rupture of a bulla (there is usually a previous history).

Pathophysiology

- This occurs when air, either from the outside or from within the lungs, enters the pleural space resulting in collapse of the underlying lung.
- It may be a:
    - Partial pneumothorax: especially when underlying disease tethers part of the layers of the pleura together.
    - Complete pneumothorax
    - Tension pneumothorax
    - Bilateral pneumothorax.

Symptoms/signs

- Pain:
    - This may be central or pleuritic.
- Increasing dyspnoea, respiratory distress, and cyanosis.
- Chest movement:
    - This may be reduced or unequal.
- Surgical emphysema
- Percussion note will be hyper-resonant.

Note: - The patient with emphysema may also show hyper-resonance.

Tension pneumothorax

Pathophysiology

- Air enters the pleural cavity during inspiration, via a tear in the lung or chest wall, which acts as a one way valve, but cannot go out, resulting in a pneumothorax.
- With each inspiratory breath, more air is drawn into the space; and so the pneumothorax gets larger with each inspiration.
- As the pneumothorax gets larger; it may cause progressive displacement of the mediastinum resulting in impaired cardiac function due to reduced venous return.

Symptoms/signs

- Tracheal deviation and mediastinal shift towards the unaffected side.
- Respiratory embarrassment:
    - Increasing dyspnoea
    - Tachypnoea
    - Expiratory grunting
    - Distension of the neck veins
    - Possible cyanosis
    - Hypoxia with a reduced SaO_2.
- Reduced air entry (breath sounds) on the affected side on auscultation.
- Hyper-resonance over the affected side.
- Tachycardia.

Management

- This depends on the clinical condition of the patient.
- May be:
    - Oxygen
    - Tube drainage with a Heimlich valve or chest drainage bag
    - Pain relief.

Tube drainage

Indications
- Life threatening tension pneumothorax
- Chest injury, requiring positive pressure ventilation or air transportation.

Sites
- Anterior:
    - Over the second intercostal space, 1 inch lateral to the mid-clavicular line. Insert the drain outwards and upwards.
- Lateral (*best*):
    - Over the fourth or fifth intercostal space, anterior to the mid axillary line.
- Posterior:
    - In the auscultatory triangle, just below the tip of the scapula with the arms abducted.

Needle decompression
- This may be performed to:
  - Establish the diagnosis
  - Relieve the symptoms while a chest drain is prepared for insertion.

Method
- Administer high flow oxygen via a mask or airway
- Identify the site for insertion
- Clean the site with antiseptic, and infiltrate with local anaesthetic down to the pleura:
  - Lignocaine 1% (with or without adrenaline).
- Use a wide bore intravenous cannula with a 20-30 ml syringe.
- Penetrate the parietal pleura and aspirate air (if unsuccessful, seal the puncture site and observe the patient for the possible development of a pneumothorax).
- Proceed to chest drain insertion.

Complications
- Local cellulitis
- Local haemotoma
- Pleural infection
- May cause a pneumothorax, if one is not already present.

Chest drain insertion

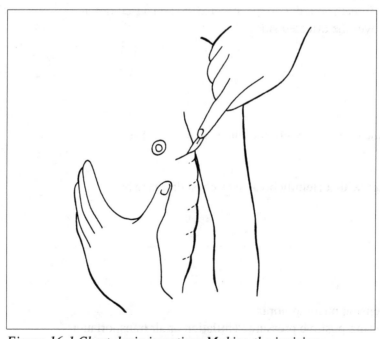

Figure 16-1 Chest drain insertion: Making the incision

Method
- Make a generous (2-3 cm) cut with a sharp ended scapel, parallel to the ribs. Be careful not to go too near the inferior border of the ribs (risk of damage to the intercostal nerve and artery).
- Insert blunt artery forceps, and spread them out in the middle of the space.
- Put a gloved index finger through the chest wall and into pleural space, and perform a finger sweep to identify adhesions, blood clots, etc.
- Remove the trochar of the chest drain, and attach artery forceps to the distal end.
- Insert the drain into the chest with the forceps, using your finger as a guide and aiming towards the apex of the lung.

Note: - If there is surgical emphysema, be careful to insert the drain far enough.

- Look for "fogging" of the chest tube with expiration, or listen for air movement out of the tube (often difficult in the Immediate Cate situation).
- Attach the end of the tube to a one way Heimlich valve or drainage bag/valve and secure it with two strong (0/00) purse string sutures.
- Use a single purse string suture to close the incision (this should be cut and *not* tied).
- Apply a dressing and airtight tape around the tube and tape the tube to the chest.
- Following the procedure, check the patient and sit them up at 45°.

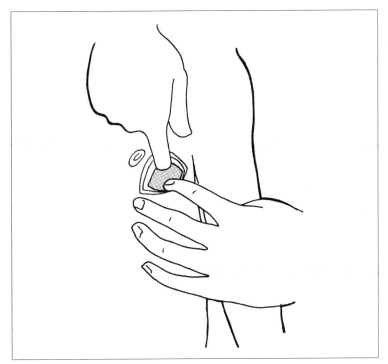

Figure 16-2 Chest drain insertion: Opening the pleura

Complications
- Allergic reaction to the surgical skin preparation or anaesthetic (unlikely in Immediate Care as there is usually little time for surgical preparation).
- Damage to the intercostal nerve artery or vein:
    - May convert pneumothorax into haemopneumothorax.
    - May cause intercostal neuralgia/neuritis later.
- Damage to the internal mammary vessels if anterior puncture is too medial, resulting in haemopneumothorax.
- Damage to intrathoracic or intra-abdominal organs (this can be avoided by using the finger technique before inserting the tube).
- Subcutaneous emphysema at insertion site.
- Incorrect tube positioning.
- Persistant pneumothorax:
    - Air leak.
    - Failure of apparatus:
        - Tube kinking
        - Blood clogging or freezing the Heimlich valve.

Drainage
- This may be direct Heimlich valve or chest drainage bag.

Haemothorax

Pathophysiology

- This is caused by haemorrhage from the intercostal and pulmonary arteries and veins or their branches and may result in the loss of a considerable volume of blood into the pleural space. This may cause profound hypovolaemia and shock.

Symptoms/signs

- Profound shock.
- Dullness to percussion in the dependant areas of the chest.

Management

- Any patient with a chest injury and signs of significant hypovolaemia, needs aggressive fluid replacement and treatment of hypovolaemic shock.
- Oxygen administration.
- Intravenous infusion: colloid.
- Insertion of chest drain.

Injuries to the trachea and main bronchus

Incidence

- Rare.

Aetiology

- Usually associated with other major injuries.
- In road traffic accidents may be caused by the steering wheel rim: ruptured bronchus, trachea and larynx.

Symptoms/signs

- Respiratory distress.
- Surgical emphysema.

Management

- Oxygen.
- If there is:
    - Surgical emphysema: be very careful about intubating.
    - Absolute tracheal obstruction: perform a cricothyrotomy.

The great vessels

Incidence

- Rupture of the thoracic aorta is a relatively common injury in high velocity deceleration road traffic accidents, especially in the young.

Aetiology

- Rapid deceleration.

Pathophysiology

- Complete rupture:
    - This results in rapid death.
- Partial rupture:
    - Patients may survive for several hours before going rapidly into profound shock, as the rupture becomes complete.

Symptoms/signs

- Central chest pain, especially radiating through to the back.
- Hypovolaemic shock.

Management

- Oxygen.
- Aggressive infusion of colloid (but be careful not to push the systolic pressure >100 mmHg, as this may induce further haemorrhage).
- Pneumatic anti-shock garment (PASG).
- Careful monitoring of the patient's haemodynamic state.

The heart

- Myocardial damage is usually fatal.

Incidence

- Injury to the heart is rarely encountered.

Aetiology

- The commonest cause is a stab wound.
- Myocardial contusion may also occur due to deceleration in road traffic accidents.

Pathophysiology

- Penetrating myocardial injury may result in cardiac tamponade:
    - This is due to the collection of blood in the pericardial space from haemorrhage into it from the coronary vessels.
    - This results in impairment of cardiac contraction.
- Blunt injury may result in myocardial contusion.

Symptoms/Signs

- Increasing dyspnoea.
- Cyanosis.
- *Distension of the neck veins.*
- *Tamponade: muffled heart sounds.*   } *Beck's triad*
- *Hypovolaemic shock with rapidly falling blood pressure.*
- A narrow pulse pressure.
- Kussmaul's sign: a rise in venous pressure with inspiration indicates tamponade.

Note: - If the patient is also hypovolaemic, the neck veins may *not* be distended.

Management

- Oxygen.
- Aggressive intravenous infusion if there is any evidence of hypovolaemic shock.
- Careful monitoring of the pulse rate, blood pressure, etc.

Pericardiocentesis (pericardial aspiration)

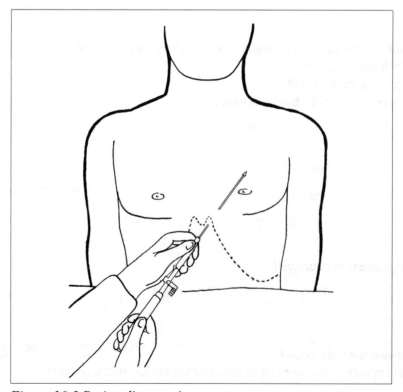

Figure 16-3 Pericardiocentesis

Indications
- Cardiac tamponade (stab wound where there is no evidence of a pneumothorax and no improvement in the patient's condition with oxygen).

Monitoring
- This procedure should be performed only with careful monitoring of the patient's vital signs and ECG before, during and after the procedure.

Method
- The patient should be on oxygen and have a large bore intravenous infusion in place.
- Obtain a long (6 inch), wide bore (16-18 SWG) intravenous cannula and attach it to a 20 ml syringe, ideally with a three way tap.
- Insert the needle into the left costo-xiphoid angle (about 1-2 cm below and to the left of the xiphisternum).
- Puncture the skin and aim the the needle cephalad towards the left sterno-clavicular joint, so as to avoid the superior epigastric vessels, at an angle of about 45º to the skin.
- Insert the needle about 4-6 cm, withdrawing the plunger until the syringe fills with blood.
- If the needle is advanced too far (into the myocardium), an injury pattern will show on the ECG monitor:
    - Extreme ST-T wave changes.
    - Widened QRS complex.
    - PVCs.
- Withdraw as much non clotted blood as possible.
- During aspiration, as blood is removed from the pericardial sac, the tip of the needle may come into contact with the inner pericardial surface overlying the myocardium. This will show as an injury pattern on the ECG monitor and the needle can be withdrawn a little.
- If the injury pattern persists or if there is no further aspirate, cease aspiration and withdraw the needle completely, keeping the cannula in place.
- Attach a three way tap and secure the cannula, so that further aspiration can take place if cardiac tamponade persists or reoccurs.

Diaphragm

Aetiology

- Rupture of the diaphragm most frequently occurs on the left side, involving the splenic flexure of the colon, the spleen and the stomach.

Symptoms/signs

- Dyspnoea.
- Profound shock.
- Bowel sounds may occasionally be heard in the left side of the chest.

Management

- Oxygen.
- Intravenous infusion.

The oesophagus

Aetiology

- There may be spontaneous rupture.
- Rupture may also be caused by:
    - External blunt trauma
    - Penetrating injury
    - Iatrogenic instrumental perforation.

Symptoms/signs
- Severe retrosternal chest pain.
- Subcutaneous and mediastinal emphysema.

Management

- Treatment of shock.

Thoraco-abdominal injuries

- Consider injury to the liver, spleen, stomach, duodenum, etc.

Differential diagnosis of chest injury

- Over transfusion.
- Aspiration pneumonia.
- Shock lung.

17

Abdominal and pelvic injuries

Abdominal and pelvic injuries

Abdominal injuries

Incidence

- Serious intra-abdominal injuries are relatively rarely encountered in Immediate Care, accounting for only 1% of hospital admissions for trauma.
- The majority are the result of road traffic accidents, and are usually associated with serious injuries to other areas, e.g. head, chest, pelvis and limbs.
- In the UK, blunt trauma is much more common than penetrating injury.

Aetiology

- Penetrating injury occurs as a result of:
    - Stabbing
    - Shooting
    - Explosions: producing high velocity fragments
    - Impaling injury.
- Blunt injury:
    - Rapid increase in intra-abdominal pressure:
        - Direct blow
        - Restraint, e.g. car seat belt.
    - Direct compression of organs.
    - Rapid deceleration or acceleration.
- Ejection injury.
- Crush injury.

Pathophysiology

Penetrating abdominal injury

Stab wound
- There is a 25% chance of damage to major viscera.
- Adjacent structures (including intrathoracic) are often involved.

Shooting/explosion injury
- There is a 75% chance of damage to major viscera, usually: bowel, liver and diaphragm.
- Many non adjacent organs may be damaged.

Blunt abdominal injury

- May result in damage to: liver, spleen, retroperitoneal area, kidney, bowel and bladder.
- May occur as a result of several different mechanisms acting alone or together.

Direct blow
- This may result in visceral injury with or without compression of the organs against the vertebral column.

Compression injury (e.g. car seat belt injury)
- Produces compression combined with deceleration.
- Incidence of injury increases with incorrect usage.

Rapid deceleration or acceleration
- This results in shearing or tearing forces.
- These are proportional to the mass and mobility of the organs concerned, e.g. liver, spleen, kidneys and mesenteries.

Assessment

- Evidence of abdominal injury is often overshadowed by other more obvious injuries, e.g. head injury, or may be masked by alcohol.
- 20% of those with serious intra-abdominal injuries will show no evidence of these injuries on initial examination.
- Any examination therefore should include assessment of the mechanism of injury and any patient sustaining a significant deceleration injury or a penetrating abdominal wound should be assumed to have an abdominal visceral injury.

History

- It is important to obtain a clear history as to the mechanism of injury if possible, e.g. in road traffic accidents:
  - Time of accident
  - Mechanism of vehicle impact and patient injury
  - Use of seat belts
  - Injuries to other vehicle occupants.
- It is also important to obtain the nature and time of any recent meal, and when urine was last passed, as distended organs are more liable to rupture than empty ones.

Symptoms/signs

- Often unreliable in the Immediate Care situation: up to 25% of significant injuries may be missed initially (50% if the patient is unconscious).
- Depend on the structure involved.
- Consider any injury in conjunction with injuries to associated areas: chest, pelvis, spine.

Examination

- Most reliable: abdominal pain or discomfort with localised tenderness, rebound tenderness, and guarding
- Unreliable: the presence or absence of bowel sounds, serial girth measurement.
- Shoulder tip pain: indicates diaphragmatic irritation.
- Pattern bruising (usually indicates significant injury even if physical examination is unremarkable).
- Loss of normal abdominal wall contour.
- Evidence of hypovolaemic shock: especially if there are indications of splenic or hepatic injury.

Diaphragmatic injury

Incidence
- A relatively common injury and is often overlooked.

Aetiology
- Injury to the upper abdomen:
    - Blunt trauma (most commonly found in RTAs), when it is associated with other major injuries including intrathoracic injury.
    - Penetrating injury (stabbing).

Pathophysiology
- The most common injury involves the left postero-lateral hemi-diaphragm.

Duodenum

Incidence
- An unusual injury.

Aetiology
- Classically encountered in the unrestrained intoxicated car driver involved in a frontal impact.

Symptoms/signs
- Bloody nasogastric aspirate.

Liver

Incidence
- Relatively common in severe blunt trauma.

Aetiology
- Usually caused by trauma to the right hypochondrium.

Symptoms/signs
- Pattern bruising, localised tenderness.
- Hypovolaemic shock.

Spleen

Incidence
- A relatively common injury.

Aetiology
- Usually caused by blunt trauma to the lower left ribs, the left loin and the lateral left hypochondrium.

Symptoms/signs
- Pattern bruising.
- Localised pain/tenderness.
- Hypovolaemic shock:
  - This may not develop immediately, as initial haemorrhage may be controlled by tamponade within the splenic capsule.

Pancreas

Incidence
- A relatively unusual injury.

Aetiology
- Most often results from a direct epigastric blow, compressing the pancreas against the vertebral column.

Kidneys

Incidence
- A fairly common injury

Aetiology
- Blunt trauma:
  - Usually caused by a blow to the loin or posterior lower ribs (usually severe enough to result in a fracture).
- Penetrating injury:
  - May also be caused by penetrating trauma of the loin.

Symptoms/signs
- Localised pain/tenderness.
- Haematuria.

Management

- Follow the usual guidelines:

    - **Primary survey/initial management:**
        - Airway with stabilisation of the cervical spine
        - **B**reathing
        - **C**irculation
        - **D**isability
        - **E**xposure.

    - **Secondary survey/management:**
        - Chest injury
        - Adominal injury
        - Head injury
        - Spinal injury.

- If there is:
    - Evidence of hypovolaemia:
        - Secure two intravenous lines with wide bore cannulae.
        - If the anticipated blood loss is considerable, then consider application of a PASG.
    - Obvious external bleeding:
        - Control with direct pressure.
        - Exposed or prolapsed viscera:
            - Cover with saline soaked towels (Hartmann's solution will do).

Pelvic injuries

Pelvic fractures

Incidence

- Pelvic fractures are relatively commonly encountered in accidents resulting in major injuries, and are associated with severe head, chest and abdominal trauma.
- Have a significant morbidity and mortality:
    - Open pelvic injuries have a mortality rate of more than 50%.

Aetiology

- Most severe pelvic injuries are associated with high velocity accidents or those involving massive forces, e.g. car-pedestrian, motorcycle or high fall accidents.
- May be trivial or complicated.
- 20% of pelvic fractures result in intraperitoneal problems.

Pathophysiology

- Usually caused by direct injury or by forces transmitted along the femur.
- Isolated fractures:
    - Any part may be affected especially the pubic rami.
- Unstable fracture:
    - Two or more fractures with loss of the integrity of the pelvic ring.

Complications
- Vascular:
    - Rarely, the common iliac artery may be damaged.
    - Haemorrhage into soft tissue/bone: this may be very considerable (6-10 units of blood).
- Neurological:
    - Common where there has been major pelvic disruption:
        - The sciatic nerves may be damaged.
- Visceral:
    - There may be associated abdominal/visceral injury.
- Bladder:
    - Disruption of the symphis pubis, or penetration by a bony spike.

Symptoms/signs

- An unstable pelvis:
    - Does the pelvis feel firm or is there bony crepitus? (pelvic springing by itself is not a good predictor of pelvic fractures).
- Urethral bleeding.
- Rectal bleeding.

Management

- Stabilisation of the pelvis: with triangular bandages, Frac Straps or a PASG.
- Treatment of complications:

Blood loss

- Adequate volume replacement:
    - Secure two intravenous infusions using wide bore cannulae.
- Careful haemodynamic monitoring.
- If the patient remains haemodynamically unstable, consider application of a PASG.

Bladder rupture

Incidence

- A relatively rare injury, usually occurring in accidents involving severe force.

Aetiology

- There are two distinct causes:
    - Sudden severe compression will result in rupture of a full bladder.
    - Rupture by a bony spike.

Pathophysiology

- Pelvic disruption/bony penetration:
    - Anterolateral tear.
- Compression:
    - Tear along peritonealised posterior wall.

Symptoms/signs

- If the rupture is intraperitoneal, these may be delayed.
- Lower abdominal and pelvic pain and associated tenderness.
- Loss of desire to micturate and inability or pain on attempting to void.
- Associated hypovolaemic shock.

Urethral rupture

Incidence

- Occurs in approximately 10% of pelvic fractures.

Aetiology

- Common in disruption of the symphysis pubis.
- Damage to the bulbar urethra usually results from straddle injuries, i.e. falling astride.

Symptoms/signs

- Unable to void or pain on attemped voiding.
- Blood at the urethral meatus (not always).
- High riding prostate on rectal examination.

External genitalia

Incidence

- Injury is uncommon.

Aetiology

- Blunt trauma:
    - Kick or sporting injury.
- Lacerations.
- The most severe injuries occur as a result of missile or blast trauma.

Notes

18

Skeletal injuries

Skeletal injury

Introduction

- Skeletal injuries are probably the commonest type of injury encountered in Immediate Care, and their management is something with which all those involved in Immediate Care should be fully competent and experienced in managing.
- It should not be forgotten, however, that they are rarely immediately life threatening, and that assessment and management of the airway, breathing, circulation and abdominal and pelvic injuries, head, and facial injuries come first.

Incidence

Age

- Fractures are encountered at all ages but:
    - The very young have very flexible bones, so fractures are unusual except where very considerable force is used.
    - Children are very active and prone to injury. Their bones are still relatively supple and so they may only sustain a "Green stick" fracture where the bone is only buckled or there is an incomplete break in the bone cortex.
    - The elderly have relatively brittle bones which are relatively easily fractured.

Sex

- Boys are usually more adventurous than girls and are more prone to injury.
- Post-menopausal women may often suffer from osteoporosis, which results in thinning of the bony cortex and their bones are more susceptible to fractures especially of the hip and wrist.

Aetiology

- Fractures are caused as a result of bones being exposed to abnormal forces or because the bones are unable to withstand normal forces because they themselves are weak, e.g. in osteoporosis.

Forces

- These may be:
    - Direct
        - Angulation force/impact results in a transverse fracture.
        - Usually results in greater soft tissue injury.
        - Usually associated with open fractures.
    - Indirect/transmitted:
        - Compression fracture.
        - Twisting force results in a spiral fracture.

Pathophysiology

- Fractures may be:
    - Open/compound:
        - Where the bone penetrates the skin.
    - Closed/simple:
        - No skin penetration.
    - Complicated, involving:
        - Blood vessels resulting in vascular injury.
        - Nerves.
        - Viscera.
    - Comminuted:
        - Multiple fractures at the same site.
- Blood loss following bony injury may be considerable (see chapter on Shock).

Assessment

The history/mechanism of injury

- This may or may not be obtainable, but the experienced Immediate Care doctor should be able to read the wreckage, predict the likely injuries, and seek them out.

Symptoms/signs

- Pain/loss of function:
    - In immediate care the patient may not or can not complain of quite significant injuries.
- Suspect a fracture, if there is:
    - Deformity.
    - Swelling.
    - Visible bruising.
- There is a definite fracture if there is:
    - Gross deformity.
    - Bony crepitus.
    - Abnormal mobility.

- Suspect vascular damage if there is:
  - Skin discolouration:
    - Looks pale, blue.
  - Reduced skin temperature:
    - Feels cold.
  - Reduced capillary return.
  - Poor or absent peripheral pulses.
  - Reduced peripheral SaO_2.
- Suspect nerve injury if there is reduced or absent sensation or voluntary movement.

Management

- Immobilisation:
  - Sling or splint.
- Traction:
  - By application of a traction splint. This is a modified version of the Thomas splint with its own self contained method of applying traction (usually to a hitch attached to the ankle).
- Reduction:
  - Depending on the type and location of the fracture, this may be possible and will minimise the complications and tissue damage following a fracture.
  - Is specifically indicated where there is impaired circulation or sensation, distal to the fracture or when the skin is at risk.
  - Polaroid photographs should be taken before and after reduction.
  - The peripheral pulses, peripheral SaO_2, sensation and movement should be monitored before and after fracture reduction.
  - The patient should be given adequate analgesia (although sometimes none is necessary).
- Prevention of complications, e.g. haemorrhage, vascular and nerve injury.
- Skin injury:
  - Preserve as much skin as possible.
  - In compound or degloving injuries:
    - Seal the wound with a Betadine dressing or spray, after taking polaroid photographs.
- Bone loss:
  - Collect any large extruded bone fragments and send with the patient to hospital.

Splinting/immobilisation

Triangular bandages

- A triangular bandage used as a sling is the method of choice for supporting most upper limb injuries.
- May be folded to make ties suitable for immobilising the lower limb.

Splints

Inflatable splints

- Used to provide immobilisation and support for fractures of the forearm and wrist, and upper and lower limb.

Mode of action
- Immobilisation
- Reduction of haemorrhage by tamponade.

Disadvantades
- May produce impairment of the distal circulation.
- May be punctured.

CONCLUSION: Only used if no better splint is available.

Box splints
- Used to provide support and splintage for lower limb injuries from (and including) the knee to the foot.
- May also be used to immobilise upper limb injuries.

Advantages
- Quick and easy to apply.
- Effective.

Disadvantages
- Do not apply traction.

CONCLUSION: Splint of choice for lower limb injuries when traction splintage is contraindicated or inappropriate.

Traction splints
- Developed from the Thomas splint.

Aims
- To reduce blood loss.
- Minimise pain.
- Prevent fracture movement, usually by fracture reduction.
- To reduce neurovascular complications.

Mode of action
- Reduce and immobilise the fracture.
- With a fractured femur:
    - The splinting effect of the bone is lost and the muscle bunches up causing the fractured bony ends to override.
    - This increases the local diameter of the muscle and initially allows a greater space into which blood can escape.
    - Further extensive blood loss may result in a compartmental syndrome with an increase in the intracompartmental pressure eventually resulting in:
        - Pressure necrosis of nerves.
        - Tamponade of the arterial blood supply and muscle necrosis.
        - Impairement of the venous return.
- Reduction results in restoration of the normal anatomical configuration and hence prevents this initial blood loss.

Indications
- Closed/simple fracture of the femoral shaft.
- Closed/simple fracture of the tibia/fibula (except undisplaced fractures of the proximal shaft of fibula).
- Open/compound fractures of the femoral shaft, tibia and fibula.
- With minimal traction:
    - Dislocation of the hip
    - Fractures around the knee.

Contraindications
- Fracture dislocation of the knee.
- Ankle fractures.

Method of application
- Administer analgesia: Entonox.
- Expose the whole of the injured leg from groin to toes by removing clothing.
- Examine the whole leg especially the peripheral pulses, colour, temperature, SaO_2, sensation, and motor power distal to the fracture.
- Prepare the splint.
- Apply a dressing to any wounds (if the fracture is open, this *must* be recorded on the patient report form).
- Apply manual traction to the ankle.
- Attach the ankle hitch to the ankle.
- Position the splint and attach the ankle hitch to the traction device hook.
- Position padding as necessary and gently apply traction (up to 15 lbs for an adult male).
- Re-examine the limb distal to the fracture.

CONCLUSION: Method of choice for most lower limb injuries.

Upper limb fractures

Clavicle

Incidence
- A relatively common injury in teenagers.

Aetiology
- Often caused by falls from horses and motorcycles.
- Fall onto the shoulder, less commonly a fall onto the outstretched hand.

Pathophysiology/complications
- Severely displaced fractures of the clavicle, or posterior dislocation of the sternoclavicular joint may cause:
    - Pressure on the subclavian or innominate arteries, and the trachea. This can be life threatening and requires urgent reduction.
    - Pneumo- or haemothorax.

Management
- Sling.
- If there is severe posterior displacement:
    - Reduce the fracture immediately by applying traction to the arm.

Scapula

Incidence
- This is a relatively rare injury.

Aetiology
- Usually caused by direct force.
- Often associated with fractures of the underlying ribs.

Symptoms/signs
- May be very painful.
- Localised tenderness.

Management
- Analgesia, as required.

Shoulder

Dislocations

Anterior dislocation of the shoulder

Incidence
- Anterior dislocation is the most common.

Aetiology
- Usually caused by a fall onto the outstretched hand.

Pathophysiology/complications
- The axillary nerve may be damaged.

Symptoms/signs
- Is usually very painful.
- Loss of the shoulder contour.
- Paraesthesia/numbness in the distribution of the axillary nerve.

Management
- Sling
- Analgesia

Posterior dislocation of the shoulder

Incidence
- Relatively rare.

Aetiology
- Caused by a direct blow to the shoulder, electric shock or epileptic fit.

Pathophysiology/complications
- Injury to the top of the shoulder, accompanied by forced lateral flexion of the head in the opposite direction, may cause a brachial plexus injury.

Symptoms/signs
- May not be obvious and is often missed.

Management
- Sling.
- Immediate reduction is not indicated in the Immediate Care situation.

Note:- Beware of converting a dislocation to a fracture.
- Analgesia as required.

Humerus

Head of humerus

Pathophysiology/complications
- Fractures of the humeral head may involve the axillary artery.

Neck of humerus

Incidence
- Often occurs in the elderly.

Aetiology
- Usually a fall onto the shoulder, resulting in impaction.

Symptoms
- There may be some function and not a lot of pain.

Greater tuberosity

- Similar to the above.

Shaft of humerus

Incidence
- Usually the middle third is affected.

Aetiology
- Direct force: transverse fracture.
- Twisting force: spiral fracture.

Pathophysiology/complications
- May result in radial nerve damage:
  - Usually a contusion; rarely a complete division.

Management
- Immobilisation with a sling.

Elbow

Supracondylar fracture

Incidence
- Usually occurs in children/adolescents.

Aetiology
- Caused by a fall onto the oustretched hand.

Pathophysiology/complications
- Brachial artery injury:
    - This can rapidly result in avascular necrosis of the forearm muscles.
    - Always check the radial pulse if this injury is suspected.

Management
- If the radial pulse is absent:
    - Attempt to straighten the elbow, with careful monitoring of the radial pulse, or peripheral circulation with a pulse oximeter.
- If the radial pulse is present:
    - Immobilisation using a broad arm sling with the angle between the upper arm and forearm at the elbow greater than 90°.

Condylar fracture

Incidence
- Uncommon, usually occurs in children.
- The lateral epicondyle is most usually fractured.

Management
- Sling.

Epicondylar fracture

Incidence
- Uncommon, usually occurs in children.

Aetiology
- Caused by direct violence and a fall onto the outstretched hand (avulsion).

Pathophysiology/complications
- Usually the medial epicondyle is fractured:
    - This may result in damage to the ulnar nerve:
        - Signs:
            - Inability to extend the fingers fully.
            - Tingling/loss of sensation in the little and ring fingers.

Elbow dislocation

Incidence
- Common both in children and adults.

Aetiology
- Caused by a fall onto the outstretched hand.

Pathophysiology/complications
- The dislocation is usually posterior.
- Rarely the brachial artery or ulnar nerve may be damaged.

Management
- Sling.

Forearm, wrist and hand

Olecranon process

Incidence
- Usually found in adults.

Aetiology
- Caused by a fall onto the point of the elbow.

Management
- Sling.

Head of radius

Incidence
- A very common injury, usually occurring in young adults.

Aetiology
- Caused by fall onto the outstretched hand (indirect force).

Symptoms
- Local pain.

Signs
- Local tenderness.
- Reduced elbow flexion.
- Reduced wrist pronation/supination.

Management
- Application of a collar and cuff.

Radius/ulna

Incidence
- A relatively common injury.

Aetiology
- Caused by a direct blow or transmitted force from a fall onto the outstretched hand.

Pathophysiology
- Is usually a greenstick fracture in children.

Signs
- Obvious deformity.

Management
- Sling or box splint.

Lower end of radius (Colles') fracture

Incidence
- This is the most common type of wrist fracture.
- Very common in:
    - Those over 40 and female (especially if there is associated osteoporosis).
    - The winter months: snow and ice.

Aetiology
- Caused by a fall onto the outstretched hand.

Pathophysiology
- Usually a greenstick fracture or epiphyseal injury in children.

Signs
- The classic dinner fork deformity (this may be reversed in a Smith's fracture).

Management
- Immediate reduction and splinting.
- Application of a sling.

Fingers

Incidence
- Fractures:
    - Not very common.
- Dislocations:
    - More common.

Management
- Immediate reduction is usually possible, followed by neighbour strapping.

Lower limb injuries

Hip

Incidence
- A very common type of injury, affecting up to 46,000 people per year in England and Wales, especially the elderly and female (with osteoporosis) of whom about 25% die as a result.

Aetiology
- Direct force:
    - Fall.
- Indirect force:
    - Blow to the knee.

Posterior dislocation of the hip

Incidence
- The commonest hip dislocation.

Aetiology
- It is usually caused by a blow to the knee causing a force to be transmitted along the femoral shaft, e.g. from the front shelf of a car. The femur is driven backwards out of the acetabulum or its fractured posterior wall.

Pathophysiology/complications
- May result in injury to the sciatic nerve.
- Will result in avascular necrosis of the femoral head, if it is not treated as soon as possible.

Symptoms/signs
- Internal rotation with shortening of the leg, hip and knee flexion, and internal rotation of the ankle.
- Sciatic nerve palsy: distal sensory loss, pain, and foot drop (detect by asking the patient to dorsiflex the foot).
- May be extremely painful.

Management
- Allow hip to remain in flexion (do *not* apply traction splintage).
- Analgesia (may require very strong analgesia).

Anterior dislocation of the hip

Incidence
- Rare.

Aetiology
- Very forceful abduction and then lateral rotation:
    - Road traffic accidents.
    - Aircraft accidents.

Management
- Apply gentle traction.

Femur

Neck of femur

Incidence
- Very common in the elderly and female with osteoporosis.

Aetiology
- Usually caused by a direct blow or a fall onto the hip.

Symptoms/signs
- Shortening, external rotation of the ankle.
- The wider the displacement the greater the degree of rotation.

Pathophysiology/complications
- Displacement of the femoral neck will result in damage to the blood supply of the head of the femur and subsequent avascular necrosis, which requires arthroplasty.
- Minimal displacement can be treated by internal fixation.

Management
- The object is to prevent any further damage to the vascular supply to the femoral head.
- Apply gentle traction splintage.
- Tie both feet together in a figure of eight, to prevent further external rotation.

Shaft of femur

Incidence
- Common injury in the young, especially motorcyclists.

Aetiology
- Usually caused by a direct blow.

Complications
- Fractures of the lower third may involve the femoral artery.
- Intramuscular haemorrhage: blood loss may be considerable (up to four units).
- Damage to the sciatic nerve.
- Pressure on the popliteal artery may be caused by:
  - Supracondylar fracture:
    - Gastrocnemius rotates the distal fragment.

Management
- Traction splinting is the method of choice (with great care if the fracture is near the knee, as the distal fragment is usually tilted posteriorly and impinges on the popliteal vessels).
- Fluid replacement to prevent hypovolaemia.
- Tight trousers may be left on the patient as they may reduce the amount of intramuscular haemorrhage by tamponade (but may make full evaluation of the injury difficult).
- Analgesia, especially if the fracture is comminuted.

Knee

Aetiology
- May be caused by direct blow:
    - Intrusion of wheel arch, shelf.
    - Collision whilst skiing.

Complications
- Disruption of the knee ligaments.
- Nerve injury:
    - Popliteal nerve.
- Vascular injury:
    - Popliteal artery.

Patella

Incidence
- A relatively rare injury.

Aetiology
- Fracture:
    - Usually caused by direct pressure, e.g. from front shelf, or sudden violent contraction of the quadriceps muscle.
- Dislocation:
    - Usually caused by indirect twisting pressure, e.g. in football.

Management
- Immediate reduction of subluxation/dislocation.
- If the subluxation has occurred with the knee flexed, the knee must be extended as the patella is pushed back medially (otherwise reduction is very difficult to do!).

Tibia/fibula

Incidence
- This is a common injury in motor cyclists and front seat car occupants, where there has been a significant amount of wheel arch intrusion.
- Also commonly seen in car drivers where the feet/ankles have become trapped by the control pedals.

Aetiology
- Usually caused by direct pressure.

Pathophysiology/complications
- Vascular damage:
    - The bifurcation of the popliteal artery or posterior tibial vessels in:
        - Fractures of the upper tibia in adults.
        - Fractures of the mid-shaft of the tibia.
        - Injury to the upper tibial epiphysis in children.
    - It is vital to observe the peripheral circulation in the feet.
- Nerve damage:
    - Common peroneal nerve or tibial nerve just below the knee.
    - Tibial nerve:
        - Fractures of the lower quarter of the tibia.

Management
- Traction:
    - Put all fractures on traction, but pay attention to the circulation in the foot.

Ankles

Incidence
- Found relatively often in all types of accident:
    - Sport
    - Road traffic accidents.

Aetiology
- May be similar to fractures of the lower leg:
    - Inversion or eversion of the ankle.

Complications
- Avascular damage to the skin, especially in bimalleolar fractures:
    - Pay careful attention to the skin over the medial malleolus.

Management
- Reduction:
    - It is probably best to attempt to reduce a subluxation of the ankle, as soon as possible after the injury, as this will minimise vascular problems.
    - Take polaroid photographs before and after reduction.
- Splintage:
    - In a box splint

Notes

19

Spinal injuries

Spinal injuries

Introduction

-   Although spinal injuries are relatively rare (17 new cases per week in the United Kingdom); it is very important that those involved in Immediate Care are fully competent in their management, as early recognition and appropriate treatment is vital, if aggravation of severe injuries and possibly even death due to incorrect initial management is to be avoided.

Incidence

-   Relatively common in certain situations:
    -   Motorcyclists.
    -   Horse riders.
    -   Falls from heights.
    -   Ejection from military aircraft (less common with newer ejection seats and may be asymptomatic).
    -   Diving into shallow water.

Aetiology

-   The major problem following a spinal injury is due to spinal cord injury.
-   The major causes of spinal cord injury are:
    -   Road traffic accidents:
        -   Ejection
        -   Sudden deceleration (whiplash injury)
        -   Collision with another (unrestrained) vehicle occupant
        -   Motor or pedal cycle accidents
        -   There is a strong association between spinal injury and:
            -   Chest injury
            -   Sternal injury.
    -   Falls from a height onto the feet:
        -   Accidental
        -   Deliberate:
            -   Suicide attempt
            -   Under the influence of alcohol.
    -   Falls onto the head:
        -   Down stairs.

- Sporting accidents:
    - Gymnastics and trampolining.
    - Rugby football:
        - Scrum collapse
        - Due to tackling or being tackled.
    - Riding and hunting on horseback.
    - Skiing:
        - Collision between skiers.
    - Hang gliding.
    - Diving, especially under the influence of alcohol:
        - Into shallow pools.
    - Dysbarism induced spinal cord injury.
- Industrial accidents:
    - Weights falling onto the back.

Pathophysiology

Bony injury

- Spinal fractures may involve:
    - The vertebral bodies:
        - Caused by compression, flexion, extension or twisting (rotational) forces.
    - The neural arch and transverse and spinal processes:
        - Caused by direct force.

Spinal cord injury

Primary injury
- Partial (<60%) or complete transection of the cord, caused by injury to and resultant movement of some of the components of the spinal column on each other.
- Spinal cord damage results in:
    - Impaired distal motor function.
    - Impaired distal sensation.
    - Impaired distal autonomic function.
- The higher up the spinal cord, the greater the resulting disability and risk to life.

Secondary injury
- Mechanical injury:
    - Mechanical displacement of the cord between vertebrae.
    - Movement of bony fragments of vertebrae impinging on the cord.
    - Usually caused by movement of the patient in the vertical position.
    - Unlikely to be caused by careful movement of the patient in the horizontal position.
- Non-mechanical injury occurs due to:
    - Hypoxia as a result of:
        - Airway obstruction
        - Ventilatory problems: chest injury, splinted diaphragm.
    - Underperfusion due to:
        - Hypovolaemia caused by multiple injuries
        - May be exacerbated by orthostatic hypotension as a result of cord injury with autonomic dysfunction.

Symptoms/signs

- It is essential to recognise that a spinal injury may be present following certain types of injury, and one should be positively looked for in those circumstances.
- Try to assess initially whether the cord lesion is complete or incomplete. It may be possible to establish the level of motor and sensory change, which may itself alter.
- The initial symptoms may be bizarre, and should not be dismissed as being due to hysteria/intoxication:
    - Burning pain.
    - Pins and needles.
    - The feeling that the present position of the body is still that in which it was prior to the accident.
- The classical signs are:
    - Local tenderness
    - Total sensory loss below the injury.
- Hemisection of the cord (Brown-Sequard syndrome):
    - Reduction/absence of power, but relatively normal pain and temperature sensation on the same side as the injury.
    - Loss of pain, temperature and touch (pin prick), on the opposite side to the loss of power.
- In the unconscious patient, 10-15% will have some kind of spinal injury indicated by:
    - Hypotension with bradycardia.
    - Diaphragmatic ventilation.
    - Differential pain responses.
    - Flaccid tone.
    - Priapism.

Management

- The first priority is to perform primary assessment and initial life saving procedures, with care of the:
    - **A**irway with cervical spine control (see below)
    - **B**reathing
    - **C**irculation
    - **D**isability
    - **E**xposure.
- Care of the airway and cervical spine thus has the first priority in the initial management of the injured patient, as it can be difficult to provde good airway care in the presence of a cervical spine injury, which itself may be a life threatening injury.
- The aim of specific management of spinal injury is to prevent any secondary injury to the spinal cord:
    - Careful handling, which prevents further mechanical injury.
    - Adequate ventilation to maintain oxygenation of the spinal cord.
    - Maintenance of adequate tissue perfusion. This must be controlled carefully as:
        - Any fall in arterial pressure caused by, e.g. sitting or standing up, will aggravate hypoxia.
        - Any major rise in perfusion pressure caused by, e.g. excessive volume replacement, may result in a haemorrhagic infarct of the cord.

Airway
- "Think spinal, do airway".
- Maintenance of an adequate airway is vital.
- Head tilt:
    - Only move the patient's cervical spine the minimum amount necessary to achieve a clear airway (10° maximum) and apply a jaw thrust (*avoid* chin lifts).
- Avoid suctioning in the tetraplegic patient, as this may stimulate the vagal reflex resulting in aggravation of any pre-existing bradycardia or may even occasionally precipitate cardiac arrest.

Ventilation
- Oxygen (important to reduce any cord hypoxia to the minimum).
- Maintenance of effective ventilation.
- If this is inadequate and the patient has a bradycardia :
    - Consider atropine 0.3-0.6 mg intravenously, prior to the insertion of an airway, suctioning or intubation.
- If the patient is in danger of aspirating, then he should be intubated (nasotracheal intubation is preferred by many).

Circulation
- If the patient has a bradycardia (less than 50 bpm):
    - Consider prophylactic atropine as even a trivial stimulus may cause asystole due to unopposed vagal activity.
    - An isolated cord lesion requires little in the way of fluid replacement:
        - 500 ml is usually sufficient to restore the systolic blood pressure to 90 mmHg.
        - Unless other injuries dictate otherwise, fluid replacement should not exceed 1500 ml.
        - Colloid is preferred to crystalloid (which may cause cord oedema).

Analgesia
- Avoid opiod analgesics in cervical and upper thoracic injuries, especially if ventilation is impaired, due to their ability to cause respiratory depression.
- If pain is not controlled with nitrous oxide/oxygen (Entonox, Nitronox), try:
    - Intravenous or intramuscular non-steroidal anti-inflammatory drugs, e.g. diclofenac, ketoprofen.
    - Small doses of opioids carefully titrated to patient response and avoiding respiratory depression.
- Avoid using buprenorphine, because its effects are only partially reversed by naloxone, if respiratory depression develops.

Moving the patient
- The patient should be moved as little as possible, and only:
    - Away from danger to a place of relative safety.
    - If needed to manage other serious injuries.
- Their injured spine should be immobilised with gentle in-line stabilisation before any movement is attempted.
- If they are wearing a helmet, this should be removed whilst still maintaining in-line stabilisation of the cervical spine.

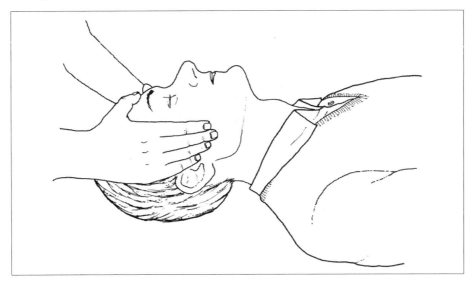

Figure 19-1 Immobilisation of the neck with gentle in-line cervical stabilisation

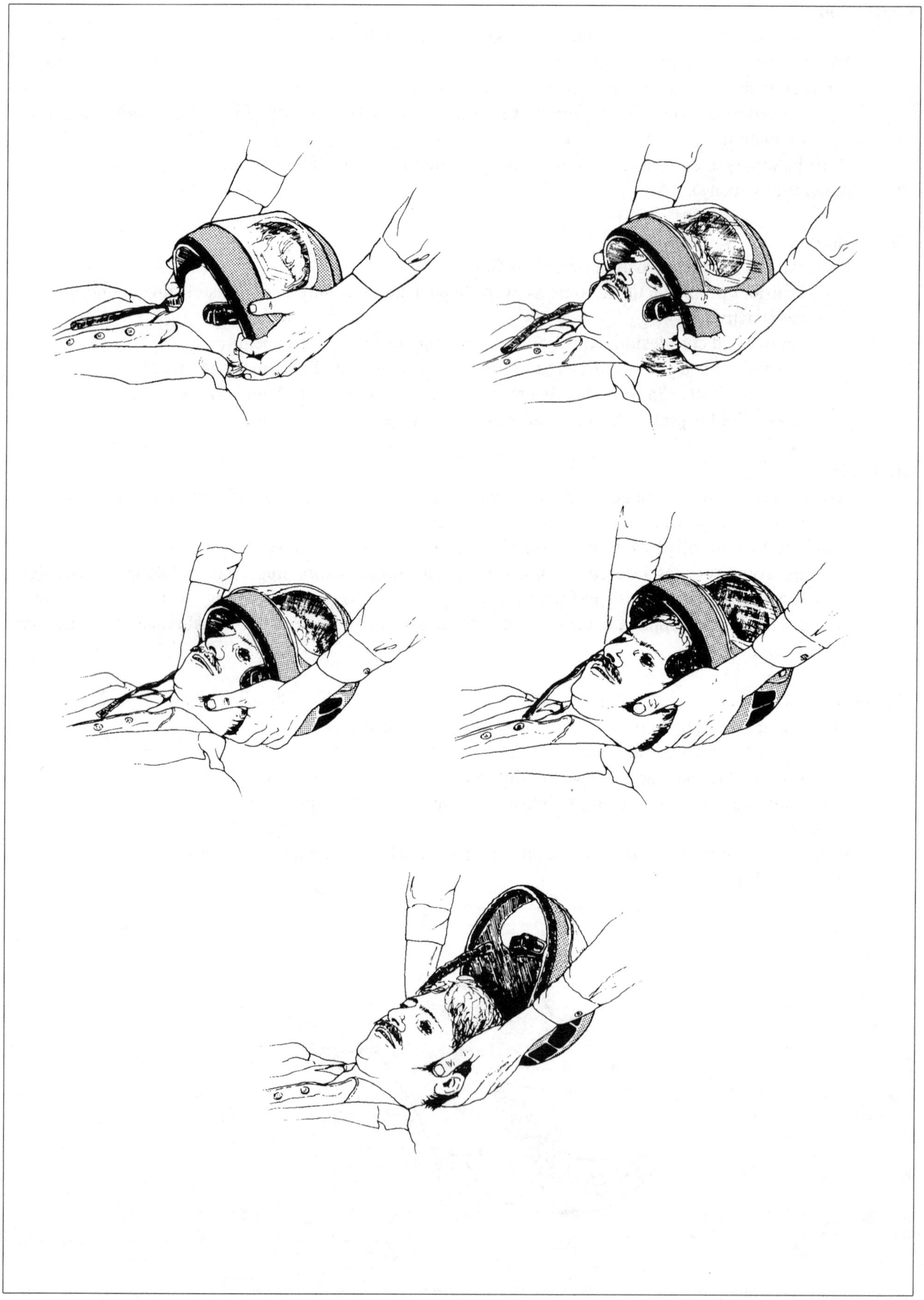

Figure 19-2 Helmet removal maintaining in-line cervical stabilisation: Single rescuer

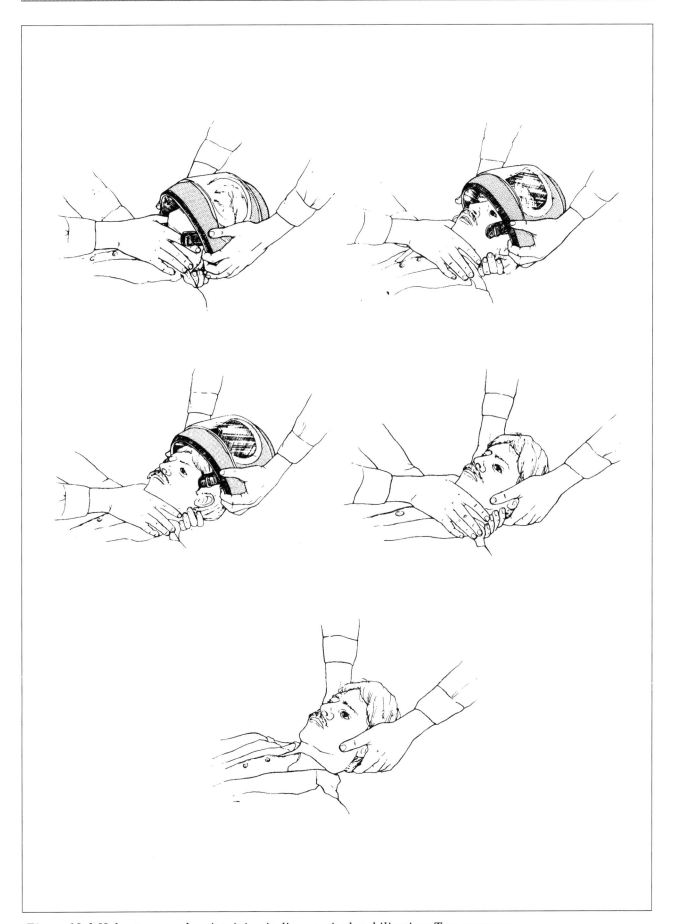

Figure 19-3 Helmet removal maintaining in-line cervical stabilisation: Two rescuers

Immobilisation
- The patient's spine should be stabilised and immobilised before any movement is attempted.
- Loading, transportation and conveyance should be carried out with the minimum of unnecessary movement.
- A scoop stretcher or Donway lifting frame (if available) should be used for transferring the patient onto the ambulance trolley (which ideally should have a vacuum mattress on it), and then from the ambulance trolley onto the hospital examination couch.

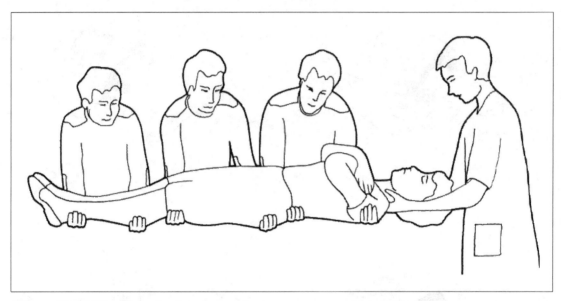

Figure 19-4 Lifting the spinal patient without a scoop stretcher or lifting frame

Position
- The conscious patient should be transported on his back, so as to avoid any respiratory embarrassment caused by splinting the diaphragm by gas, air, or blood from any thoraco-abdominal trauma.
- The patient should *not* at any time be stood or sat up.

Turning the patient onto the back
- If the patient needs turning onto his back, this should be done using the "log roll" method.

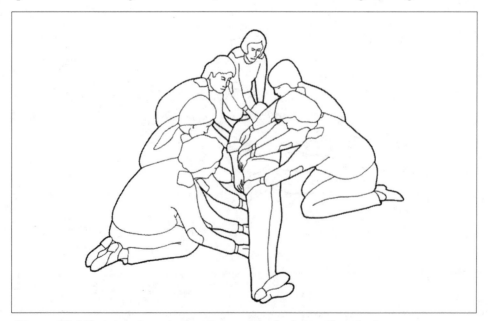

Figure 19-5 Turning the spinal patient using the log roll method

- An alternative method involves using two scoop stretchers.

Method
- With the casualty lying on one scoop stretcher, place another upside down on top of him. The two stretchers are then tied together using triangular bandages along their lengths and the patient is turned.

Turning the patient onto his side:
- It may occasionally be necessary to turn the patient onto his side, as long as breathing is adequate, to prevent an aspiration pneumonitis:
  - The patient's head and neck must always be under the control of a skilled operator, and a rigid cervical collar of the correct size used as an adjunct.
  - The turn is effected, keeping the head in neutral, with the neck and back in a straight line, and providing three point stability at the shoulder, pelvis and knee.
  - One hemidiaphragm should be kept clear of the ground so as to allow adequate ventilation (chest expansion).

Method
- Place the patient's arm nearest your assistant at a right angle to their body, putting the other arm across the chest and bending the furthest knee to a right angle.
- Support the patient's head with your nearest hand, grasp the patient's body at the hip and roll him towards your assistant, who should be positioned kneeling close to the patient.
- The uppermost knee should then be adjusted for stability, and the hand providing head support, is carefully substituted for the other hand, taking care to leave the hand nearest the patient's abducted arm, free to adjust it.
- The elbow of this arm is then bent, bringing the hand close to the patient's chin or even under his head.
- The patient's other arm is then adjusted to interlock in the triangle formed between the lower arm and the head and neck.

Note: - Before turning the patient, make sure that keys, coins, etc. have been removed from his pockets, and that there is no debris or folded clothes under him, as denervated skin may be easily damaged.

Cervical spine injury

Incidence
- This is probably the most common injury to the spinal cord, as the cervical spine is the most vulnerable to injury.

Aetiology
- Occurs most often in unseated motorcyclists, pedal cyclists and horseriders.
- Results in the most severe disability.

Pathophysiology
- Mechanism of injury:
  - Usually caused by an indirect force, e.g. a severe blow to the head, as a result of ejection and the subsequent impact with the ground.
- May be caused by excessive movement in any direction:
  - Flexion.
  - Extension.
  - Lateral flexion.
  - Rotation (in fact it is often a combination of these).

- Flexion alone:
    - Wedge compression fracture: posterior ligament/interspinous ligament rupture.
- Flexion/rotation:
    - Subluxation, dislocation or fracture dislocation (this is the most common cause of spinal cord injury resulting in paralysis).
    - This may also cause massive displacement of an intervertebral disc without any bony injury.
- Hyperextension:
    - Fracture of the neural arch, especially of the atlas or axis.
    - Fracture of the odontoid peg of the axis.
    - May rupture the anterior longitudinal ligament and the annulus fibrosus, forcing the vertebrae apart anteriorly (extension subluxation).
    - Spinal cord damage may be caused in arthritic cervical vertebrae, in which the spinal canal is already narrowed by osteophytes.
- Vertical compression:
    - This may cause a fracture of the atlas (if the pressure is applied from the skull).
    - May result in a burst fracture of the vertebral body.

Assessment
- Often associated with head injury.
- It is frequently impossible to diagnose in the unconscious patient in the field.
- *A cervical spine injury in the unconscious patient following trauma should be presumed until proven otherwise.*

Symptoms/signs
- In the conscious patient there may be:
    - Reduced or absent power distal to the injury.
    - Reduced or absent sensation distal to the injury.
    - Priapism.
- There may be a boggy swelling along the dorsum of the cervical spine.

Management
- It is not usually possible to tell whether or not a fracture is stable or unstable initially (only 1 in 300 deceleration victims who are unconscious have biomechanical instability), so any suspected neck injury should be immobilised in a neutral position, in a cervical splint such as the Hines, or a cervical collar of the correct size such as the Stiffneck, Necklok or Vertebrace, until it can be X-rayed.

Method
- The cervical spine should be supported in a neutral position and a rigid cervical splint carefully applied
- Any applied traction should be minimal, as excessive force can cause a traction injury to the spinal cord in high cervical injuries.
- If the patient is wearing a helmet; this must be removed with care before immobilisation in a rigid collar or splint is attempted (see diagram).
- *If in doubt immobilise the entire spine.*

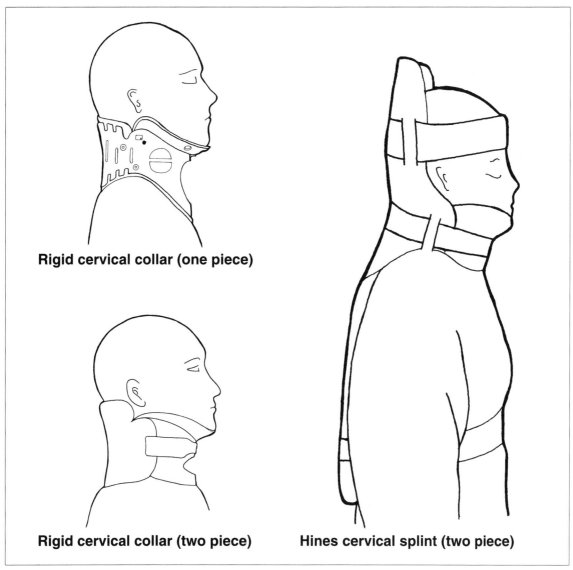

Rigid cervical collar (one piece)

Rigid cervical collar (two piece)

Hines cervical splint (two piece)

Figure 19-6 Rigid cervical collars and cervical splint

Thoracic and lumbar spine

Incidence

- This is a relatively uncommon injury.

Aetiology

- It is usually caused by a direct blow to the back, e.g. as a result of a fall onto a bar, impact from behind.

Pathophysiology

- Flexion (the major cause):
    - Burst fracture
    - Wedge fracture
    - Shear fracture.

- Flexion/rotation:
    - Dislocation of the intervertebral joint, with forward displacement of the upper vertebra on the lower, resulting in spinal cord injury.
- The spinal cord ends at the level of L1.
- Below this it becomes the cauda equina, injury to which carries a much better prognosis than injury to the spinal cord itself.

Symptoms/signs

- Local pain.
- Prominent spinous process, tenderness, or step in the normal contour (may be the only sign in the unconscious patient).
- Painful limitation of movement.
- Reduced or absent power distal to the injury.
- Reduced or absent sensation distal to the injury.
- Sometimes priapism.

Management
- Immobilisation on a spinal board, or if available a spinal immobilation device, before movement is attempted.
- Careful monitoring of any neurological loss, and general condition.

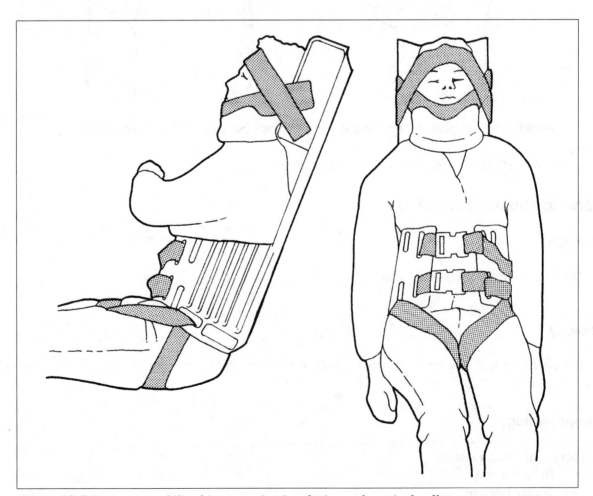

Figure 19-7 Patient immobilised in an extrication device and cervical collar

20

Gunshot and blast injuries

Blast and gunshot injuries

Introduction

- Whilst gunshot and blast injuries are relatively rarely seen in the civilian practice of Immediate Care, their incidence is increasing due to terrorism, and their effective management forms a major part of the role that those practising military Immediate Care are trained in.
- In rural areas, accidental shotgun injuries do occasionally happen, and there is a regrettable increase in the tendency of the use of firearms by the criminal fraternity.
- Unfortunately, there has also been an increase in the type of incident, when a large number of innocent civilians are shot at random as occurred at Hungerford.

Missile injuries

Aetiology
- The missiles may be bullets, or fragments from an explosive device such as a bomb.
- Bullets are aerodynamically far more stable, and have higher kinetic energy than bomb fragments and therefore travel further and can be aimed.

Pathophysiology
- The effect is the same regardless of whether the missile penetrating the skin is a bullet or a fragment.
- In missile injuries there will always be some tissue damage of some extent along the wound track.
- If the damage is confined to this track, it is classified as being a *low energy transfer wound.*
- In some wounds, however, there is tissue damage outside the track caused by the transfer of excess kinetic energy from the missile: this injury is classified as being a *high energy transfer wound.*
- The kinetic energy of a missile is proportional to the product of its mass and the square of its velocity.
- In general bullets from:
    - Rifles and machine guns have a high initial velocity (often up to three or four times the speed of sound) and a resulting high kinetic energy, and usually cause *high energy transfer wounds.*
    - Hand guns and most bomb fragments have subsonic velocities and as a result have a lower kinetic energy and cause *low energy transfer wounds.*

- The amount of energy transferred for any given bullet will depend on:
    - Its position in flight or angle of yaw:
        - This varies during flight, and can affect the amount of kinetic energy transferred to the tissue by a factor of up to 200, depending on the angle at which the bullet strikes the skin. Thus:
            - The same weapon firing identical rounds may have different effects.
            - In some circumstances a very fast bullet may produce a small energy transfer wound, whilst a slow bullet may produce a high energy transfer wound.
    - The weapon firing it.
    - The type of target struck.
- High energy transfer wound results in:
    - A very severe amount of tissue damage/loss around the missile track.
    - Massive wound contamination with a large amount of foreign material which is sucked into both the entry and exit wounds and broken into small fragments and disseminated widely. This is caused by the negative pressure occurring behind the wave of high pressure within the soft tissues and which sucks in debris from outside.
- Low energy transfer wound:
    - The missile may drag in bits of clothing into the wound as it passes, but this is confined to its track and does not cause gross contamination.

Note: - Irrespective of velocity or energy potential, any missile which penetrates the skin, may kill if its path passes through vital organs or structures

Signs/symptoms

- Patients are often unaware of their injuries initially.
- The entry wound may be surprisingly small.

Management

- Whilst an understanding of the pathophysiology of injury is important, it does not usually affect the Immediate Care of the patient, unless evacuation is very prolonged.
- Initial care and management of the:
    - **A**irway, with care of the cervical spine if indicated
    - **B**reathing
    - **C**irculation
    - **D**isability
    - **E**xposure
- If chest penetration is suspected, look for a possible tension pneumothorax.
- If abdominal injury is suspected administer antibiotics and tetanus prophylaxis early.
- If hospital admission is delayed, systemic antibiotics, e.g. benzyl penicillin administered intravenously, should be started (because of the high risk of infection with organisms such as clostridium tetani and clostridium welchii).

Explosives: blast injuries

Aetiology

- Explosives account for the majority of terrorist incidents.
- Urban bombing may result in up to several hundred people being injured.

Types
- Low explosive:
    - Gunpowder.
        - Needs to be confined in an enclosed space to be explosive.
- High explosive:
    - Does not rely on burning.
    - Explodes immediately, but needs more power to set it off, i.e. a detonator.

Pathophysiology

- Injuries can be caused by:
    - Blast waves.
    - Missiles from an explosive device.
    - Casualties being thrown into the air.
- Explosive method:
    - Point explosion.
    - Cloud explosion:
        - May occur with a chemical or gas explosion.
- The explosive blast in a conventional explosion is caused by the very rapid expansion of hot gases, which may propel missiles, but also has three primary effects:
    - The formation of a *blast shock wave*.
    - The release of radiant heat to cause burns.
    - The production of rapidly moving columns of gas and debris in the surrounding air: *the blast wind*.

Primary blast shock wave

Aetiology
- This is a wave of high (over) pressure which spreads out (like the ripples in a pond when a stone is dropped into it) from the centre of the explosion, travelling at just over the speed of sound.
- The power of this high pressure wave may be increased many times when it is reflected from solid objects such as walls, and it therefore causes much more serious injuries when it hits people in an enclosed space.

Pathophysiology
- On hitting a human target, some of the shock wave is reflected, some is deflected, but the majority enters the patient's tissues. Initially the wave entering the patient's tissues is dammed up and increases in strength until it is sufficient to break down the skin and pass through it.
- The wave passes through the tissues producing its greatest effect/damage where there is a change in tissue density.
- Most tissue damage therefore occurs where there is a tissue/gas interface, e.g. in the:
    - Upper and lower respiratory tract.
    - Gastrointestinal tract and abdomen.

Tympanic membrane rupture

Incidence
- This is a very common injury following exposure to an explosive force.

Pathophysiology
- The tympanic membrane is the most susceptible part of the body to damage from high pressure waves (and is a useful indicator that a significant explosion has occurred).
- Unfortunately the converse is not true:
    - The absence of such an injury does *not* exclude exposure to a serious blast wave/over pressure, as the main determinant is the incident angle at which the shock wave hits the tympanic membrane.
- The resultant perforation usually heals spontaneously.
- Higher levels of overpressure may result in additional direct sensineural damage to the cochlea, resulting in deafness similar to that produced by severe acoustic barotrauma.

Symptoms/signs
- Impaired hearing.
- *Always examine the tympanic membranes of anyone who has been near an explosion.*

Olfactory nerve injury

- In the nasal air passages, there may be damage to the olfactory nerve endings resulting in anosmia.

Lung damage: "blast lung"

Incidence
- May occur in up to 5% of those injured in explosions.

Pathophysiology
- The damage produced is:
    - Alveolar and alveolar membrane rupture with intra-alveolar haemorrhage.
        - This haemorrhage causes acute respiratory failure, and produces features similar to the adult respiratory distress syndrome (ARDS).
        - This may result:
            - Immediately
                - Severe respiratory failure: massive contusion.
            - After up to 48 hours:
                - Diffuse less severe lung damage.
        - Even moderate excercise may have an adverse effect.
    - Pulmonary AV shunt damage with air entry into the pulmonary circulation, producing small arterial emboli, which may in turn produce secondary damage.
        - Multiple air emboli may cause occlusion and infarction in the:
            - Coronary circulation resulting in cardiac arrest.
            - Cerebral circulation resulting in bizzare neurological symptoms/signs.
        - Pulmonary air emboli:
            - May also result in pneumothoraces with or without tension.

Symptoms/signs
- The lung damage presents clinically in two ways:
    - Sudden, usually fatal, respiratory failure (with no evidence of external injury).
    - Symptoms may be delayed for up to 48 hours; patients may develop symptoms similar to those in the adult respiratory distress syndrome:
        - Increasing respiratory failure.
- Air emboli:
    - Sudden cardiac arrest (due to coronary artery air emboli)
    - Symptoms similar to stroke
    - Air in the retinal vessels on fundoscopy
    - Pneumothorax.

Management
- If the patient requires ventilation:
    - Intermittent positive pressure ventilation should be avoided if possible, and positive end expiratory pressure (PEEP) should not be used, due to the danger of causing micro air emboli.

Abdominal injury

Pathophysiology
- Massive damage to abdominal organs may occur, but is rarely seen in the survivors of blast injury.
- The most common injuries seen in survivors are:
    - Multiple contusions, with haemorrhage.
    - Intestinal perforation due to necrosis secondary to ischaemia at the site of the haematomas. This may be acute or delayed (up to 5 days).

Symptoms/signs
- Diffuse abdominal pain and tenderness

Blast wind

Aetiology
- Blast wind is a column of gas, initially generated by the explosion, and later by air displaced by the explosion, which moves outwards at very high speed.

Pathophysiology
- Blast winds are often channelled by surrounding features, e.g. furniture, and as a result injuries are totally unpredictable, and may range from very severe to none.
- The injuries produced may be bizarre and very severe:
    - Close to the blast:
        - Total destruction and atomisation may occur with victims being torn apart.
    - On the periphery:
        - Traumatic amputations often occur, with different tissues and structures being avulsed at different levels.
        - Nerves are often avulsed at a much higher level than other tissues.
- The wind may pick up and carry individuals, resulting in injuries when they land.

Management
- A tourniquet may be life-saving.
- Remove any non-viable tissue.

Flash burns

Aetiology
- Depending on the type of explosive, the sudden release of energy may release a wave of hot gas, which may be hot enough to cause flash burns and smoke inhalation injury in those nearby.

Pathophysiology
- Injuries may include superficial burns to the hands and face.
- Smoke inhalation injury may result in delayed symptoms.
- The patient's condition may get worse if he is allowed to exercise.

Management
- All patients should be admitted to hospital.
- All patients must rest.
- Administer oxygen if smoke inhalation injury is suspected.
- Because of the possibility of the delayed onset of respiratory failure due to either blast lung or smoke inhalation and systemic microemboli, a high index of suspicion is required and a conservative attitude adopted to the early discharge of victims home.

Fragment injuries

Incidence
- More often cause injuries than bomb explosions.

Aetiology
- Fragments from the explosive device travel at high speed and may be:
    - Pieces of bomb casing
    - Fragments from near the device
    - Buckshot from a shotgun
    - Bullets from small firearms
- This is a major cause of injuries, as each fragment/missile acts like a independent bullet.
- May cause multiple penetrating missile injuries.

Symptoms/signs
- Patients may be unaware of their injuries initially.

General management

Approach
- Be very careful with your approach to the injured:
    - There may be more explosives around.
    - In a terrorist situation, there may be armed security personnel around.
    - Beware of a secondary device; therefore *do not go near the incident until you are told that it is all clear, and do NOT use your radio!* (may trigger off the device).
- Do *not* touch or move anything except that necessary to provide care of the injured.
- Do *not* disturb any dead bodies except the minimum necessary required to confirm death.
- Be aware of the risk of:
    - Secondary panic: hysteria; myocardial infarction, etc.
    - Terrorists may attempt to kill the survivors later, e.g. in the Intensive Care Unit.

Initial treatment
- Care and management of the patient's:
    - Airway
    - Breathing
    - Circulation, etc.

Specific injuries

Thorax/Thoracic cavity
- Very good at deflecting bullets.
- Beware of tension pneumothorax.
- Close any open wound after first inserting a chest drain.
- Monitor respiratory state continuously.

Head
- Note the patient's neurological state, and their response to the injury.
- Often patients with a significant injury may *not* be unconscious.
- The prognosis for penetrating injuries of the brain caused by missiles is far more accurately related to the neurological status after the injury, than in closed injury: unconsciousness is a grave sign and carries a very poor prognosis.

Forensic responsibilities

- Doctors have a duty to assist in the investigation of crimes as well as obtaining information that may assist in the patient's management.
- They should therefore be aware of the need to obtain information and retain material for forensic investigation of the incident.
- All material pertaining to the incident should be preserved and labelled, with its origin noted and recorded:
    - Debris from wounds.
    - The patient's clothing.
    - Fragments of missile, explosive.
- Examination of the patient should also include noting and recording (and photographing if possible):
    - The entry wound:
        - Ring of contusion.
    - The exit wound:
        - Neat hole or ragged edge.

21

Impalement and penetrating injuries

Impalement and penetrating injuries

Introduction

- The importance, significance, and severity of these injuries may not be appreciated initially, especially by the inexperienced. They require aggressive and effective Immediate Care, if the high morbidity and mortality associated with them is to be reduced.

Incidence

- An uncommon, but serious injury, often but not always a complication of entrapment.

Aetiology

- Most serious if it involves:
    - Head
    - Neck
    - Thoracic cavity
    - Abdominal cavity
- In road traffic accidents often caused by:
    - Vehicle running through roadside fence.
    - Penetration of the passenger compartment by part of (lorry) load.
    - Penetration by part of vehicle.
- May also be caused by:
    - Fall onto a sharp object.
    - Entrapment in moving machinery.
- Patients often have other significant injuries.

Pathophysiology

- In general injury to underlying structures is often more severe than may be suspected at first due to elasticity of the body tissues.
- There may be little obvious haemorrhage initially, due to arterial spasm, but as the spasm wears off haemorrhage may be severe.
- If the object has penetrated one of the body cavities, haemorrhage may be hidden (not apparent) initially.
- Young men in particular may compensate very well for considerable blood loss initially and then go into profound hypovolaemic shock.

Management

Removal of impaling object

- In general *no* attempt should be made to remove the offending object, and great care should be taken not to move it any more than necessary either in transit or if it requires division to release the casualty.
- Blind removal will cause further trauma to the surrounding tissues, which may result in more serious injury, and may precipitate fatal haemorrhage.
- Removal is best carried out in an operating theatre, with full resuscitation facilities, and where the track of the penetrating object will be obvious and can be fully explored.

Hypovolaemia

- Intravenous access should be established as early as possible, preferably with two lines and large bore cannulae, and the patient's haemodynamic status carefully monitored.
- If there is evidence of hypovolaemia, either suspected from the type and location of the injury, or apparent, the patient should be transfused aggressively.

Pneumatic anti-shock garment (PASG)
- Use of a PASG should be considered.
- It may be wise to put patient in a non-inflated PASG prior to transport, and then it is ready to be inflated should the need arise.

Analgesia

- Intravenous analgesia is usually required during release of the casualty, or while the impaling object is divided to facilitate transportation.
- Impaled limbs may require regional anaesthesia.

Notes

22

Amputation and crush injuries

Amputation

Introduction

- Both traumatic amputation, and the need for field amputation are situations which most of those involved in Immediate Care dread, but, thankfully, only experience rarely. Nonetheless the Immediate Care doctor must be familiar with this subject.

Traumatic amputation/avulsion

Aetiology

- This is a relatively rare injury.
- May result from road traffic accidents, industrial accidents, etc.
- Is usually associated with other severe injury, except in industrial accidents, when partial or complete amputation may be the only injury.

Pathophysiology

- Immediately after amputation/avulsion there may be little blood loss due to arterial spasm. As this wears off there may be profuse haemorrhage.
- Owing to advances in microsurgical techniques, it may be possible for the severed limb, etc. to be replanted. This depends on:
    - The level of the amputation.
    - Duration of ischaemia.
    - Type of injury:
        - Amount of bone and tissue loss.
    - Age of patient: fitness to undergo surgery and ability to rehabilitate.
    - Patient's occupation: how important is the severed limb to their job.
    - Severity of associated injuries, and fitness to undergo prolonged surgery.

Management

The patient
- Asessment and management of the patient's:
    - **A**irway, with care of the cervical spine
    - **B**reathing
    - **C**irculation:
        - Prevention of haemorrhage:
            - Tourniquet, arterial clamps.
        - Treatment of hypovolaemic shock:
            - Intravenous infusion of colloid: aggressive fluid replacement may be indicated.
            - It may be possible to cannulate a major vein, which has been left exposed directly.
    - Consider application of a PASG.

The severed limb, etc.
- Should be placed in a clean dry plastic bag, put inside another bag, and kept cool with an instant cool pack, etc. in the outer bag (prolongs ischaemic life).
- If the patient is trapped: the severed part should be sent immediately to the hospital to which the patient will be sent, so that it can be further cooled and prepared for replantation.

Emergency amputation

Incidence

- Very rarely has to be performed at the scene of an accident.

Management

- Unless other dangers dictate the need for immediate rescue, it is best performed by a surgical team from the appropriate district hospital.
- The decision to amputate should never be taken lightly and is best made by two doctors.
- If there is a need for immediate amputation, it is also best performed by two doctors:
    - One to provide analgesia/anaesthesia.
    - One to perform the amputation.

Method
- Establish an intravenous infusion, preferably with two lines and large bore cannulae.
- Administer analgesia:
    - Intravenous opiates.
    - Regional anaesthesia.
    - Ketamine anaesthesia.
- Consider sedation:
    - Midazolam, diazepam.
- Apply a tourniquet and amputate as low as possible with all tissues being divided in the same plane.
- If possible tie off all bleeding vessels.
- Apply a pressure dressing, and elevate the limb (it should then be possible to remove the tourniquet).

Note: - Minimum desirable equipment:
- 6 inch amputation knife.
- 4 inch finger saw.
- Artery forceps and sutures.

Elective dismemberment

Incidence

- Very rarely has to be performed.

Aetiology

- May be necessary:
    - To facilitate the release of other live but trapped casualties.
    - To allow removal of the deceased.

Management

- To facilitate the release of live trapped casualties:
    - Establish an intravenous infusion, if not already done:
        - For management of haemorrhage
        - For administration of drugs.
    - Appropriate anaesthesia should be provided:
        - Ketamine
        - Local/regional anaesthesia.
- To allow removal of the deceased:
    - Death should always be confirmed first.
    - If possible, local guideliness should be discussed with the local Coroner and senior police officers (preferably before the event!).
    - If there is any suggestion of foul play, then if time permits, a forensic pathologist, or if he is not available the local police surgeon, should be called in for his opinion.
    - If possible a photographic record of the circumstances should also be kept (if time permits, the police will call in a Scenes of Crimes Officer (SOCO) to photograph events).
- Disarticulation through the appropriate joint using an amputation knife, scalpel, etc. is the preferred method.

Crush injuries

Introduction

- Crush injuries are relatively rarely encountered in Immediate Care, but their correct management is vital, if patients are going to survive what may be a very serious injury.

Aetiology

- Significant limb compression may occur:
    - When accidents produce prolonged entrapment, e.g.:
        - Inside or under a motor vehicle.
        - Beneath fallen masonry following building collapse due to gas, terrorist activity, earthquake.
        - Industrial accidents when limbs are trapped in machinery.
    - When there is prolonged unconsciousness following:
        - Overdosage.
        - Cerebral vascular accident.
    - Overinflation of a PASG.

Crush injury

Pathophysiology
- Local compression causes:
    - Muscle necrosis due to direct pressure injury and ischaemia.
    - Vascular injury resulting from:
        - Blunt trauma to the limb causing:
            - A rise in pressure in the limb compartments causing external compression of the blood vessels supplying the limb.
            - The muscle damage results in oedema which in turn raises the intracompartmental pressure, causing embarrassment of the venous return.
            - This results in increased swelling and a further rise in compartmental pressure and so a vicious cycle develops.
            - Later, the intracompartmental pressure may be so high that the arterial supply to the comparment is compromised, resulting in further ischaemia and necrosis.
        - Direct arterial injury with intimal vessel injury which may result in occlusion by flaps of intima or by reactive thrombus.

Symptoms/signs
- Petechial haemorrhages: especially of the face and chest.
- Swelling: this is usually severe with tense, shiny skin.
- Significant injury may not always be apparent.
- Absent/reduced peripheral pulses (the presence of a distal pulse does *not* exclude a dangerously high intracompartmental pressure).
- Skin mottling:
    - This is a bad prognostic sign, but if capillary blanching on direct pressure is present, the outlook may not be so gloomy.
- Pallor, cold skin.

- Sensory changes:
    - Reduced sensation/anaesthesia; this may be patchy unless a nerve is damaged.
- Muscle weakness.
- Severe pain on passive stretching of the affected muscles.

Crush syndrome

Pathophysiology
- Death and necrosis of muscle cells results in the release of toxic intracellular constituents into the circulation, after the trapped limb is released, causing:
    - Myoglobinaemia which results in:
        - Myoglobinuria, which causes renal failure (this occurs in 50 % of patients with a crush injury; 100% of those who receive inadequate early fluid replacement).
    - Hyperkalaemia:
        - Arrhythmias and cardiac arrest.
    - An increase in plasma uric acid.
    - An increase in plasma phosphate.
    - An increase in plasma creatinine phosphokinase.
    - A decrease in plasma calcium.
    - A metabolic acidosis.
- Hypovolaemia: due to capillary leakage.

Symptoms/signs
- Neuropsychiatric disturbance: behavioural problems.
- Respiratory distress: Adult Respiratory Distress syndrome.
- Hypovolaemic shock.
- Acute renal failure: oliguria.
- Disseminated intravascular coagulation.
- Stress induced upper gastrointestinal tract ulceration.

Management
- Airway support and oxygen.
- Breathing: ventilatory support.
- Circulation:
    - Aggressive intravenous fluid infusion:
        - Crystalloid is best as it helps produce a diuresis, which helps prevent the kidneys from being damaged by absorbed toxin, by protecting the distal tubules.
- Analgesia:
    - Nitrous oxide/oxygen.
    - Opiates.
- Consider amputation:
    - *Only* if the limb is non viable, or to expedite release from a hazardous environment:
        - Fire, toxic fumes, rising water level, collapsing building, etc.
    - The best anaesthetic is probably ketamine.
- Sedation: diazepam/midazolam
- Apply adequate splintage.

23

Burns

Burns

Introduction

- Severe burns are relatively rarely encountered in Immediate Care, but they can be amongst the most severe injuries encountered, and require appropriate and effective Immediate Care if patients are going to survive them.

Incidence

- Most common in the very young and the elderly.
- Burns are the second most common cause of accidental death in children in the UK.
- Account for 10000 hospital admissions per year in England and Wales, of whom 1000 (>10% of children and >15% of adults) suffer from hypovolaemic shock. Of these up to 30% can be expected to have an inhalational injury.

Aetiology

- Usually hot liquids under the age of 3 years.
- Careless smoking and hot liquids in the elderly.
- Accidents with flammable liquids: adults.
- RTAs and house fires: adults.

Pathophysiology

The insult
- The insult causing damage to the skin may be:
    - Heat/cold/friction.
    - Electricity:
        - There may be associated cardiorespiratory arrest/cardiac arrythmias.
        - Electrical burns are usually full thickness, with considerable underlying tissue damage.
    - Chemicals:
        - Acids
        - Alkalis
    - Radiation.

Burn oedema

-   Shortly after the burn, plasma begins to pool beneath the damaged area, as a result of the altered capillary permeability, and there is fluid (plasma) shift from the intravascular space to the extravascular space.
-   There will be a rise in haematocrit, as more plasma is lost from the intravascular to the extravascular space.
-   If more than 15% of the body surface is burnt, progressive fluid loss from the circulation will result in hypovolaemic shock:
    -   Critical % levels:
        -   Child: >10%
        -   Adult: >20%
        -   Elderly: >10%

Depth of burn

-   This is determined by:
    -   The nature of the agent: temperature, concentration.
    -   The length of contact.
    -   The tissues' resistance to injury:
        -   Skin: vascularity, thickness.

Classification of burns

Partial thickness

-   Involving the epidermis and the superficial dermis.
-   Often caused by flash burns, scalds in adults.

Full thickness

-   Damage extending through the dermis to the subcutaneous tissues.
-   Caused by flames, burning clothing and scalds in young children.
-   Usually there is a combination of both full and partial thickness burns.

Symptoms/signs

Partial thickness burn

-   Pain, erythema, blistering.
-   Tenderness, blanching with applied pressure.

Full thickness burn

-   Dull red, grey-white.
-   Painless, insensitive, does not blanch with pressure.

Assessment of area of burn

-   This is done roughly using the "rule of nines" (but not for children):
    -   The body is divided up into eleven areas, each representing 9% of the total body surface.
-   A Lund & Browder chart gives a more accurate assessment.

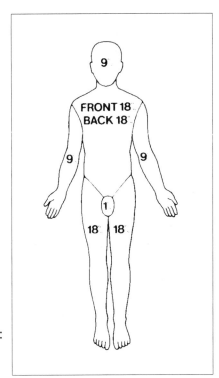

Figure 23-1 Rule of nines

Initial management

Heat burns

- Remove the casualty from the source of the danger:
    - Fire, heat, etc.
- Lie the casualty down, and smother any flames (flames travel upwards, and may cause burns of the face and head).
- If there is smoke or toxic fumes:
    - Remove the patient into fresh air.
- Clothing:
    - If it is still smouldering: douse with water.
    - If it is saturated with hot liquids: remove or cool with water.
    - Other than this, especially if clothing is adherent to skin: leave it on.

Chemical burns

- Remove the chemicals:
    - Usually by applying copious fluids, especially to the eyes and face, and continue applying for as long as possible.
- Remove any contaminated clothing.
- Note the identity of the chemical.

Electrical burns

- Domestic:
    - Unplug the appliance involved and/or if possible switch off the mains electricity.
    - Remove the patient from the source of electricity, with a non conducting object.
- Begin Basic Life Support immediately, and defibrillate if appropriate.
- Treat the dermal injury (see below).

Specific injuries

The airway

General

- Oxygen:
    - Put the patient in a respirable atmosphere, especially when they have been exposed to smoke and noxious gases.
- If unconscious:
    - Make sure that the patient has an adequate airway.
    - In electrical burns/electric shock, be prepared to begin expired air ventilation.

Upper airway injury: laryngeal oedema

Aetiology
- May be caused by:
    - Burns
    - Scalds to the face
    - Inhalation of flame, hot gases or steam.

Pathophysiology
- Acute tissue injury resulting in oedema and swelling, which may eventually obstruct the airway.
- The more severe the thermal injury, the earlier obstruction will be apparent.

Symptoms/signs
- Facial burns especially around mouth, nose and neck.
- Soot in the nostrils.
- Singed nasal hairs.
- Pharyngeal oedema.
- Laryngeal oedema:
    - Hoarseness.
    - Stridor.

Management
- Airway:
    - Maintain a satisfactory position for the head/neck.
    - Administer humidified air or oxygen if available (consider using a nebuliser).
    - Endotracheal intubation:
        - Should be performed on a conscious patient using a local anaesthetic (lignocaine) spray.
        - Perform early, using a smaller tube than usual, as intubation may be difficult later due to laryngeal oedema.
    - Cricothyrotomy:
        - For severe facial injury.
        - If endotracheal intubation is not possible.
    - Inhaled beclomethasone may help reduce inflammation and make the patient more comfortable.

Lower airway injury

Aetiology
- Injury may be caused by:
    - Fire in an enclosed space.
    - Facial burns.
    - Inhalation of smoke or steam (may cause a severe thermal injury).
    - Noxious gases:
        - Hydrogen cyanide
        - Isocyanates
        - Isocyanides
        - Nitrogen dioxide
        - Sulphur dioxide
        - Hydrogen chloride ⎫ given off when
        - Phosgene ⎬ PVC burns.
        - Phenol
        - Toluene
        - Carbon monoxide.

Pathophysiology

- Damage to the lung parenchyma is due to a combination of:
  - Poor tissue perfusion of the lungs, secondary to hypovolaemia.
  - The corrosive effect of chemicals, rather than heat (with the exception of steam).

Symptoms/signs

- Perioral burns/soot in the nostrils.
- Pharyngeal oedema.
- Hoarseness/loss of voice/stridor.
- Wheezing
- Soot in the sputum.
- Bronchorrhea.
- A reduced peak flow.
- A reduced SaO_2, but beware of over optimistic readings, as a pulse oximeter probe is unable to distinguish carboxyhaemoglobin from oxyhaemoglobin.
- Altered level of consciousness.

Management

Airway (see above)

Breathing: ventilation
- Intermittent positive pressure ventilation.
- Bronchospasm:
  - Nebulised β_2 agonists (salbutamol).
  - Steroids are of no immediate value.
- If circumferential burns of the chest are interfering with effective ventilation by restricting chest expansion, consider:
  - Escharotomy.

Circulation
- Cardiac arrest:
  - Begin external chest compressions immediately.
- Fluid replacement:
  - Aggressive fluid replacement should be started as soon as possible:
    - Rate of infusion in the first hour post burn: 1 ml/%burn/10 kg body weight.
  - Use two large bore cannulae: 12/14/16 gauge.
  - The best veins for this are:
    - Antecubital fossa veins
    - Forearm veins
    - Jugular veins.
  - An intravenous cutdown may be necessary, but may not require local analgesia due to damage to the sensory nerve endings (there may also be damage to the superficial veins).
  - Blood samples should be obtained if possible.
  - Crystalloid is preferable to colloid initially.
- Keep the patient warm.

Note:- Sites distal to the burn may be shut down, and those under the burn may be fried.

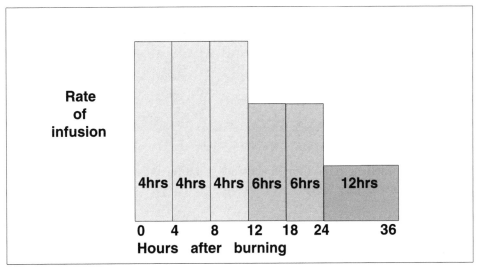

Figure 23-2 Infusion for burns using the Muir and Barclay formula: each block represents an equal volume of plasma. The volume of plasma to be infused in each block is 0.5 ml/kg/% burn.

Pain

- There may be less pain than expected in full thickness burns.
- Analgesia:
    - Entonox.
    - Morphine, preferably combined with an antiemetic.
- Sedation of the burnt patient:
    - Consider chlorpromazine:
        - Potentiates narcotics.
        - Antiemetic.
        - Sedative.
        - (Also long acting).

Dermal injury

Assessment of the severity of burns

- Nature.
- Depth.
- Area: "rule of nines"or calculated from Lund and Browder chart.

Management

Dressings
- Cover the burns with sterile dressings:
    - Cling film (ideal)
    - Polythene bags.
- If the travelling time to hospital is more than 1 hour consider using Roehampton burns dressings or similar.
- Minor/small injury:
    - Cooling with water may be very useful.

Note:- - Do not burst blisters.
- - Do not apply cream, e.g. Flamazine, as this can make subsequent assessment of the burn difficult.

Infection
- - Avoidance of unnecessary contamination.
- - Antibiotics:
  - - Erythromycin
  - - Flucloxacillin.
  - - May not be practical in the Immediate Care situation and should only be used if the travelling time to hospital is very long.

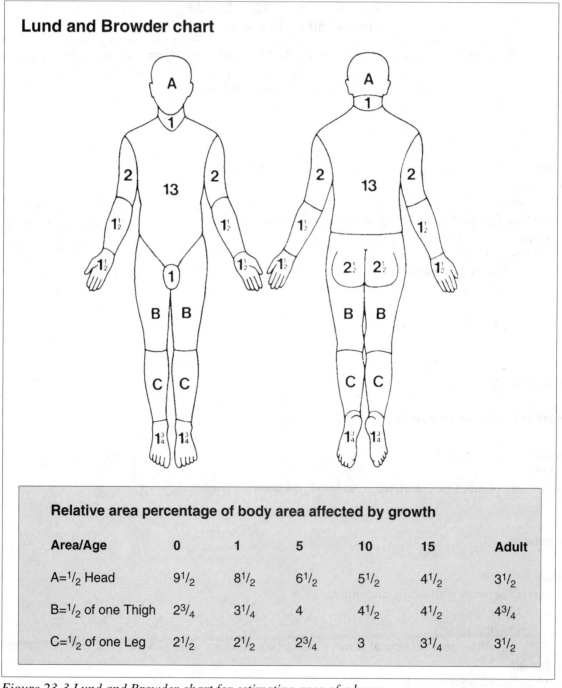

Lund and Browder chart

Relative area percentage of body area affected by growth

Area/Age	0	1	5	10	15	Adult
A=$^1/_2$ Head	$9^1/_2$	$8^1/_2$	$6^1/_2$	$5^1/_2$	$4^1/_2$	$3^1/_2$
B=$^1/_2$ of one Thigh	$2^3/_4$	$3^1/_4$	4	$4^1/_2$	$4^1/_2$	$4^3/_4$
C=$^1/_2$ of one Leg	$2^1/_2$	$2^1/_2$	$2^3/_4$	3	$3^1/_4$	$3^1/_2$

Figure 23-3 Lund and Browder chart for estimating area of a burn

24

Obstetric emergencies

Obstetric emergencies

Introduction

- A knowledge of the Immediate Care of obstetric emergencies is a prerequisite for those in General Practice involved in Immediate Care, especially with the recent run down of obstetric flying squads, and the current proposals that the ambulance service supported by BASICS' doctors take over this role.

Antenatal problems

Vaginal bleeding in pregnancy

Miscarriage

Incidence
- Approximately 10-15% of confirmed pregnancies end in miscarriage/spontaneous abortion.
- Most often occurs at about 8 weeks and again at about 12 weeks from the first day of the last menstrual period.
- Less commonly, it may occur later in pregnancy, i.e. up to 28 weeks due to:
    - Cervical incompetence.
    - Rarely:
        - Congenital uterine abnormality.
        - Severe maternal illness.

Aetiology
- The precise cause for most miscarriages is unknown, but may include:
    - Fetal abnormality.
    - Failure of implantation and malimplantation "placenta praevia".
    - Cervical incompetence.
    - Uterine abnormality.
    - Maternal illness.
- Many threatened miscarriages may progress to an established pregnancy and the successful delivery of a normal infant.

Pathophysiology

Threatened miscarriage/abortion
- There is some vaginal bleeding, which may or may not be retroplacental.
- The pregnancy may continue to term.

Inevitable miscarriage/abortion
- Complete:
  - More likely after 16 weeks.
  - This occurs when the cervix dilates and the products of conception are extruded into the cervical canal.
  - The uterus expels its contents completely and the cervical os is open.
- Incomplete:
  - More likely before 16 weeks.
  - The blood loss may be considerable.
  - The cervix is open and the uterus contracts, expelling some, but not all, of its contents. Some decidua is retained, so the miscarriage is incomplete.

Septic abortion
- This occurs following an incomplete or induced abortion, when, due to non-sterile conditions, pathogenic organisms ascend from the vagina into the uterus.
- The commonest organisms involved are *E. coli* and *Streptococcus faecalis,* which may cause endotoxic shock.

Symptoms/signs
- Known to be pregnant or late with a period.
- History of a recent spontaneous miscarriage.
- Vaginal blood loss:
  - This may be either light or heavy.
  - Will be offensive in septic abortion.
- Lower abdominal pain:
  - There may be no pain initially, or there may be colicky lower abdominal pain similar to dysmenorrhoea (it may be less or more severe).
- Hypovolaemic shock.
- Toxic shock.

Management
- If the blood loss is:

Minor (threatened miscarriage/abortion)
- Bed rest for 48 hr.
- Consider sedation.
- If the vaginal loss continues:
  - Perform a speculum examination of the cervix to exclude:
    - Cervical polyps
    - Severe cervical erosion
    - Carcinoma of the cervix.
- Arrange an urgent outpatient assessment:
  - For probable ultrasound scan.

Note:- Digital vaginal examination is not advisable.

Moderate
- Set up a precautionary intravenous infusion.
- Arrange immediate hospital admission (there is little justification for examination).

Severe (indicates an inevitable abortion)
- Set up an intravenous infusion of colloid.
- Examine vaginally.
- Remove any products of conception from the cervical os.
- Evacuate the vagina (send all fetal material to the hospital with the patient if possible).
- Administer:
    - Ergometrine and oxytocin (Syntometrine) intramuscularly or intravenously.
- Transfer to hospital immediately.

Septic shock
- See chapter on Circulation Care: Bacteriological Shock.

Hydatidiform mole

Incidence
- Occurs in approximately 1:2-3000 pregnancies.

Pathophysiology
- Chromosomal changes in the fertilised oocyte lead to degeneration of the blood vessels in the villi in very early pregnancy, resulting in vesicles being formed inside the uterus (usually no fetus is found).
- 10% progress to become an invasive mole or choriocarcinoma.

Symptoms/signs
- May present at 8-10 weeks with symptoms similar to a threatened miscarriage.
- The uterine size is usually larger than the dates would suggest.
- Vomiting may be severe.
- The signs of pre-eclampsia may develop with hypertension and proteinuria.
- No fetal heart is heard and no fetal parts are palpable.

Management
- Treatment of complications, e.g. vomiting, eclampsia.
- Hospital admission.

Ectopic pregnancy

Incidence
- 1:200 pregnancies and is increasing.
- The death rate from this complication is falling, due to increased awareness and improved early diagnostic facilities.

Aetiology
- Most often occurs due to tubal damage caused by previous:
    - Infection:
        - Salpingitis
        - Pelvic inflammatory disease.
    - Tubal surgery.
- Other precipitating factors include:
    - IUD use.
    - Use of the progesterone only oral contraceptive pill.
    - History of infertility.

Pathophysiology
- An ectopic pregnancy may develop outside the uterine cavity; most (96%) occur in the fallopian tube.

Tubal ectopic pregnancy
- May either:
    - Rupture through the tubal wall, resulting in a brisk intra peritoneal haemorrhage *or*
    - Leak a little blood from the fimbrial end of the tube, which causes irritation in the peritoneum pouch of Douglas.

Symptoms/signs
- The diagnosis may be difficult: 40% are missed by the first doctor.
- Sudden collapse at home (unusual as the initial presentation).
- Pain:
    - Lower abdominal pain in either iliac fossae:
        - Stabbing
        - Colicky
        - Cramping.
    - Usually precedes the vaginal loss (other causes usually result in vaginal loss followed by the onset of pain).
- Vaginal bleeding:
    - Only present in 75%.
    - May be scanty, dark brown (like prune juice).
- Symptoms of early pregnancy (sometimes):
    - Frequency.
    - Breast tenderness.
- Signs of hypovolaemic shock.
- Anaemia:
    - There may have been blood loss for some time.
- Localised lower abdominal tenderness with the signs of peritonism:
    - Guarding.
    - Shifting dullness.
    - Evidence of infective shock.
    - Shoulder tip pain.
    - Pyrexia.

- On vaginal examination:
    - Cervical excitability is characteristic.
    - Tenderness in the pouch of Douglas or in either adnexa.

Differential diagnosis
- Abortion:
    - The vaginal loss is more profuse, with fresh blood.
- Salpingitis:
    - Swelling and bilateral lower abdominal pain, pyrexia.
- Appendicitis:
    - The area of tenderness is usually higher.
- Torsion of ovarian cyst.

Management
- Initial resuscitation, if there is evidence of hypovolaemic shock:
    - Set up an intravenous infusion(s) of colloid using a wide bore cannula.
- Carry out careful monitoring of the pulse and blood pressure.
- Consider:
    - Application of a PASG.
    - Calling for the assistance of a flying squad, or another Immediate Care doctor, if they can be on the scene very rapidly.
- Arrange for immediate admission.

Cyst accidents

Incidence
- Rare

Aetiology
- Torsion of an ovary containing a functional, e.g. luteal, or neoplastic cyst.

Symptoms/signs
- Collapse
- Vomiting
- Pain in the region of the sacro-iliac joint or iliac fossa.

Differential diagnosis
- Tubal pregnancy (very difficult to distinguish from this).
- Renal colic.
- Infection.
- Dysmenorrhoea.
- Appendicitis.

Management
- Treat symptomatically and admit.

Antepartum haemorrhage   (bleeding after 28 weeks of pregnancy)

Incidence
- Occurs in 3% of pregnancies.

Pathophysiology
- If the placenta separates before delivery, the denuded placental bed will bleed profusely.
- The amount of placental separation may only be small, but if it is large, the placental circulation may be compromised and fetal death may ensue.

Placental abruption
- Occurs when the placenta is situated in the upper uterus.
- The blood from the placental bed is confined initially between the placenta and the uterine wall.

Placenta praevia
- Occurs when the placenta is in the lower segment.
- The blood from the placental bed is released into the vagina.

Aetiology
- May be caused by:
    - Bleeding from the cervix from cervical erosion, polyps or carcinoma.
    - Placenta praevia.
    - Placental abruption.

Assessment
- This must be rapid: rely on the physical signs:
    - General maternal appearance:
        - Signs of hypovolaemic shock.
    - Vaginal bleeding:
        - *Do not perform a vaginal examination.*
        - Minimal examination only is indicated.
    - Uterine irritability.
    - Adominal pain/tenderness.
    - Increasing fundal height.
    - Evidence of fetal distress:
        - Fetal heart rate.

Management
- All patients need admission.
- How quickly depends on:
    - The amount of blood loss.
    - Whether or not resuscitation is needed first.
- Minor blood loss:
    - Intravenous infusion.
    - Transfer to hospital.
- Major blood loss:
    - Hypovolaemic shock:
        - The patient needs fluid/blood as soon as possible:
            - Set up two infusions of colloid.
            - Use a large cannula: 14/16 gauge.
            - Take blood for group (if not already done), cross match and clotting factors.
            - Infuse rapidly.

- Pain relief:
    - There may be little or no pain with a placenta praevia.
    - If there is an abruption, there may be very considerable pain, consider:
        - Administration of morphine.
- Monitor the fetal heart.
- Transfer the patient quickly to hospital (an accurate diagnosis is irrelevant).

Pain in pregnancy

Differential diagnosis

- Abruption: see above.
- Renal colic:
    - Acute loin pain radiating to the groin, haematuria.
- Fibroids:
    - Torsion.
    - Red degeneration: acute pain, vomiting, tenderness, pyrexia at 24-30 weeks.
- Ovarian cysts:
    - Torsion: acute pain, tenderness, vomiting and often pyrexia.
- Uterine rupture:
    - Rupture of old LSCS, myomectomy or hysterotomy scar: obvious on palpation.
    - In high parity.
- Aneurysm:
    - Rupture.
- Appendicitis:
    - The point of tenderness is usually higher than normal.
    - Nausea.
    - There is a reduced response to inflammation.
- Cholecystitis:
    - Tenderness in the right hypochondrium.
- Toxaemia: may also present as abdominal pain (see below).

Fits: Pre-eclamptic toxaemia/eclampsia
- More likely to be fatal outside hospital due to poor recognition.
- More likely to be fatal the earlier it occurs in pregnancy.

Incidence

Pre-eclamptic toxaemia
- Commonest antenatal problem in pregnancy affecting up to 10% of all pregnancies (20% first).
- More likely to develop into eclampsia in concealed pregnancy due to failure to recognise the significance of the symptoms.
- Usually occurs in the third trimester, but may be as early as 20 weeks or occur a few days after delivery.

Eclampsia
- Occurs in about 1:1,500 deliveries (UK 1992)
- Results in the death of about 1000 babies and 10 women each year in the UK.
- Less common now than it used to be because of improvements in antenatal care (27 deaths in the period 1985-7 in England and Wales).
- Pregnancy-induced hypertension is responsible for 25% of cases of low and very low birth-weight.

Aetiology

- The precise cause is unknown, but predisposing factors include:
    - Maternal:
        - First pregnancies
        - Lower socio-economic class
        - Short stature
        - Increasing maternal age
        - Diabetes mellitus
        - Previous history of eclampsia and renal disease
        - Pre-existing or pregnancy induced hypertension
        - Obesity.
    - Fetal:
        - Multiple pregnancy
        - Hydatidiform mole
        - Hydrops.

Pathophysiology

- The disease is not fully understood, but is primarily a placental disorder:
    - Abnormal invasion of the uterus by the trophoblast, with absence of the second phase in which the trophoblast usually invades the spiral arteries.
    - The spiral arteries retain their muscular coat and their responsiveness to myotonic stimuli.
    - There is abnormal fibrin deposition in the placenta with acute atheroma deposition.
    - Vascular endothelial damage activates the coagulation cascade resulting in an increase in platelet aggregation.
    - There is a failure of adequate dilation of the maternal spiral arteries feeding the placenta resulting in placental ischaemia, and maternal and fetal illness.
    - Arteriolar constriction results in:
        - Fitting
        - Secondary pulmonary and cerebral oedema
        - Cerebral haemorrhage (cause most of the maternal mortality associated with eclampsia)
        - Cardiac, hepatic and renal failure
        - Secondary blood clotting disorder
        - Intrauterine growth retardation
        - Placental abruption
        - Fetal hypoxia and intrauterine death.

Symptoms/signs

- Pre-eclampsia is diagnosed when a pregnant woman of 20 or more weeks gestation has a blood pressure greater than 140/90 mmHg, and she has proteinuria +, or more, on dipstick testing.
- Headache, vomiting and itching in the mask area of the face.
- Visual disturbance:
    - Spots in front of the eyes.
    - Angular flashes at the periphery of the visual fields.
    - Loss of vision in some areas.
- May be jittery, hyperreactive/hyperreflexic before the onset of fits.
- Upper abdominal pain (usually epigastric or right sided):
    - Due to sub-capsular hepatic haemorrhage or peritoneal stretching over an oedematous liver.
- Oedema and weight gain.
- Hypertensive retinopathy (in a few cases).

Management

- If not fitting:
    - Establish an intravenous infusion.
    - Sedate with intravenous or rectal diazepam (stesolid).
- If there is imminent risk of fitting:
    - Sedate with diazepam.
    - Arrange immediate hospital admission.
    - Carry out careful and continuous monitoring of the patient's condition before and during transfer to hospital and on arrival.
- If there is fitting, manage as for epilepsy:
    - Airway maintenance
        - Position on their side
        - Oxygen
        - Consider intubation to protect the airway from the risk of gastric aspiration (a common cause of maternal death).
    - Prevent self injury during fits.
    - Stop fits:
        - Diazepam: 10-40 mg:
            - Intravenous: Valium
                          Diazemuls (better as less irritant).
            - Rectal: Stesolid.
        - Midazolam: 5-10 mg administered intravenously.
        - Consider a diazepam infusion.
    - Monitor the fetal heart.
    - Transfer to hospital immediately.
    - Consider administration of a hypotensive, e.g. a β-blocker.
      (Delivery is the ultimate treatment for eclampsia).

Problems during labour

Labour at home

Aetiology
- May be:
    - Unplanned: concealed pregnancy.
    - Early labour.
- Rapid labour.
    - Complicated delivery.

Assessment
- History.
- Is the patient:
    - In labour?
    - Bleeding?
- Is the blood pressure elevated or depressed?
- Is the fetal heart rate satisfactory?

Management
- Decide whether patient should:
    - Stay at home.
    - Be transferred to hospital.

Uncomplicated
- Deliver and then transfer to hospital.

Complicated delivery
- Delay in the second stage:
    - Admit to hospital.
- Fetal distress:
    - Deliver rapidly or if this is not possible arrange immediate admission to hospital.
- Cord prolapse:
    - If there is *no* detectable fetal heart:
        - Allow the patient to deliver.
    - If there *is* a good fetal heartbeat:
        - Consider an attempt to reduce the cord back into the vagina with a pack, as this will keep it warm and moist, and will reduce the risk of cord spasm and avoids any unnecessary handling.
        - Put the patient in the knee elbow position with elevation of the buttocks.
        - Convey to hospital for probable LSCS.
- Breech presentation:
    - If in the second stage:
        - Control delivery with the patient in the lithotomy position using an effective episiotomy.
        - Maintain jaw flexion, exert gentle shoulder traction to the aftercoming head, allowing controlled delivery.
- Shoulder dystocia:
    - Deliver with the patient lying on her left side with a large episiotomy.
    - Pull the head back to allow the anterior shoulder to escape beneath the symphysis pubis.

Neonatal resuscitation

- Full paediatric resuscitation equipment should always be available.
- For full method: see chapter on Neonatal Resuscitation.

Management (brief summary)

Airway
- Suction; aspiration of the oropharynx.
- Oxygen.

Breathing
- Ventilation with a bag and mask.
- Intubation if necessary.
- Keep the baby as warm as possible (neonates lose heat very rapidly).

Pulmonary embolism of amniotic fluid

Incidence
- This is very rare, usually occuring as a complication of surgical induction, and therefore almost unknown outside hospital.
- It is usually fatal; often the diagnosis is only made at postmortem.
- If the patient survives the initial shock a coagulation defect is inevitable.

Aetiology
- May occur as a result of:
    - Surgical induction
    - Placental abruption
    - Multiple pregnancy
    - Polyhydramnios.

Pathophysiology
- Amniotic fluid or trophoblast tissue enters the maternal circulation, where the thromboplastins provoke disseminated intravascular coagulation, which leads to depletion of plasma fibrinogen.

Symptoms/signs
- May occur immediately after amniotomy, but is usually preceded by strong uterine contractions.
- Pulmonary embolism: intense dyspnoea.
- Severe shock with total circulatory collapse.
- If caused by abruption, there may be loss of fetal movement and heartbeat.

Management
- Treat shock aggressively:
    - Oxygen.
    - Administer intravenous fluids.
    - Consider application of PASG.
- Arrange for immediate conveyance to hospital.

Post-partum problems

Post partum haemorrhage

Incidence
- Uncommon outside hospital.

Aetiology

Primary
- Retained placenta.
- Atonic uterus.

Secondary
- Retained placenta (more likely to happen at home with the current vogue for early discharge).
- Post LSCS: infected placental site or incision site.
- Uterine inversion.
- Infection.

Management
- Assess the blood loss (it is easy to over estimate this).
- Establish an intravenous infusion.
- Administer intravenous oxytocics: ergometrine.
- Treat the cause:
  - Haemorrhage:
    - Stop the bleeding by applying bimanual uterine pressure after first emptying the bladder (if possible).
  - Uterine inversion:
    - Needs to be corrected immediately, as this condition may be fatal very rapidly due to irreversible shock.
  - Retained placenta:
    - Attempt removal (empty the bladder first).
- Apply controlled cord traction.
- Transfer the patient to hospital immediately.

Obstetric pharmacology

Introduction

- The drugs used in obstetrics are smooth muscle stimulants, and cause uterine contraction.
- Those doctors involved in Immediate Care should carry one drug rather than the whole range of drugs.

Ergometrine maleate

Indications
- Active management of the third stage of labour, post-partum haemorrhage.

Contraindications
- 1st and 2nd stages of labour.
- Vascular disease.
- Impaired pulmonary, hepatic or renal function.

Cautions
- Toxaemia
- Cardiac disease
- Hypertension
- Sepsis.

Side effects
- Nausea, vomiting
- Transient hypertension
- Peripheral vasoconstriction.

Presentation
- Ergometrine 500 μg per ml: 1 ml ampoule.

Dosage
- Intramuscularly: 200-500 μg: (onset 5-7 minutes, duration about 45 minutes).
- Intravenously (emergency control of haemorrhage): 100-500 μg (onset 1 minute).

CONCLUSION: The oxytocic of choice for the management of post-partum haemorrhage.

Oxytocin (Syntocinon)

Indications
- Induction and augmentation of labour.
- Management of incomplete and missed abortion.

Contraindications
- Severe toxaemia.
- Predisposition to amniotic fluid embolism.

Cautions
- Hypertension.
- High parity.

Side effects
- Violent uterine contractions.
- Maternal hypertension and subsequent subarachnoid haemorrhage.
- Cardiac arrhythmias.
- Water intoxication.

Presentation
- Oxytocin: 5 units/ml: 1 ml ampoules.
            10 units/ml: 1 ml ampoules.

Dosage
- Missed abortion:
    - 10-20 units/500 ml given at a rate of 15 drops per minute and adjusted according to response.

Ergometrine maleate/oxytocin (Syntometrine)

Properties

- Combines the rapid action of oxytocin with the more sustained action of ergometrine, both of which cause uterine contraction.

Indications
- The active management of the third stage of labour.
- The prevention of post-partum haemorrhage, following delivery of the placenta.
- To control post-partum haemorrhage.

Presentation
- Ergometrine 500 μg/5 units oxytocin per 1 ml: 1 ml ampoule.

Dosage
- 1 ml intramuscularly or 0.5-1.0 ml intravenously (if there is a high risk of post-partum haemorrhage).

CONCLUSION: The oxytocic of choice for the active management of the third stage of labour and controlling haemorrhage due to incomplete abortion (ergometrine and oxytocin may be used alone for the management of haemorrhage due to incomplete abortion, but have less effect on the early pregnant uterus).

Notes

25

The accident scene

The accident scene

Introduction

- Although almost every incident is unique, the procedures and guideliness to be followed are basically the same, and with experience should be instinctive.
- It requires a lot of self discipline to adhere to them and not to be distracted into doing either what others expect, or what your emotions tell you.
- In particular, it is best to be relatively slow and sure, although a great deal of pressure may be put on you to do things either too quickly or not at all.
- A few minutes doing things properly may save much time and even life, later on.

Preparation

- Your **vehicle** should be:
    - Well prepared and maintained with:
        - Clean headlights.
        - Regularly checked brakes, tyres, oil level, etc.
        - A full petrol tank.
    - Highly visible: white or red, possibly with reflective strips.

- Your **equipment** should be:
    - Well maintained, and expendable items replaced immediately after use (you never know when the next incident will be).
    - All expendable items should be checked for expiry.
    - Stowed neatly, so that it is readily accessible for use, and easy for others to find. Similar boxes/ cases should be clearly labelled or colour coded according to their contents.

PRACTICAL POINT
- *It is advisable to have:*
    - *An arrangement with your local ambulance service/hospital for the replacement of medical gases.*
    - *An arrangement with your local ambulance crews for the return of equipment after use.*
    - *An arrangement with your local Accident and Emergency Department and Ambulance Service for replacement of expendable or date expired items.*

Before setting off

- Ascertain the correct location of the incident before setting off, but do not waste too much time with this, as further directions are usually obtainable over the radio.
- Log in with the local ambulance service.

Getting there

- Get there rapidly, but safely, and without hazarding or inconveniencing other road users.
- Your **vehicle**:
    - Visible warning:
        - Green beacons: rotating light, strobe or light bar.
            - It may be magnetic or permanently mounted, depending on the frequency of callout.
        - Dipped headlights only should be used except in very heavy traffic, when rapid flashing of headlights may be permissible (a special unit can be fitted to your car for this purpose).
        - Fog lights should only be used in very poor visibility, i.e. fog, very heavy rain.
    - Audible warning devices/sirens:
        - Should only be used if prior permission for their use has been obtained from the Police to do so.
        - Twin tone horns/siren, may be mechanical or electric.
        - These should be used with care as they can cause as many problems as they solve.
    - Driving:
        - Do not take any unnecessary risks, and expect the unexpected.
        - Driving training with your local traffic police is highly recommended.

PRACTICAL POINT
  - *The absence of oncoming traffic may mean that the road ahead is blocked, and may indicate a serious accident.*

On arrival at the scene

Self protection

Protective identifying clothing
    - Put on appropriate protective clothing preferably before setting off (especially if the accident/incident is on the motorway) or immediately on arriving at the scene.
    - It should be:
        - Protective, waterproof, warm, highly visible (fluorescent green/yellow).
        - Identifying with "DOCTOR" on the back and front.
        - Chemical/fire resistant.
        - Easy to clean
        - Allow you to "breathe".
        - Meet current regulations/standards for reflectivity/visibility.
    - Consider: Helmet, goggles, jacket, tabard, gloves, over trousers, boots, etc.

Hazards
- Do not expose yourself needlessly to any hazards, and look for those which may not be immediately obvious:
  - Oncoming traffic
  - Fire
  - Electricity
  - Dangerous chemicals/gases
  - Falling masonry
  - Strong water currents.

Protecting the scene

Parking at the scene
- *Always park under police supervision.*
  - This should be as near to the incident as possible, so that you have all your equipment accessible, but do not obstruct any ambulances or fire appliances.
  - If necessary, particularly if you are the first on the scene, and there is poor visibility, park so as to protect the scene and minimise the chances of other vehicles colliding with any of the vehicles, etc. involved in the accident. Consider parking in the fend off position.

The fend off position
- This is when a vehicle parks at an angle of about 45 degrees to the direction of travel.
- It has the advantages that:
  - It makes a vehicle more visible to the oncoming traffic, as it displays a greater (side) area.
  - If the parked vehicle is hit by another, it should tend to go in the direction in which its wheels are pointing, and not into the accident site.
- The green beacon should be left on, and the hazard warning lights switched on.
- If there is a danger of approaching vehicles not seeing the incident until too late and you are the first vehicle on scene, consider putting out a warning triangle, cones, etc.

PRACTICAL POINT
- *Leave the ignition keys in the vehicle, so that it can be moved if necessary.*
- *Leave the engine running, so that you do not end up with a flat battery ("quitting" a vehicle, i.e. leaving it with the engine running, is permissible in these circumstances).*

Motorways

- These are particularly hazardous due to the high traffic density, and speed of vehicles, so special procedures have been agreed for the parking of emergency vehicles, using the ACECARD system (see diagram below).

Parking

Procedure:- Doctors attending an emergency on the motorway should:
- Put on protective clothing and safety helmets before proceeding to the incident or immediately on arrival.
- Make sure of the location of the incident and access points onto the motorway.
- Do *not* use emergency crossing points unless under police supervision (most have now been closed due to some bad crossover accidents).
- En route, check the motorway marker posts against the distance from the incident.
- Park the vehicle as follows:

- *Police first in attendance*
  - At most motorway incidents the Police will be in attendance before the arrival of the doctor, and will probably have placed "Police Accident" warning signs in position. Reflective cones and/or flashing lights may also be in use. A police vehicle should already have been parked 50 m on the approach side of the accident within the coned off area .
  - The first doctor to arrive should park beyond the accident and first ambulance; leaving his green light and hazard warning flashers on.
  - If an ambulance has not already arrived, he should leave room for an ambulance to park between the accident and his car.
  - Reinforcing doctors should overtake the accident area and park 100 m beyond it on the hard shoulder displaying hazard lights but not green lights.

Motorway accidents: vehicle parking: either lane blocked

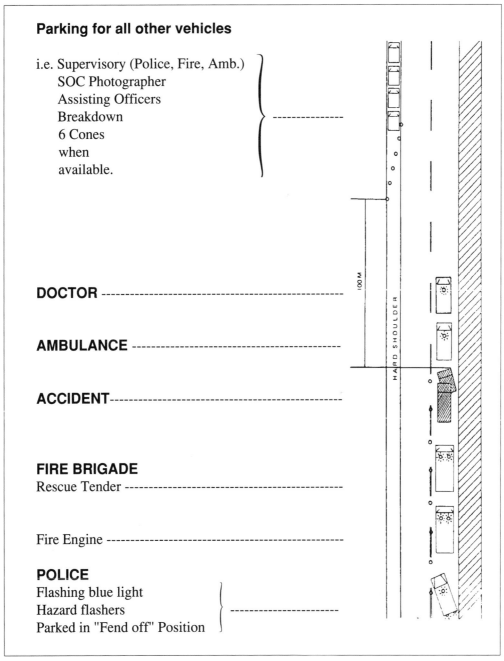

Parking for all other vehicles

i.e. Supervisory (Police, Fire, Amb.)
    SOC Photographer
    Assisting Officers
    Breakdown
    6 Cones
    when
    available.

DOCTOR

AMBULANCE

ACCIDENT

FIRE BRIGADE
Rescue Tender

Fire Engine

POLICE
Flashing blue light
Hazard flashers
Parked in "Fend off" Position

Figure 25-1 Motorway parking

- If it is not possible to pass the accident area, the initial police vehicle in attendance will have stopped short of the accident, leaving enough space between itself and the accident for fire appliances, ambulances and doctors to pull into.

- *Doctor first in attendance*
    - Should he be the first to arrive, and part of the carriageway is still open, the first doctor should still park just beyond the incident.
    - To protect the scene, immediately place reflective cones, flares and flashing lights if carried at the rear of the accident site, i.e. nearest the oncoming traffic. If possible, one flare or flashing light should be positioned approximately 300 metres in advance of the accident. This should be on the hard shoulder if the accident is on the near side, and on the central reservation if the right hand lane is blocked.
    - Vehicle lights, hazard warning lights and green beacons should be left on.
    - Any reinforcing doctors should park in the positions as detailed previously.

- *Liaison*
    - Where other services are in attendance, report to the officer in charge for information, and in particular liaise with the first ambulance crew or ambulance officer if he/she is in attendance.

- *Leaving the scene*
    - When leaving the scene, switch off hazard warning lights and green beacon and drive off under police direction to enable safe merging with any passing traffic.

Guidelines for patient management at an accident

Initial scene assessment

Primary survey
- Initial triage of patients
- Initial patient assessment
- Initial patient management: resuscitation.

Review of the scene/reading the wreckage
- Injury prediction

Secondary survey
- Secondary triage.
- Secondary patient assessment
- Secondary patient management
- Monitoring and recording the patient's condition

Monitoring
- Reassessment/review of management:
    - On the stretcher (with triage)
    - In the ambulance (with triage)
    - In transit.

Initial scene assessment

General principles
- Do not rush headlong into the incident towards those who are making the most noise, but inspect the scene carefully and methodically so as to get an overall picture.
- This should be done rapidly without becoming over involved in the management of any individual casualties, except to carry out rapid life saving procedures.

Specific points

Liaison
- Make contact as soon as possible with the ambulance crew in attendance.
- Liaise with the senior ambulance, police, and fire officers present.

The incident
- What has happened?
- What type of incident is it?

The casualties
- How many are there?
- What kind of injuries do they have?
- How severely injured are they?
- Are they trapped?

Are there any hazards?
- Weather:
    - Cold
    - Snow
    - Wind
    - Rain
    - Heat.
- Dangerous chemicals (Hazchem code markings).
- Fire/explosion risk;
    - Petrol
    - Gas
    - Explosives
- Unstable vehicles, buildings.
- Electrocution from electricity power lines.

PRACTICAL POINT
- *It is normal practice for power supply companies to restore the power supply following a short, after about 20 minutes, without investigating the cause (most are apparently due to bird strike).*
- *It is therefore vital that they are informed* as soon as possible, *so as to avoid the accidental electrocution of rescuers and rescued.*

What is the geography?
- Are there any problems with access?
    - Ditches
    - Water
    - Woods
    - Ploughed fields.
    - Buildings/building sites.

Briefly examine the vehicles
- The road:
    - Skid marks
    - Trail of wreckage, etc.
- Exteriors:
    - For deformity.
        - This will give an idea of the collision/deceleration forces involved.
- Interiors:
    - For intrusion into and deformity of the passenger compartment.

Priorities in patient management
- Treat those patients who will die if not treated immediately, in particular:
    - The unconscious patient with an obstructed airway.
    - The patient with a cardiac arrest.
    - Patient with severe haemorrhage from a major vessel.
- Consider searching for ejected casualties and others whose presence may not be obvious initially especially in conditions of poor visibility, e.g. at night and in rough terrain, e.g. motorway embankments, ditches, hedges and in adjacent fields. This is best done by line searching (using a line of searchers who move forward together one step at a time).

Maximise medical/ambulance resources
- Use those doctors with the greatest expertise to treat those patients who most need those skills.
- Identify ambulance personnel with special skills and make sure that they are used appropriately.

Have other services been alerted?
- The Fire service:
    - Trapped patients.
    - Dangerous chemicals/petrol.
    - Fire/fire risk.
    - Illumination of the scene.
    - Heavy lift.

Medical/ambulance backup
- Are more doctors/ambulance personnel with extended skills needed?
- Is a surgical team required? (for field amputations).
- Is special medical equipment necessary?:
    - Pneumatic anti-shock garment (PASG)
    - Extrication devices
    - Blood.
- Is helicopter evacuation required?:
    - Spinal injuries
    - Severe burns   } for rapid evacuation to a specialist unit
    - Injuries requiring immediate in-hospital management
- Are more ambulances required due to the number or severity of injuries of the casualties? (liaise with the ambulance crews (or ambulance officer if present).

The wreckage
- Do not interfere unnecessarily with any wreckage or debris from the accident site, which may be needed later by the police for forensic purposes.

The dead
- Do not interfere with any dead casualties, but after confirming death in the presence of a police officer, leave them where they are until a police Scenes of Crimes Officer (SOCO) has arrived to examine the scene and take photographs.
- It is advisable to note the date and time of confirmation of death, together with the name and number of the police officer dealing with the incident, for future reference, in case the coroner requires a statement.
- Photographs of the deceased, taken with police permission, may also be useful.

Triage

- Sort the casualties into various categories according to their needs for:
    - Immediate treatment.
    - Special resources:
        - Experienced doctors
        - Extended trained ambulancemen
        - Splints.
    - Early evacuation.
    - Evacuation to special (hospital) facilities.
- If necessary label them according to their triage category, and be prepared to change their category according to any significant changes in their condition.
- Triage should be dynamic, i.e. continuous and changeable.

Primary survey and resuscitation (see chapter: Guidelines for Immediate Medical Care)

Guidelines

- This is the simultaneous assessment, identification and management of immediate life threatening problems, followed by an assessment of the potential for developing other serious life threatening problems or complications.

- **A**irway with care of the cervical spine
- **B**reathing
- **C**irculation with control of haemorrhage
- **D**isability
- **E**xposure

Reassessment of the scene/reading the wreckage (see below)

- Examine the scene
- Examine the wreckage
- Work out the mechanism of injury
  (You have already examined the patient)
- Relate the two to each other
- Do they correlate or might you expect injuries that you have not yet found
- If so look for them whilst doing the secondary survey

Secondary survey and management

Subjective interview

Objective examination

Head
- *Scalp*
- *Neurological state*
- *Base of skull*
- *Face*

Neck

Chest
- *Chest wall and lungs*
- *Heart*

Abdomen/pelvis

Extremeties

Spine
- *Back*

Pain
- Analgesia

Medical history

Monitoring/reassessment of the patient

Monitoring

Trending

Reading the wreckage/determining the mechanism of injury

Introduction

- Examination of the wreckage helps to predict the kind of injuries that the patient may be suffering from, and they should be positively looked for, although they may not be obvious or even complained of initially.
- *Example:-* A common situation is one in which the driver of a vehicle anticipates the impending impact and produces endorphins to provide his own pain relief, enabling him to ignore his own pain and therefore injuries in the first few hours after injury. A notable historical example was the Marquis of Anglesey who had a leg shot off during the battle of Waterloo, but didn't realise it until the battle was over.
- The Police, for forensic purposes, and the Road Research Laboratory, who carry out research into the causes of accidents and the mechanisms of injury, have a lot of experience in analysing the mechanism of injury from studying post-mortem reports and the wreckage from serious accidents.

Examination of the accident scene

- Why did the accident happen?:
  - Was the driver asleep?
  - Was alcohol involved?
  - Is the driver diabetic or epileptic?
  - Did the driver have a myocardial infarction?
  - Was there:
    - Too much speed?
    - A fault with one of the vehicles?
    - Adverse weather conditions?
- How did the accident happen?:
  - What hit what? and what happened then?
  - What were the road conditions?
- Assess:
  - The speed of impact.
  - The forces involved (force = mass x acceleration), and their direction.

Examination of the vehicle wreckage

- The type of impact:
  - Was it frontal, side, rear, or rollover, etc.
- Look for:
  - Deformity of the exterior of the vehicle:
    - Shortening of the front of the vehicle.
    - Rearward displacement of the wheels, doors and body panels.
    - Buckling of the vehicle's floor or roof.
- The degree of deformity can give a good idea as to the velocity of impact:
  - Intrusion into the passenger compartment:
  - Backwards displacement of the front wheel arch.
  - Inwards displacement of the doors, roof and rarely the floor pan.

- Deformity of the interior of the vehicle caused by the occupants, e.g. damage to the:
    - Windscreen (head).
    - Steering wheel (chest).
    - Front parcels shelf (knees), etc.
- The human body is softer than metal, and where there is major distortion of metal, it can be predicted that there will be even greater damage done to the human body involved.
- Was a seat belt worn and did it lock?
- Was there any movement of objects inside the vehicle?:
    - Forward movement of seats.
    - Unrestrained rear seat passengers.
    - Loose luggage, etc.
- Examine a motor/pedal cyclist's helmet for signs of impact/damage.

Examine the injury pattern of the patient
- Look for pattern bruising.

Injury prediction

- From consideration of all the above it should be possible to predict the injuries that the patient is likely to be suffering from.
- In road traffic accidents, there are impacts involving:
    - The vehicle(s).
    - The patient(s).
    - The patient's internal organs.
- Determine the mechanism of injury:
    - How was the patient injured?
    - What forces were involved?
    - What injuries would you expect?
- Was deceleration rapid or gradual? (the more rapid the deceleration, the more serious the injuries are likely to be).
- Relate the mechanism of injury to the clinical findings.
- Look positively for injuries that the patient may not yet be aware of, but you may suspect from your examination of the scene/vehicle.

Injuries in road traffic accidents

Car occupants

Frontal impact (80%)

- Occurs when the front or front corner of the vehicle collides with another vehicle or a stationary object, causing it to come to an abrupt halt.
- This results in severe deceleration of the vehicle and anything contained within it, including its driver and any passengers.
- The unrestrained car occupant will move forwards, with extension of the lumbar spine, hitting their knees on the front parcels shelf, then upwards hitting their head on the vehicle's roof and forwards flexing the neck, followed by the head hitting and breaking the windscreen and in the case of the driver hitting the chest and neck on the steering wheel.
- Restrained occupants tend to flex their cervical spine more and hit the windscreen with their heads.

Front seat occupants:
- Will be thrown forward unless they are wearing seat belts.
- The front seat passenger often suffers more severe injuries than the driver, as they are often less prepared for the impact than the driver who may anticipate the impact and can use the steering wheel to reduce forward movement.
- There may be impact with:
  - Rear view mirror:
    - Person in the front right hand seat:
      - Laceration of the left side of the forehead.
      - Injury of the left eye.
    - Person in the front left hand seat:
      - Laceration of the right side of the forehead.
      - Injury to the right eye.
  - Windscreen glass/frame or side pillars:
    - Injuries of the forehead and neck (rare since the introduction of seat belts, which have dramatically reduced this type of injury).
    - May also cause head, neck and facial injuries to unrestrained rear seat passengers who are ejected forwards.
  - Steering wheel:
    - Chest injuries: especially of the ribs, sternum and heart.
    - Facial injuries in the belted driver.
    - Abdominal injuries especially of the liver, particularly in lorry drivers.
  - Front parcels shelf:
    - Knee injuries:
      - Patella
      - Dislocation (popliteal artery injury).
    - Backwards displacement (posterior dislocation) of the hip, fractured shaft of femur.

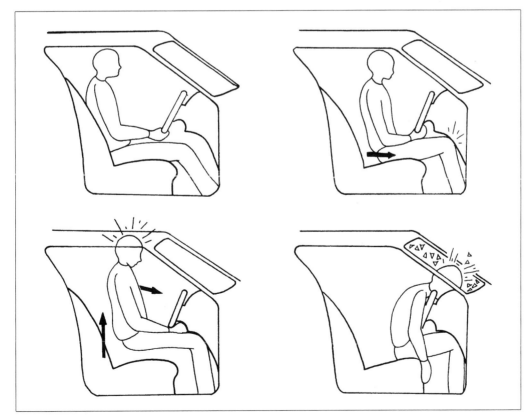

Figure 25-2 Mechanism of injury: Unrestrained driver

- Front wheel arch:
  - Fractured ankles/lower legs (more common and more severe in car drivers, as their feet and ankles can become tangled around the control pedals, especially the right ankle, which is used for braking).
- Seat belts:
  - Restrain the patient reducing forward movement and ejection.
  - Spread the deceleration forces over a considerable area, reducing the force applied per unit area.
  - Stretch during severe deceleration increasing the time interval before the body ceases forward movement, and reduces the force of deceleration.
  - May cause some injuries (which are much less severe than if no seat belt was worn):
    - Chest strap:
      - For those in the right front seat:
        - The line of injury may extend down across the chest from the right shoulder to the left costal margin and loin, and may result in:
          - A fractured right clavicle
          - A subluxed acromio-clavicular joint
          - Fractured sternum
          - Fractured left lower ribs
          - Injury to the spleen and left kidney.
      - For those in left front seat; this pattern will be reversed with injury to the liver rather than the spleen.
      - Injury to the neck may be caused by a seat belt which is anchored too high up.
    - Lap strap:
      - Injury to the lower abdominal viscera and bladder.
- The doors may burst open and the driver or passenger may be ejected (see below).

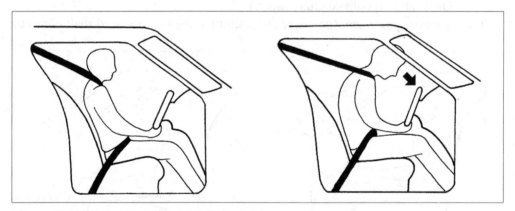

Figure 25-3 Mechanism of injury: Belted driver

Rear seat occupants
- Injuries are usually less severe than those of the front seat occupants.
- Unrestrained rear seat passengers will be thrown forwards:
  - Colliding with front seat passengers causing them:
    - Head and neck injuries
    - Back injuries (collide with the back of the front seats).
  - Colliding with front seat passengers resulting in:
    - Neck injuries
    - Knee injuries.
  - Collision with the windscreen:
    - Neck and facial injuries.
  - Ejection through the windscreen.

- Restrained rear seat passengers may sustain:
  - Injury to the lower abdominal viscera and the bladder.
  - More likely to be a severe injury, if the only belt securing the patient is a lap belt (centre rear passenger).
  - Facial and knee injuries (collision with the back of the front seats).
  - Severe cervical spine injury: lap belt secured passenger, involved in high speed frontal impact, flexes forward, hitting their head on the seat in front of them.
- In side impacts may be:
  - Injured by side intrusion (door fittings, etc.)
  - Ejected through a burst door.
- Ejection:
  - If the casualty is ejected because he/she was either not wearing a seat belt, or it was loose:
    - Severe facial and neck injuries (see below).

Rear impact
- Whiplash (hyperextension) injury to the cervical spine.
- Seat belt injuries.
- Rear seat passengers may also have:
  - Spinal injury: rear intrusion.
  - Knee/femoral injury: impact with front seat.

Side impact
- The injuries sustained depend on the side of impact:
  - Left side:
    - Mid door (impact with car front):
      - Ruptured spleen, left kidney or ruptured left lung and associated rib fractures.
      - Fractures of the left upper limb.
    - Low door (impact with front wheel of motorcycle):
      - Left pelvic and lower limb fracture.
  - Right side:
    - As left side apart from:
      - Ruptured liver, right kidney, etc.
- The car occupant on the opposite side to that which sustains the impact may be ejected sideways (seat belts are designed to prevent forward movement only).

High speed frontal impact
- Results in massive deceleration causing:
  - Ruptured thoracic aorta (especially in the young), which may not be obvious initially.

Rollover accidents
- Injuries are usually multiple and depend on the points of impact between car and occupant:
  - May be:
    - Spinal, head and neck injury.
- The severity of injury varies depending on the amount of deceleration.
- There is a significant risk of ejection, especially of unbelted occupants:
  - Front seat occupants are most frequently ejected through a side door.
  - Rear seat occupants are most frequently ejected through the rear window.

Motor cyclists

- Most major injuries are due to ejection of the motorcyclist onto the road or adjacent surfaces or objects, due to the inherent instability of the vehicle and its frequent high speed.
- Lower limb injuries are particularly common, occuring in up to 50% of motorcylists attending hospital, of these 50% are of the lower leg.

Frontal impact
- Sudden deceleration resulting in ejection:
    - Head and cervical spine, chest and abdominal injury.
    - Bilateral fractured femurs (impact with the handlebars).
- Collision with back (tail-gating), or side of lorry:
    - Hyperextension injury of cervical spine.
    - Decapitation.

Side impacts
- Usually caused by direct impact with a car:
    - Fractures of the femur (most common), lower leg and ankle.
- May result in entrapment of the lower limb between the machine and the struck object:
    - The upper leg is usually trappped by the petrol tank and car wing (less common).
    - The lower leg is usually trapped between the motorcycle gearbox and the front bumper or corner of the car (most common).

Note: - Following the initial impact, if the motorcyclist is not ejected, the motorbike may fall over onto the motorcyclist's legs resulting in further injury.
- A pedal/motor cyclist's helmet should always be inspected and sent with them to hospital.

Pedal cyclists

- The mechanism of injury is generally similar to that of motor cyclists, but their velocity is usually considerably less, and injuries are consequently less severe.
- Uniquely the skin fom the lower leg may be stripped (avulsed) from the lower leg due to the limb being forced between the wheel spokes.

Pedestrians

Primary injury
- The primary impact/injury is due to collision with the vehicle.
- The injuries depend on the size of the casualty and of the vehicle.

Adult pedestrian
- The car bumper usually hits the patient first, resulting in:
    - Injuries to the front or side of the knee/lower leg.
- The radiator grille, lamps or bonnet often cause further primary injury to the thigh or hip.
- If the vehicle is large (lorry or bus):
    - The primary injuries may be at a higher level: on the chest, arms, or head.
- The patient is usually knocked forwards or obliquely sideways (impacts are usually caused by impact with the front or front corner of the vehicle).
- Pedestrians may be thrown into the air on impact:
    - At low speeds (20 kph), the body may be thrown violently away.

- At higher speeds (60-100 kph), the patient may be ejected up into the air and may travel a considerable distance before hitting the ground or other object, resulting in "secondary injuries", which may be more severe than the primary injury.
- At speeds over 25 kph, "scooping up injury" may also occur (cars only):
  - The patient has their feet knocked out from under them and they are thrown up onto the bonnet of the car, resulting in their head impacting with the windscreen (sometimes going through the glass) or windscreen pillar.
  - Once on the bonnet, the patient assumes the same velocity as the vehicle, but seldom stays there before being flung:
    - Sideways onto the road, sustaining severe secondary injuries, and are at risk of being run over by passing cars.
    - Over the roof of the car (at high speeds) hitting the road behind the vehicle.

Child pedestrians
- Impact with the bumper will result in fractures of the femur and pelvis.

Secondary injury
- Due to collision with the ground or other object resulting in:
  - Skidding causing "brush" abrasions.
  - Head injury (most common) including scalp laceration, skull and facial fractures, meningeal haemorrhage and cerebral contusion.
  - Spinal injury especially of the cervical and thoracic regions with spinal cord involvement.
  - Chest and pelvic injuries.
  - Fractures of the femur and tibia.
- The severity of the injury depends on the surface on which the patient lands or the object with which they collide, and their velocity at the time of impact.

Running over injury
- Occurs when a wheel passes over the patient.
- May result in injury to the:
  - Head causing gross distortion and very severe injury.
  - Chest resulting in a flail chest with fractured rigs, sternum, spine and severe lung contusion.
  - Abdomen and pelvis, causing rupture of the internal organs.
  - Severe damage to the skin and subcutaneous tissue (usually of a leg, arm or the scalp), where the wheel (usually from a large vehicle, e.g. lorry or bus) rotates the body on the ground ripping the skin off, "flaying injury".

Examples of other injuries

Falls from heights
- The severity of the injury depends on:
  - The height of the fall.
  - The type of surface on which the patient lands.
  - The part of the body which impacts with the ground.
- Onto heels/feet:
  - Fractured calcaneii
  - Fractured/ dislocated hips
  - Compression fracture of lumbar and thoracic spine.
- Onto hands:
  - Bilateral colles fractures.

Entrapment

- Entrapment is a situation commonly encountered at the roadside but may also be a problem in industrial, recreational, aircraft, train, and domestic incidents.
- May be absolute, or relative.
- Is usually but not always associated with significant injury.
- In road traffic accidents entrapment is usually associated with extensive deformity of the vehicle, with intrusion into the passenger compartment.
- There are usually problems with gaining access to the patient, both for assessing injuries, monitoring vital signs and treatment (initial resuscitation, followed by splinting, etc.).
- Almost always results in delay in full assessment and management of injuries, and evacuation to hospital may be delayed for several hours.
- May result in prolonged exposure to hazards/hostile environment.
- Special rescue equipment may be required to obtain the release of the casualty, and special medical equipment may be required for their actual removal, e.g. an extrication device.

Complicated entrapments

- Entrapment may be prolonged due to:
    - Impaction.
    - The patient's injuries.
    - Impalement.
    - The need for amputation.

Guidelines for the management of the trapped patient

Introduction

- This should follow the usual guidelines, but in a slightly modified form because of the problems associated with lack of access for examination and management of the patient.
- It may not be possible to examine and treat some parts of the patient until they have been released.
- The aim of management is to:
    - Save life
    - Prevent and treat complications
    - Extricate the patient rapidly, without aggravating any injuries.
- It should be remembered that the management of the trapped and injured patient is a team effort, everyone involved has their own special role and the more everybody works together as a cohesive unit, the greater the benefit will be for the patient.
- The whole situation is dynamic:
    - The cause of the patient's injuries may still be present and may continue to cause injury (unlike the patient in hospital, when the cause of injury has usually been removed).
- There may be more than one patient who is trapped and injured.
- The guidelines below shows features to be considered in entrapment, which are additional to the usual guidelines, and do not replace them.

Initial assessment of the scene

Primary survey and resuscitation
- Initial triage of patients
- Initial patient assessment/management: resuscitation.

Reassessment of the scene/reading the wreckage

Secondary survey and management
- Secondary patient assessment/management
- Monitoring and recording the patient's condition
- Secondary triage.

Overview of the scene

Monitoring
- Reassessment/review of management:
    - During extrication
    - On the stretcher
    - In the ambulance (with triage)
    - In transit.

Assessment of the entrapment scene

- Scene assessment:
    - What is the cause of entrapment: why?
    - What is the method of entrapment: how?
- If trapped, is entrapment:
    - Relative? e.g. in the unconscious.
    - Absolute? e.g. in the impacted casualty.
- Are any special resources required to rescue the patient?

Primary survey and resuscitation in entrapment

- Identify the "time critical" patients (triage):
    - Those whose injuries and condition are such that they have priority for rapid extrication.
- Determine the need for any additional medical support.
- Liaise with the Fire Service especially over:
    - Safety and access to the patient during the extrication.
    - The release of trapped limbs, etc.
- Liaise with the ambulance service over:
    - The use of medical equipment
    - The method of patient removal, etc.

Airway
- Potential problems:
    - Access to the patient for:
        - Assessment.
        - Management:
            - Cricothyrotomy
            - Intubation.

Breathing
- Potential problems:
    - The position of the patient may inhibit breathing.
    - Access to the patient for:
        - Assessment:
            - Monitoring the colour of the patient may be difficult due to poor lighting conditions.
        - Management:
            - Difficulty with carrying out practical proceedures:
    - Oxygen may be contraindicated due to the risk of explosion.

Circulation
- Potential problems:
    - The patient's position may impair the circulation.
    - The environment:
        - Cold:
            - May cause peripheral circulatory shutdown.
            - May precipitate shock.
            - Certain intravenous fluids may freeze and heat retaining cases and fluid warming devices may be necessary.
    - Access/adequate light for:
        - Assessing the patient.
        - Management:
            - Putting up an intravenous infusion.

Disability
- Potential problems:
    - Cerebral hypoxia resulting in confusion; consider:
        - Sedation, ventilation.
        - This may also cause problems with extrication.

Exposure
- Not usually appropriate in the entrapment situation, except for:
    - Assessment of major injuries.
    - Management of:
        - Life threatening injuries
        - Open injuries/lacerations:
            - Application of dressings/protection.
- Be careful not to let the patient get cold:
    - Cover with blankets, etc.

Secondary survey and management in entrapment

- The full secondary survey is usually best left until the patient has been removed from the place of entrapment to a "place of relative safety", usually the ambulance.
- Depending on access, a modified secondary survey and management should be performed.

Bony injury
- Potential problems
    - Access for:
        - Assessment:
            - Fractures
            - Peripheral pulses
        - Management:
            - Access for applying a splint.
            - Position:
                - May not permit formal splint application.
                - (Consider temporary splinting with: frac straps, bandages).

Analgesia/sedation
- Potential problems in administration of:
    - Entonox:
        - Risk of fire
        - Room for the gas cylinder
    - Intravenous opiate
    - Intravenous midazolam } difficult intravenous access.
    - Intravenous diazepam

Overviews of the scene

- Stand back and review:
    - The patient.
    - The scene.
    - The extrication process.
- Review/repeat regularly.

During extrication

- Anchor equipment securely, e.g. intravenous lines, splints.
- Liaise closely with the ambulance crew and Ambulance Incident Officer (if present).
- Prepare:
    - The patient (for haemorrhage, pain).
    - For extrication:
        - Carrying sheet
        - Extrication device.
    - The stretcher, e.g.:
        - Lay out PASG
        - Traction splints.

Assessment/management on the stretcher

- Take advantage of any open access to thoroughly reassess the patient if practicable, but be careful not to expose him/her unnecessarily or for too long to a hostile environment, e.g. the cold, wet or extreme heat.
- Perform any procedures which may be difficult to perform in the confined space of an ambulance or helicopter, e.g. stabilisation or splinting.
- Package/prepare the patient for loading making sure that all attached equipment is secure and accessable where necessary.
- Liaise with the ambulance or helicopter crew to determine the most appropriate loading method and position of the patient in the ambulance or helicopter taking into account:
    - The patient's injuries, splinting, monitoring equipment, etc.
    - Any special characteristics of the ambulance's or helicopter's patient compartment.

Assessment/management in the ambulance

- Reassessment of the patient prior to departure: take advantage of the stable platform, better lighting (if it is dark outside), and warm environment to thoroughly reassess the patient and perform any necessary practical procedures that it was not possible to perform whilst the patient was trapped:
    - *Primary survey and resuscitation*
        - Airway care:
            - Intubation
        - Breathing: ventilatory care
        - Circulation:
            - Furher intravenous lines
            - Application of PASG
        - Disability
        - Exposure:
            - Remove all clothing to facilitate a full secondary survey
    - *Secondary survey and management*
- Triage: Identify the "time critical" patient ("scoop and run" vs "stay and stabilise").
- Select the hospital appropriate to the patient's injuries and medical condition according to local policies:
    - A hospital with a Burns Unit for those severely burnt.
    - A hospital with a Neurosurgical Unit for head injuries.
    - A major hospital for those with multiple serious injuries.
- Determine any treatment required in transit.
- Determine the need to travel yourself.
- Determine the need for a police escort:
    - If traffic is heavy or the patient's condition is critical.
- Brief the ambulance crew whether you are travelling with the patient or not.

Note: - In the case of motor/pedal cyclists, their crash hat/helmet should always be sent with them to hospital.
   - Keep the ambulance's doors closed to:
        - Conserve heat.
        - Enable life saving procedures to be performed in private.
        - Spare anxious relatives unnecessary distress.
        - Keep all unnecessary personnel out.

Assessment/management in transit

- Continuously monitor the patient's:
    - Airway
    - Breathing
    - Circulation
    - Dysfunction: neurological status
- Review the equipment in use and the patient positioning.
- Radio the patient's clinical details to the hospital as necessary (according to local policies).
- Stop the ambulance if necessary to treat the patient:
    - To modify any splinting, etc.
    - To carry out defibrillation.

Triage decision guidelines for hospital selection

1. *If:*
- The Glasgow coma scale score: <13.
- The systolic blood pressure: <90 mmHg.
- The respiratory rate: <10 or >29 bpm.
- The Triage Revised Trauma Score: <11

Then:
- Take the patient to a major hospital.

2. *If not:*
- Assess the mechanism of injury, and the patient's actual injuries.
- If the patient has:
    - A penetrating injury to the head, neck, chest, abdomen, pelvis or groin.
    - Fractures of two or more proximal long bones.
    - Burns totalling 15% or more, or burns to the face or burns involving the airway.
    - A flail chest.
    - Evidence of a high energy impact, e.g.:
        - Falls of 20 ft or more.
        - An impact velocity of more than 20 mph.
        - 20" deformity of front of vehicle or 30" if involving less than 2/3 of front of vehicle.
        - Rearwards displacement of the front axle.
        - 15" intrusion of the passenger compartment of the vehicle on the patient's side.
        - Ejection of the patient.
        - Vehicle rollover.
        - Death of an occupant in the same car.
        - A pedestrian hit at 20 mph or more by a car, or at more than 10 mph by a heavy vehicle, e.g. a lorry or bus.

Then:
- Take the patient to a major hospital.

3. *If not:*
- If:
    - The patient's age is <5 or >55 yrs.

    or:
    - There is a known history of cardiac or respiratory disease, and moderate injury severity.

Then consider:
- Taking the patient to a major hospital.

If in doubt take the patient to a major hospital.

Classification of hospitals

Major hospital

- A large District General Hospital (DGH), or Regional Centre, with full facilities for patient investigation (CT scanner, etc.), and treatment (ITU and a full range of surgical specialities).

Minor hospital

- A small DGH or peripheral unit with full time medical staff, but without the full range of facilities for patient investigation, no ITU and limited surgical resources.

Community/GP hospital
- A small hospital with a minor casualty department only and no surgical resources.
- Only suitable as a staging post for assessment and stabilisation of the patient prior to evacuation to a major hospital in remote areas and where the nearest major/minor hospital is a long travelling time away.

26

Reporting from the scene

Reporting from the scene

Introduction

- Reporting from the scene using report forms, photography, and any other relevant material will give the receiving doctor as much information as possible to help him determine how best to further treat and investigate the patient.
- All doctors are taught, to a certain extent, to ignore what the other doctor has found and to examine the patient for themselves, but in Immediate Care they do so at their peril.

Report forms

Purpose

- To inform the receiving doctor of:
    - The patient's identity:
        - Name, address and date of birth.
    - The type of accident:
        - RTA
        - Industrial
        - Domestic
        - Recreational
    - The history of the accident:
        - Alcohol?
        - Knocked out?
        - Vomited?
    - The mechanism of injury:
        - Driver/ front/rear seat passenger.
        - Wearing/not wearing seat belt.
        - Motorcyclist wearing/ not wearing helmet.
        - Pedal cyclist, pedestrian, etc.
        - Details of the type of impact.
    - The patient's suspected injuries.
    - The patient's initial (baseline) condition:
        - Vital signs:
            - Glasgow coma scale.
            - Trauma score.

- Changes in that condition (trends):
    - During extrication.
    - In transit.
    - In response to the treatment carried out.
- Treatment carried since the time of injury:
    - Airway care:
        - Adjuncts used:
            - Airways.
            - Intubation.
            - Oxygen.
    - Breathing:
        - Ventilation
        - Chest drain.
    - Circulation:
        - Intravenous infusion.
    - Analgesia:
        - Entonox, morphine.
    - Splinting:
        - Spine, limb.
- The time intervals involved:
    - From first call (approximate time of accident) to first attendance.
    - Duration of any entrapment.
    - The time taken to stabilise the patient's condition.
    - The time spent in transit.
- Any significant/relevant past medical history if available.
- The patient's triage category:
    - Major incidents.
- By whom the patient was examined and treated.
- To help predict the likely patient outcome (trauma scoring).
- To act as a guide as to which hospital the patient should be sent and treatment priority (triage).
- For audit/research: for the ambulance service, Immediate Care doctors and the hospital.
- To act as an aide memoire.
- To act as a record for medico-legal purposes.
- To be a training aid.

Requirements

- Any report form should:
    - Provide all the above information.
    - Be user friendly:
        - Easy to understand.
        - Easy to carry, etc.
    - Be quick and easy to fill in:
        - Requiring the minimum of writing; with most questions answered by a tick.
        - Should only contain space for observations and measurements which are readily obtainable in the field, e.g. pupil sizing is unreliable in the field where the lighting conditions can vary considerably, and so the terms: large, medium and small should be used.

Note: - Consideration should be given as to whether any report form should be A4 size (or even A3 size), which is fairly large, but will show lots of information clearly or A5 size, which is more convenient and may fit into a pocket, but may be too small for all the information to be shown clearly).

Patient Report Form

BASICS — BRITISH ASSOCIATION FOR IMMEDIATE CARE

INJURY ASSESSMENT/PRIORITY

Critical/Immediate	☐
Serious/Urgent	☐
Minor/Delayed	☐

CALLSIGN: Ambulance | **Dr.**

Date	**Time** Call		Surname		Forename
Location	Arrival		**M/F d.o.b.**		Address
	Depart				
Hospital	Arrival		Vehicle No.		

ASSESSMENT ☐ RTA ☐ Work ☐ Home ☐ Organised Sport ☐ Leisure ☐ Other (Specify)

If RTA: ☐ Driver ☐ Front/Rear Passenger ☐ Pedestrian ☐ Motor-cyclist ☐ Cyclist

Seatbelts? ☐ Yes ☐ No ☐ Not known | Vomited? ☐ Yes ☐ No | Alcohol? ☐ Yes ☐ No ☐ Not known

Crash helmet? ☐ Yes ☐ No ☐ Not known | Ko'd? ☐ Yes ☐ No | Trapped? ☐ Yes ☐ No How Long?

PRIMARY SURVEY

Airway: ☐ Clear ☐ Obstructed

C. Spine ☐ Normal ☐ Possible injury

Breathing: ☐ Spontaneous ☐ Problem

Circulation/Haemorrhage: ☐ External ☐ None/slight ☐ Possible Internal ☐ Moderate ☐ Severe

Disability: ☐ Alert   Responds to ☐ Visual stimuli ☐ Pain ☐ Unresponsive

Exposure/Injuries

C# Closed Fracture
O# Open Fracture   L   Laceration
B   Burn (shade area)   A   Abrasion
F   Foreign body   E   Eccymosis (bruising)

PRIMARY MANAGEMENT

Airway ☐ Oropharyngeal ☐ Nasal ☐ ET Tube
☐ C/Thyrotomy ☐ Oxygen ☐ Suction
C. Spine ☐ C. Collar ☐ Hines

Breathing: ☐ Ventilated ☐ Chest drain

Circulation Cannula size: Rt............ Lt............
IV Fluids   Volume   Time
☐ H'mans/N.Saline _____ _____
☐ H'maccel/G'fusine _____ _____

SECONDARY MANAGEMENT

Analgesia ☐ Entonox   Dose   Time
Drugs ☐ _____ _____ _____
(specify) ☐ _____ _____ _____

Splinting ☐ Frac straps ☐ Inflatable ☐ Traction
☐ Box ☐ Other (specify)_____

OBSERVATIONS   Time   1)   2)   3)

	1)	2)	3)
Respiratory Rate			
Oxygen Saturation: Sa O$_2$%			
Blood Pressure	-----	-----	-----
Pulse Rate			

SECONDARY SURVEY

Eye Opening	Spontaneous	4 ☐	☐	☐	
	To voice	3 ☐	☐	☐	
	To pain	2 ☐	☐	☐	
	Nil	1 ☐	☐	☐	
Best Verbal Response	Oriented	5 ☐	☐	☐	
	Confused	4 ☐	☐	☐	
	Inappropriate	3 ☐	☐	☐	
	Incomprehensible	2 ☐	☐	☐	
	Nil	1 ☐	☐	☐	
Motor Response	Obeys command	6 ☐	☐	☐	
	Localises pain	5 ☐	☐	☐	
	Withdrawal (pain)	4 ☐	☐	☐	
	Flexion (pain)	3 ☐	☐	☐	
	Extension (pain)	2 ☐	☐	☐	
	Nil	1 ☐	☐	☐	

Pupils   React R   ☐ ☐ ☐
(✓ or X) L   ☐ ☐ ☐

1   o Constricted   Size R _____ _____ _____
2   o Normal
3   O Dilated   L _____ _____ _____

Trauma Score: Time   1)   2)   3)

COMMENTS:

Signed Crew | **Dr.** | **Nurse**

Figure: 26-1 Patient report form

- Have space for serial observations.
- Allow easy information retrieval:
    - Both clinical and research.
- Show uniformity:
    - Should use commonly understood terms and internationally agreed categories between ambulance services, Immediate Care schemes, and hospitals.

Procedure

- Any report form should be initiated by the first person attending the patient; ambulance personnel or Immediate Care doctor, be added to as necessary, especially if there are any serial observations, and go with the patient in the ambulance to the hospital casualty department, where they should be incorporated into the patient's notes.
- Ideally there should be three copies; one each for the:
    - Ambulance service
    - Immediate Care doctor
    - Hospital.

The Coma Scale

Introduction

- This was developed with the objective of indicating the patient's neurological injury and probable outcome following serious head trauma.

Glasgow coma scale		
Eye opening	Spontaneously	4
	To verbal command	3
	To pain	2
	No response	1
Best motor response	To verbal command: Obeys	6
	To painful stimulus: Localises pain	5
	Flexion/withdrawal	4
	Flexion decorticate	3
	Extension decerebrate	2
	None	1
Best verbal response	Orientated/converses	5
	Disorientated/confused	4
	Inappropriate words	3
	Incomprehensible sounds	2
	Nil	1
	Total	**(3-15)**

Trauma scoring

Introduction

- This is a method of measuring (scoring) the physiological state of the patient, in an effort to predict the outcome on a statistical basis.
- It should be understood that as it is a statistical tool, it does not accurately estimate the outcome for a particular patient, but purely predicts the average outcome for a group of patients with similar scores.
- It may be used for triaging patients at major incidents or to determine the appropriate hospital for any particular patient.
- It can also be used as an evaluation tool, e.g. in statistical analysis.
- To be of greatest value, it must use accurately obtained and recorded and repeatable measurements/ values, so as to reduce to the minimum any errors due to observer error or bias. If possible recording or measuring devices giving a clear readout and/or printout are to be preferred.

Triage revised trauma score

- The original trauma score was revised in 1987 to make scoring easier in the field, and to weigh it more in favour of the neurological state of the patient, using the Glasgow coma scale.
- Capillary return and respiratory expansion, which are difficult to see in the field, have been omitted.
- A score below 4 for any variable indicates a survival rate of less than 90%
- A score below 6 indicates a survival rate of just over 45%.

Triage revised trauma score		
Glasgow coma	13-15	4
scale score	9-12	3
	6-8	2
	4-5	1
	3	0
Systolic	>90	4
blood pressure	76-89	3
	50-75	2
	1-49	1
	0	0
Respiratory	10-29	4
rate	>29	3
	6-9	2
	1-5	1
	0	0
Total score	**(0-12)**	

Note: - A more sensitive trauma score is currently being developed, using the addition of the SaO_2 reading, but this has not yet been validated.

Paediatric trauma score

Introduction

- Introduced as the paediatric counterpart of the triage revised trauma score, but has not been validated.
- It is rather more complicated and less easy to remember than the adult score. In particular, the weight can only be guessed, unless one of the parents knows it.
- It is probably best reserved for use in the hospital, rather than the pre-hospital setting.
- A score of greater than +6 gives a predicted mortality rate of less than 1%.
- A score of less than +6 gives a predicted mortality rate of 25%

Paediatric trauma score

Weight	>44 lbs:20 kg	+2
	22-44 lbs:10-20 kg	+1
	<22 lbs:10 kg	-1
Airway	Normal	+2
	Oral/nasal airway	+1
	Intubated/tracheostomy	-1
Diastolic blood pressure	90 mmHg	+2
	50-90 mmHg	+1
	50 mmHg	-1
Level of 1 consciousness	Completely awake	+2
	Drowsy, but rousable	+1
	Comatose	-1
Open wound	None	+2
	Minor	+1
	Major or penetrating	-1
Fractures	None	+2
	Closed Fracture	+1
	Open or Multiple	-1
Total score	**(-6 to+12)**	

Problems with trauma scoring

- Lacks sensitivity
- There may not be enough time for the patient to deteriorate.
- The patient may be hypertensive.

Photography

Introduction

- This may play an important part in recording what has happened in an accident.
- If possible the time, date, and location where the pictures were taken should be recorded.
- Can help with learning to read the wreckage.

Legal and ethical aspects of photography

- There is no law of privacy in the UK and technically, taking a photograph of someone without their consent, is not an assault.
- If photographs are to be taken, however, it is good clinical practice to obtain the freely given consent of the injured or their families first, if the photographs are going to be used in lectures or for publication (in practice this is nearly always forthcoming).
- Photographs should never be released for publication before the police have informed the next of kin.
- Consideration should also be given to blanking out identifying marks, e.g. the number plates of vehicles, facial characteristics of the patient, etc.
- If the photographs are only going to be used as part of the patient's clinical (medical) records, then the obtaining of their consent is probably implied.
- Although not normally admissible as evidence, photographs may be requisitioned by the police, or asked for by the patient's solicitor.
- In some areas, hospital photographers are prepared to go out to accidents, but need to be incorporated into the callout system, and to have personal and vehicle identification.

Instant or polaroid photography

- This uses an automatic camera (autofocus, autoflash) which can produce instant pictures (Polaroid) which can be sent with the patient to hospital.

Purpose

- To inform the receiving doctor of:
    - The mechanism of accident/injury.
    - The forces involved:
        - Deformity of the exterior of the vehicle:
            - Deceleration.
        - Deformity of the passenger compartment:
            - Prediction of injuries.
    - Any special injuries:
        - Dislocations and fractures before and after reduction at the scene.
        - Degloving injuries, etc. which are best not disturbed too often.
    - Blood loss after haemorrhage.
- They may also be:
    - A legal record of the above.
    - Useful for helping the hospital staff, especially junior medical staff, to appreciate what the patient has been through and to help bridge the gap between pre-hospital and hospital care.
- Ideally the camera should be robust and small enough to fit in a pocket or emergency medical case and should form part of the first response equipment.

Method

- Pictures should be taken of:
    - The accident scene:
        - To give an idea of what happened when the accident occurred.
    - The exterior of the vehicle:
        - To show any deformity of the vehicle, including any shortening, displacement of panels, buckling of the floor pan, indentation of the roof, etc.
    - The interior of the vehicle
        - To show any intrusion into the passenger compartment, e.g. wheel arch, door panel.
        - To show any deformity caused by impact with the occupants, e.g. steering wheel.

Still photography

- This uses fully automatic compact cameras with autofocus, autoflash and a wide angle, zoom and close up (macro) facility. Those which can fit in a jacket pocket are to be preferred.
- More bulky Single Lens Reflex cameras are probably best reserved for the professional photographer or when there is plenty of time.
- They can be useful as a teaching or learning medium, but to maximise their value, details of the injuries sustained by the patients, etc. should be kept.
- In serious accidents involving the death or probable death of the injured, a police Scenes of Crime Officer (SOCO), is usually called in to photograph the scene to obtain forensic evidence as to the cause of injury or death, and can be a useful source of material.

Video recording

- This requires bulky equipment and a professional camera operator to produce a professional result.
- It can be very useful as a training aid, and is being increasingly used by the Fire Service and Police Forces (also for forensic purposes).

Other aspects of recording

- Where possible, it is advisable to send with the patient to hospital any other items which may be useful to the receiving doctor.
    - ECG recordings
    - Medication the patient may be taking
    - Poisons the patient may have ingested
    - Motor cyclists helmet, etc.

Notes

27

The emergency services

The emergency services

Introduction

- All those involved in Immediate Care, and especially doctors, should consider themselves to be part of the emergency team, whose prime role is to treat the person who is ill or injured as effectively and as efficiently as possible.
- To do so they must integrate themselves into the team, realising that each member of the team is as important in his own way as any other, and each has his own area of specialist expertise and part to play.
- To achieve this he must have an understanding of the roles of the other members of the team, together with some knowledge of their command structure, way of working, their equipment, and its uses and limitations.
- The team will need a leader, but this may not necessarily be the same person all the time provided that everybody in the team knows who it is, and recognises their authority. An example may be the motorway accident with a serious entrapment. The police will be in overall command and will direct all the other emergency services to an appropriate parking place. The fire service will usually be in control of the physical extrication process, but this may be under medical/ambulance direction if the patient's condition necessitates medical treatment before and during the extrication process. Once this is achieved the medical and ambulance services will manage the patient's treatment, before his eventual evacuation to hospital by the ambulance service. Each service will need continuous liaison with and assistance from each of the other services.

The police

Role

- To preserve and safeguard life and protect property.
- To uphold and enforce the law.
- The prevention and detection of crime and the prosecution of offenders.
- The enforcement of the road traffic law.
- To control, co-ordinate and facilitate the work of the other emergency services.
- To provide assistance for the other sevices moving to and from the scene of any incident.
- To supply information to the press at major incidents.
- To estabish and provide initial communications at the scene of any accident or incident.
- To act on behalf of the coroner:
    - Investigate sudden or suspicious deaths.
    - Arrange mortuary facilities, transport and custody of the deceased at major incidents.

Command structure

- In each County or Metropolitan Area, there is a Police Force with its headquarters; each commanded by the Chief Constable, with his staff.
- Attached to each headquarters is a Control Room and various specialist Departments:
    - Traffic
    - Scenes of Crime
    - Diving, etc.
- Each force is divided into Territorial Divisions, usually under the command of a Chief Superintendent, with a senior staff of Superintendents. Attached to each territorial division may be a number of specialist units, eg.:
    - Traffic
    - Community Service.
- In most areas, the Division is further subdivided into Sub Divisions, under the command of a Superintendent or Chief Inspector.
- Each Territorial Division or Sub Division will include a number of Police Stations, usually under the command of a Chief Inspector or Inspector.
- Each police station will usually be staffed by a number of shifts under the command of an Inspector or Sergeant.

The medical service

Role

- To prevent unnecessary death and suffering by providing assessment and medical treatment for the seriously ill or injured.
- General Practitioners have a legal duty as part of their terms of service to "give treatment which is immediately required owing to an accident or emergency" within their practice area.
- To confirm death.
- Registered Medical Practitioners are the only people legally able to confirm death.

Relationships with ambulance crews

- Immediate Care doctors need to work very closely with their colleagues in the Ambulance Service:
    - Provide support.
    - Advise.
    - Supervise.
- Once in attendance, the doctor has legal and clinical responsibility for the purely medical management of the patient, regardless of who actually treats that patient.

The ambulance service

Role

- To provide ambulance aid and where there are ambulance persons with advanced skills; paramedic ambulance aid to the seriously ill and injured.
- To provide appropriate transport to hospital for the seriously ill and injured, and to render ambulance aid en route.
- To provide appropriate transport to and from hospital for patients attending outpatient departments, day hospitals, physiotherapy departments, etc. and for non urgent admissions and discharges.
- Provide transport for interhospital transfers.
- To provide Health Service communications, logistical support and site management in close co-operation with the Police and Medical Incident officers.

Command structure

- In each National Health Service Region and Metropolitan Area, there is normally a Regional Chief Ambulance Officer, each County Ambulance Service in the Region being commanded by a Chief Ambulance Officer.
- Each Ambulance service has a Headquarters, usually situated adjacent to its control, which may also incorporate a training school, and is normally split up into three areas of activity:
    - Operations.
    - Control and Communications.
    - Support Services (Training, Fleet Transport).
- Services may be divided into Operational Divisions, which may be commanded by a Divisional Ambulance Officer.
- Each Division may be further subdivided into Sub Divisions under the command of a Subdivisional Officer.
- Each Ambulance Station or group of ambulance stations, depending on their size, is commanded by a Station Officer. Each small ambulance station may be supervised by a Leading ambulance person.

Note:- Each Ambulance Service is co-terminus with its Health Authority and its area may extend beyond the boundaries of the Police and Fire and Rescue Services within the County boundary.

The fire and rescue service

Role

- To fight fires, and protect life and property.
- To advise on fire prevention.
- To provide a rescue service for those trapped in road traffic, industrial, farming and industrial accidents or any other incident where people become trapped.
- To rescue patients from chemical incidents, and then deal with the chemicals themselves, rendering them harmless.
- To provide special equipment, e.g. Emergency lighting, pumping equipment, at incidents on request from the other emergency services.

Command structure

- In each county or metropolitan area, there is a Fire and Rescue Service, commanded by a Chief Fire

Officer, who has a Headquarters with an associated Central Control and a Headquarters staff.
- The area in which the service operates is usually divided into Divisions, under the command of a Divisional Commander.
- Each division will consist of a number of Stations, each under the command of a Station Officer.
- In each Station there will be several Watches, which man the station in turn.
- Each Watch is under the command of a Sub Officer, who has the assistance of a Leading Fireman.

PRACTICAL POINT: *It is often easier to identify firemen at an incident, by looking at their helmets. Officers above the rank of Sub Officer have white helmets, and below that rank yellow helmets. The greater the number and width of the black bands, the higher the rank.*

Rural areas

- In rural areas, where there is not enough work to justify employing full time firemen, Fire Services employ Retained Firemen, who have other full time jobs. They are alerted by long range radio pagers and proceed to the fire station, where the first to arrive form a crew and man the first fire engine or "Pump".

Inter-service co-ordination

- There are usually dedicated land lines linking the central controls of each emergency service to the other.

Rank identification in the emergency services

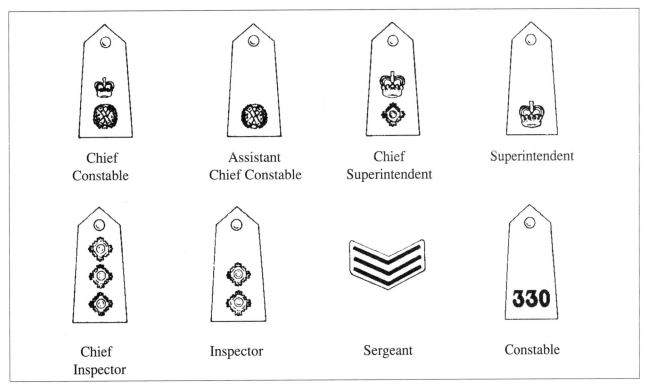

Figure 27-1 Rank identification: Police

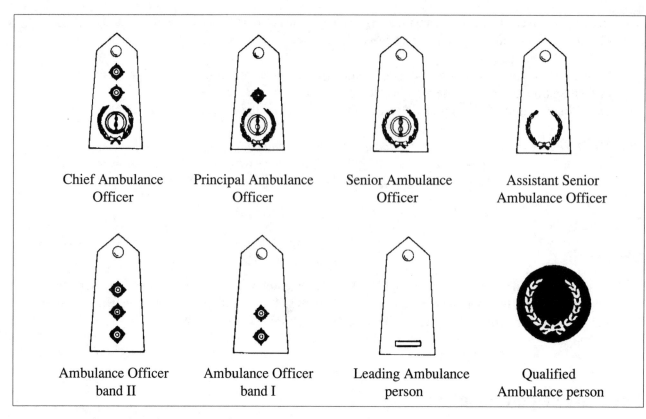

Figure 27-2 Rank identification: Ambulance service

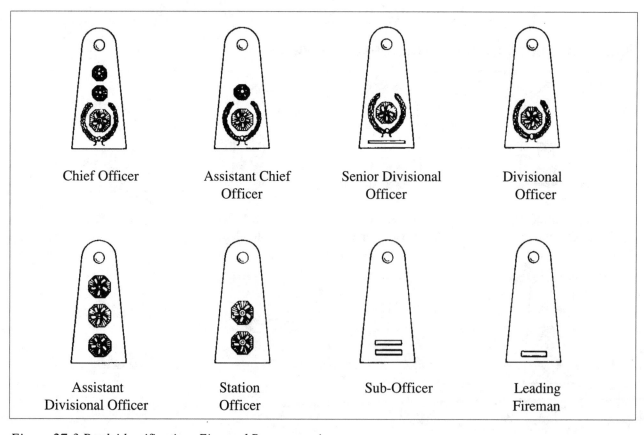

Figure 27-3 Rank identification: Fire and Rescue service

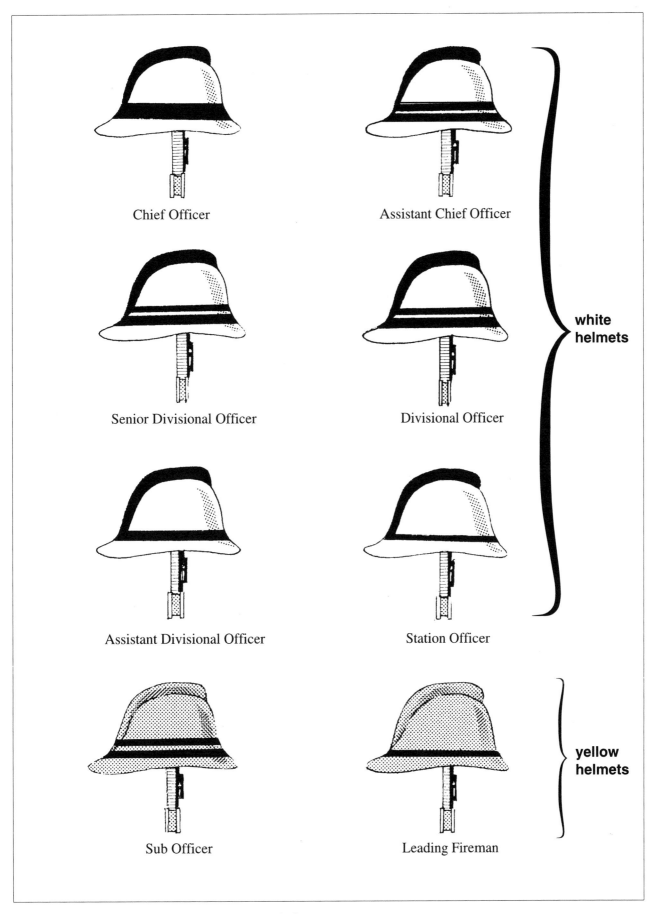

Figure 27-4 Rank identification: Fire service helmets

Notes

Dangerous chemicals

Dangerous chemicals

Introduction

- The number, quantity and variety of dangerous substances transported by road, rail or in the air is steadily increasing and with it the risk of exposure following an accident.
- The possibility of dangerous substances being involved should therefore always be borne in mind when assessing the scene of any accident.
- Hazardous substances may be:
    - Chemical.
    - Biological.
    - Nuclear (radioactive).

Chemicals

- Chemicals may be in three physical forms:
    - **Solid**
        - powder, granules, crystals, pellets or molten.
    - **Liquid**
    - **Gas**
- Chemicals may be:
    - Corrosive/non corrosive
    - Toxic/non toxic
    - Flammable
    - Lighter than air/heavier than air
    - Explosive/inert
    - Soluble/non soluble
    - Gases which can condense into liquids
    - Liquids which can solidify or evaporate as a gas or give off gaseous fumes
    - Chemical which are immiscible with water or react with water.

Labelling of chemicals

Hazard warnings: United Kingdom hazard information system (UKHIS)

- In order to provide rapid identification of individual dangerous chemicals, together with the hazard risk and method of dealing with them, all vehicles carrying prescribed dangerous substances in the UK are required to display warning labels on both sides and the rear.
- In addition companies are obliged by law to inform the drivers of tankers of the significance of the warning panels and the load carried.
- The warning labels must give the following information:
    - Hazchem scale number.
    - The name of the substance and its United Nations code number.
    - The United Nations hazard warning label.
    - The special advice telephone number.
    - The symbol or housemark of the manufacturer.

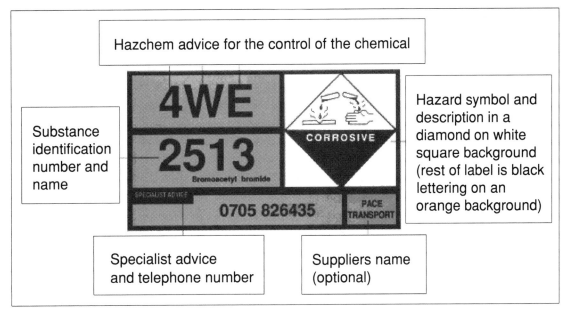

Figure 28-1 Example of a"UKHIS" board

Hazchem scale

- This gives the information necessary for the fire service to deal with the chemical:
    - The recommended dispersal method:
        - Jets
        - Fog
        - Foam
        - Dry agent.
    - The personal protection required:
        - Full body protective clothing with breathing apparatus.
        - Breathing apparatus plus protective gloves.
    - The risk of explosion.
    - The need for evacuation.
    - The method of disposal:
        - May be diluted and washed down drains.
        - Should be prevented from entering drains or water course.

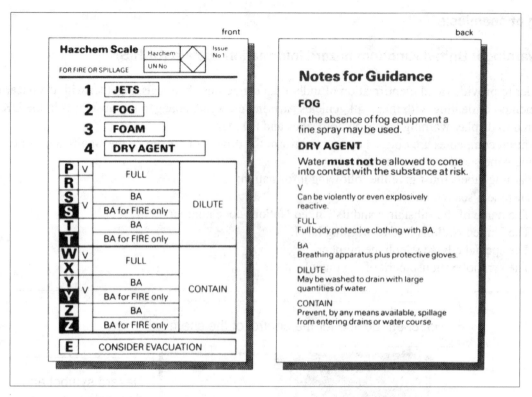

Figure 28-2 Hazchem card

Hazchem card

- This is a small card designed for fire service use which details the management of chemical spillages.
- Carried in all fire appliances and should also be carried by all Immediate Care doctors and ambulances.

United Nations warning label

- This is a diamond shaped warning label indicating the primary hazard:
  - Inflammable
  - Corrosive
  - Toxic
  - Explosive
- If there is more than one hazard, the diamond will show an exclamation mark.

United Nations number

- This number, which is used worldwide, is specific to individual substances so as to allow rapid identification.

Specialist advice telephone number

- The 24 hour emergency telephone number of the supplier or manufacturer of the chemical.

CEFIC system of transport emergency cards (Road)-TREMCARD

- This is a system developed by the European Council of Chemical Manufactures Federation and is a manual of cards designed to give the emergency services information about dealing with chemicals, before expert advice can be obtained.
- It is A4 sized and gives the following information:
    - The correct British Standard chemical name of the substance.
    - A description of the chemical's appearance and physical properties.
    - The appropriate protection to be used.
    - Advice on the immediate management of spillage or fire.
    - The first aid management of contaminated casualties.

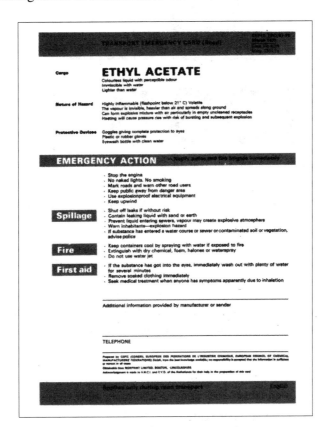

Figure 28-3 Example of a TREM card

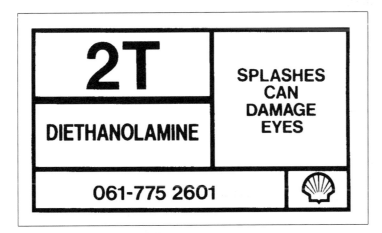

Figure 28-4 Example of a panel giving warnimg of a low hazard

ADR European Transport System

- This is a label borne on vehicles carrying hazardous substances to and from the European mainland.
- It is in two parts:
    - The upper displays the Kemler code.
    - The lower part shows the United Nations number.

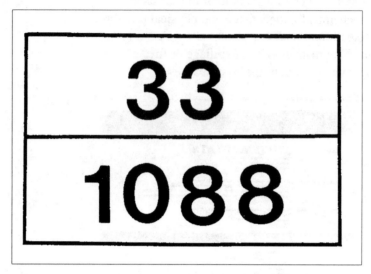

Figure 28-5 ECE-ADR "Kemler" board (black lettering on orange)

The Kemler code

- This is a numerical code using two or three digits which indicates the properties of the chemical
- The first digit indicates the primary hazard and the next two digits any secondary hazard.
- An X in front of the first number indicates do not mix with water.
- First digit:
    - 2 Gas.
    - 3 Inflammable liquid.
    - 4 Inflammable solid.
    - 5 Oxidising substance or organic peroxide.
    - 6 Toxic substance.
    - 7 Radioactive substance.
    - 8 Corrosive.
- Second digit:
    - 0 No meaning.
    - 1 Explosion risk.
    - 2 Gas may be given off.
    - 3 Inflammable risk.
    - 5 Oxidising risk.
    - 6 Toxic risk.
    - 8 Corrosive risk.
    - 9 Violent reaction risk.
- A repeated digit indicates an increased hazard, e.g. 3   flammable
                                                       33   highly flammable
                                                       333   spontaneously flammable

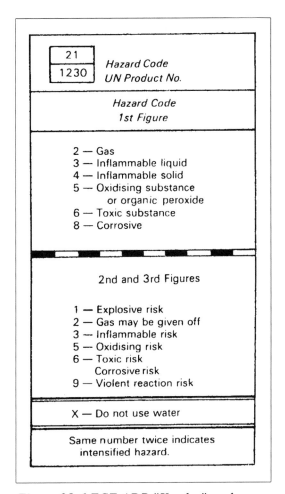

Figure 28-6 ECE-ADR "Kemler" scale

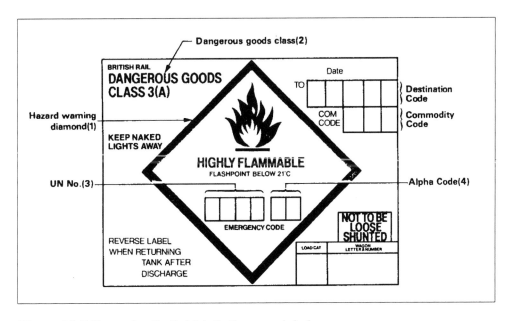

Figure 28-7 Example of a British Rail wagon label

Management of chemical incidents

Principles

- It is primarily the responsibility of the Fire and Rescue Services to deal with the rescue and decontamination of contaminated casualties, and the disposal of the chemicals involved. In the UK, most if not all Fire services have access to CHEMDATA, a computerised database, which gives advice on how to deal with most dangerous chemicals, and there is also a national centre prepared to provide assistance in identifying any chemical not in CHEMDATA.
- If dangerous chemicals are involved in an incident, you should not risk your own safety to treat seriously contaminated casualties, as you may only add yourself to their number!
- Casualties should usually only be treated after they have first been rescued and if necessary decontaminated by the Fire Service.
- Any personnel with a pre-existing skin condition or wounds involving breaches of the skin should not attend chemical incidents.

Procedure

On arrival
- If a chemical incident is suspected on arrival at the scene, you should immediately inform ambulance control and request the attendance of the Fire and Rescue Service, giving any details of the chemicals that may be immediately obvious.
- Doctors should then don protective clothing, if available, including overalls, boots, impervious gloves, "debris gloves" and eye protection.

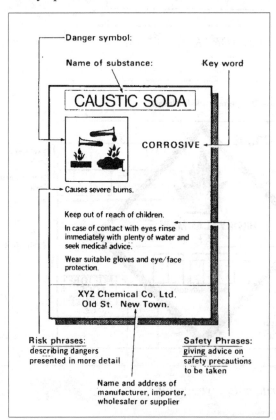

Figure 28-8 Label for dangerous goods in a package

Initial assessment
- If you are the first to arrive, try to assess the wind direction if any gases are involved, and the flow of any liquids. Always approach the scene from upwind and uphill.
- Advise anybody else in attendance to do likewise.
- Life saving procedures should be carried out during the initial assessment, provided this can be done without risking contaminating yourself.
- If you are not completely protected do not touch any chemical containers, etc., and if you are protected but contaminated do not touch anybody else especially any casualties, without first being decontaminated yourself.
- Obtain full details of the chemicals involved (see above), together with the number and severity of contamination of the casualties and convey this information to the Fire Service, Ambulance Service and Receiving Hospital immediately.
- If possible the chemicals involved should be identified, and details of the appropriate risk and immediate treatment obtained.

PRACTICAL POINT: *All Immediate Care doctors should carry a copy of:*
- *"DANGEROUS CHEMICALS: Emergency First Aid Guide".*
- *This gives the emergency treatment for most hazardous chemicals.*
- *Information about the management of contamination with chemicals not listed, can usually be obtained from the nearest Poisons Information Centre (see chapter on Poisoning).*

Chemical protective clothing

- There are two basic types of chemical protective clothing:
    - Chemical protective:
        - Plastic PVC.
    - Gas tight:
        - Very protective, vulcanised with an integral facemask and sometimes gloves.

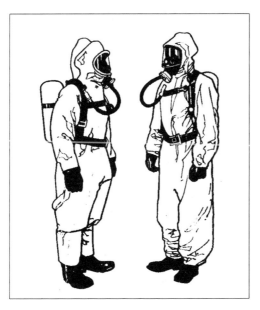

Figure 28-9 Examples of protective clothing

Breathing apparatus (BA)

- This is a pressurised air breathing system weighing 40-45 lbs and comprises:
  - A cylinder containing enough air for approximately 35 minutes working time (depending on conditions), with a reserve of just under 10 minutes.
  - An airtight face mask with a double reflex seal and an air demand valve.
  - A harness to which the cylinder is attached incorporating:
    - A warning whistle indicating that there is just under 10 minutes of air left in the cylinder.
    - A cylinder contents gauge.
    - An inlet valve for a direct air supply (used during decontamination procedures, etc.).
    - A distress signal unit, which can only be reset using the safety tag. This tag records all the user details, e.g. time of start of use, state of the cylinder, etc., and is put on a control board, on which the movements of all personnel into the contaminated area, fireground, etc. are recorded.

Decontamination

- The fire service will usually establish a decontamination area with a well defined entry and exit point, and control and perform the decontamination process on all those wearing protective clothing.
- Some industrial establishments may have their own facilities, with trained staff in attendance to assist the fire service.
- If casualties are involved, they will usually be removed from the incident as rapidly as possible. In the case of noxious gases or smoke, removal to the fresh air may be all that is necessary, but for a few highly toxic and persistant chemicals, it may be necessary to decontaminate them at the scene.
- A few authorities have vehicles specially designed for this purpose, but most do not. In this case facilities may have to be improvised, usually from the equipment used by the fire service.
- In practice, stripping and washing the patients down with either water or soap and water is all that is required in most cases.
- Rarely, dry methods of cleaning: using intrinsically safe vacuum cleaners for dry powder contamination, or scraping, when tarry or viscous substances are involved, may be necessary.
- Care must be exercised however, not to exacerbate any medical problems or injuries, and in particular shock. This can easily happen if the casualty is hosed down in the cold, and then not dried properly, which may result in him/her becoming hypothermic.
- If the patient requires a stretcher, then they should be decontaminated on a "scoop stretcher". However care should be taken not to put undue stress on the stretcher, as it is not designed for carrying heavy casualties any distance.
- In the case of female casualties, due account should be taken of their modesty, if circumstances and their condition permits. If available, female ambulance staff and firefighters should be provided.
- If possible, at least one doctor should remain at the scene, until it is declared safe, to treat any member of the emergency services who may be injured or contaminated.

Decontamination procedure

- The actual decontamination zone is usually divided into three areas:
  - Dirty:
    - This is where the initial decontamination is carried out, using wet or dry methods.
    - Wet cleaning is carried out using a portable high pressure shower unit capable of delivering 2000 litres per minute for 3 minutes. This is capable of washing off nearly all known chemicals and the high rate of water delivery results in adequate dilution of any dangerous chemicals.

- Intermediate:
    - This is where personnel have their BA and protective clothing removed and are wet or dry cleaned before donning clean overalls.
- Clean:
    - This is the area into which the cleaned personnel pass.

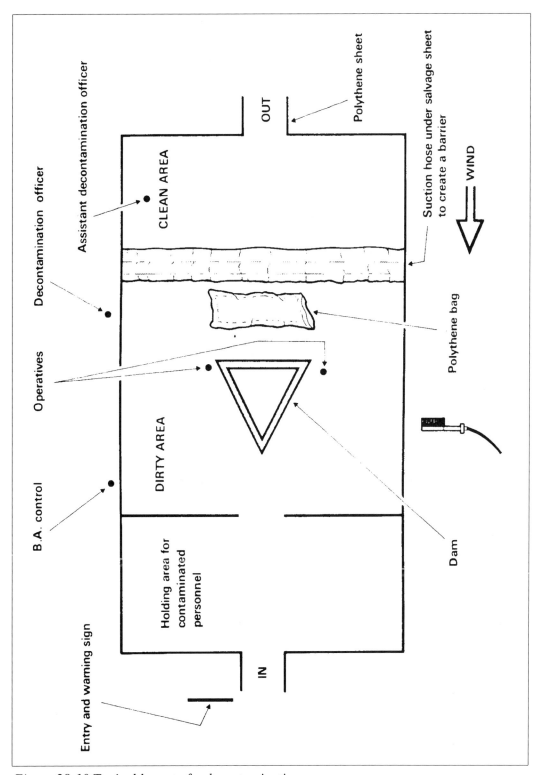

Figure 28-10 Typical layout of a decontamination zone

Reducing the risk of contamination

- It is important that, if possible, all contamination is contained, and the risk of its spread reduced to a minimum.
- Contaminated clothing and property should be sealed in polythene bags and labelled, and left at the scene.
- All vehicles leaving the scene should if possible be made clean.
- If patients are still contaminated, especially with volatile liquids:
    - They should be put feet first in plastic bags, leaving their heads clear, and if not contraindicated, given oxygen by oxygen mask.
    - The ambulance should have all its windows opened, and the connecting door between the cab and patient area, closed.
    - After use, each ambulance should be thoroughly decontaminated, before it re-enters service.

Hospital decontamination

- The hospital should provide a suitable area for receiving the patient, with adequate ventilation and air extraction systems, together with showers and trolley baths for further decontamination.
- In some cases further decontamination may be deemed necessary before severely contaminated casualties are allowed to enter the hospital.

The contaminated dead

- Ideally, the dead should be left where they lie after confirmation of death, so that forensic examination of the scene may take place, provided that to do so does not increase the risk of contamination for others.
- Following this they should be bagged up and labelled, before being decontaminated later under forensic examination.

PRACTICAL POINT: Training in the use of both Breathing Apparatus (BA), and decontamination procedures can often be arranged with your local Fire and Rescue Service.

Biological hazards

Introduction

- Contamination is caused by contact with pathogenic micro-organisms.

Management

- The basic management principles are similar to those involving hazardous chemical, and involves effective containment of the organisms or infected animals incurring minimal unnecessary exposure to the hazard in the process.

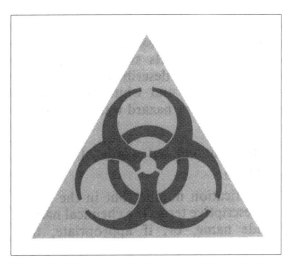

Figure 28-11 Symbol indicating a biological hazard

Radioactive contamination

Introduction

-   There is an increasing use of radioactive substances in industry, research/teaching and in medicine.

Management

-   Specific guidance on the management of such incidents is given in the document "National Arrangements for Incidents Involving Radioactivity" (NAIR).
-   The basic principles for managing radioactive materials are basically similar to those for chemical incidents with the exception that radioactivity cannot be detected or measured without special instruments and can penetrate considerable thicknesses of even dense materials.
-   Radioactive materials may exhibit different levels of radioactivity.
-   The objective of management is to remove the casualties from sources of high radioactivity and remove other radioactive substances from the patient. This can usually be achieved with soap and water.

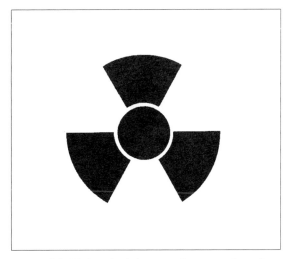

Figure 28-12 Symbol designating a nuclear hazard

Notes

29

Major incidents

Major incidents

Introduction

- Although major incidents may occur only rarely, their management is something with which all Immediate Care doctors should be familiar, as they provide the initial medical response in many areas, and in those areas are usually the first doctors to arrive at the scene.
- In some areas where there are Immediate Care Schemes, there are formal arrangements with the local hospitals for the scheme to provide not only the medical team, but also the Medical Incident Officer.
- The procedures used should be considered to be an extension of those procedures commonly used at all incidents, except on a larger scale. Everyone is good at doing what they do often, and if major incidents are treated as being something special or different, there is the danger of there being even more confusion than is inevitable.

Definitions

Major incident
- An unexpected event which overwhelms the normal resources of the unit be it Department, Hospital, Area or Region.
- A major incident for one emergency service may not necessarily be a major incident for all the emergency services.
- There is almost inevitably initial chaos and confusion.

Health circular: HC 90/25
- "A major incident arises when any occurrence presents a serious threat to the health of the community, disruption to the (health) service, or causes or is likely to cause such numbers of casualties as to require special arrangements by the health service".

Mass casualty situation
- A situation when the number and severity of the casualties overwhelms the medical resources available for their treatment.

Roles of the emergency services

General priorities

- The preservation of life.
- The prevention of further loss of life and further injury.
- The protection of property.

Police

- Exert overall command and control of the incident and the surrounding area, except in the case of a fire, chemical or radiation incident, when the fire service in overall command until that hazard is neutralised, and major aircraft accidents, when the Royal Air Force may have a co-ordinating role, especially when military aircraft are involved.
- Perform essential duties until the arrival of the specialist emergency service.
- Co-ordinate and facilitate the work of the other emergency services:
    - Plan:
        - Access/egress to the scene.
        - Location of:
            - Incident Post, Casualty Clearing Station, etc. (in consultation with the Ambulance Incidence Officer).
    - Provide the means of communication, if this is not otherwise available.
    - Act on behalf of the Coroner:
        - Obtain confirmation of death and identification of the dead.
        - Provide temporary mortuary facilities.
- Establish a Casualty Bureau:
    - Identify the injured, maintain records and inform the relatives.
- Establish traffic and crowd control, both locally, and in the general area of the incident.
- Safeguard the public:
    - Evacuate the area if necessary.
- Initiate action to provide food, warmth, clothing, and shelter for those rendered homeless by the incident.
- Safeguard any property directly and indirectly involved in the incident.
- Carry out an investigation into the causes and management of the incident.

Fire and rescue service

- Exert overall command and control of the incident in the case of fires, chemical and nuclear incidents until the hazard is neutralized, when this role reverts to the police.
- Neutralization of hazards: fire, dangerous chemicals, radiation.
- Rescue of the injured from immediate danger.
- Release of the trapped.
- (May be a useful source of manpower once their primary role is accomplished.)

Ambulance service

- Mobilise and work in close liaison with the medical services:
  - Immediately alert and mobilise the local Immediate Care Scheme, where one exists.
  - Select and alert the Receiving Hospital(s).
  - Provide transport for any hospital medical or nursing team.
  - Provide on site and site to hospital communications.
- Provide triage of, give ambulance aid to, and stabilise the injured, under medical supervision/directon if present.
- Provide accommodation and extra medical equipment for the treatment of any casualties (many ambulance services can provide inflatable tents, in which casualties can be accommodated and treated).
- Transport the injured to the receiving hospitals, and provide inter-hospital transfers to specialist care facilities, e.g. for burns, spinal injury.
- Provide transport home for those patients who are discharged early to make room for casualties from the major incident.

Medical services

- Have legal responsibility for the treatment of the injured at the scene and elsewhere.
- Provide medical triage, medical treatment and stabilisation of the injured, prior to their removal to hospital, by the ambulance service.
- Provide confirmation of death.
- Work in close unison with the ambulance service and receiving hospitals.
- Give advice on any occupation health matters or medical forensic aspects of the incident which may have a bearing on its overall management.

Organisation of the incident site

Emergency services rendezvous point

- A predetermined area where emergency service vehicles are assembled prior to their being called forward to the scene, usually by the police.
- Usually only found near special risk sites, e.g. airports, chemical complexes, nuclear sites, etc.

Incident scene

- The actual location of the incident:
  - Wrecked vehicles
  - Aircraft
  - Train
  - Buildings.
- May be spread over a very considerable area especially in aircraft, train accidents, etc. If so, it may have to be divided into sectors for management purposes.
- As far as medical services are concerned, it is the area in which casualties both dead and alive remain following the incident.

Incident control point

- A central point, readily identifiable, at which the Incident Officers and their emergency control vehicles are situated.
- It is usually some distance from the actual incident scene, but ideally overlooking it.
- In practice, the emergency control vehicles have to park a little distance apart so as to avoid mutual radio interference.
- The police incident control vehicle should remain the only vehicle displaying a blue light (in some areas the fire and ambulance emergency control vehicles may also display flashing lights (red or red and white lights in the case of the fire control point).

Ambulance/medical control point

- An ambulance emergency control vehicle providing an "on site" communications facility, which may be situated some distance from the incident scene, and is identified by a green or green and white flashing light.
- It provides a focal point for NHS/medical resources attending the incident.

Casualty clearing station/casualty treatment area

- A place of relative safety to which casualties are conveyed from the incident, and where treatment and stabilisation is carried out by doctors and ambulance personnel working together under the joint direction of a senior doctor and the Ambulance Casualty Clearing Officer prior to their evacuation by ambulance.

Ambulance (casualty) loading point

- A point near the casualty clearing station at which the casualties are loaded into ambulances under the direction of the Ambulance Loading Officer.

Ambulance parking area

- The area where ambulances are held prior to being called forward to load patients and is under the control of the Ambulance Parking Officer.

Temporary mortuary

- The place to which the deceased will be taken after confirmation of death, for initial identification purposes and forensic examination.

Site personnel

Police incident officer

- The senior police officer with overall responsibility for a major incident.

Ambulance incident officer

- The senior ambulance officer with the overall responsibility for the work of the ambulance service at the scene of a major incident.
- He liaises closely with the Medical Incident Officer to ensure effective use of the medical and ambulance resources at the scene.
- He will also be responsible for the direction and control of the St John, Red Cross and Civil Aid input into the incident.

Nursing incident officer

- The nursing officer who co-ordinates nursing activities at the scene of an incident, where more than one mobile team is required, and where the appointment of a nursing incident officer is considered necessary.
- He/she should work together with the Medical Incident Officer and should not be a member of any mobile medical and nursing team.

Medical incident officer

- The senior doctor, with overall responsibility, in close liaison with the Ambulance Incident Officer, for the medical resources at the scene of the major incident. He should not be a member of any mobile medical team.

Qualities

- He/she needs to:
    - Be known to and respected by the senior members of the other emergency services.
    - Be disciplined and experienced in and trained for the role of medical management.
    - Be familiar with likely scenario.
    - Be familiar with the organisation, role, equipment and requirements of Immediate Care and the attending medical teams.
    - Be familiar with the organisation, role, equipment and requirements of the other emergency services, especially the ambulance service.
    - Be familiar with the organisation, role, requirements and capabilities of the surrounding hospitals, and location of any special facilities, e.g. burns unit, neurosurgical unit, thoracic unit and their admissions policies.
    - Have the ability not to get involved in management/treatment of individuals.

Requirements

- He/she should:
    - Be readily identifiable, i.e. wear clothing (flourescent tabard and hat), which are clearly labelled and highly visible.
    - Have a runner.
    - Be able to communicate with:
        - Other senior doctors, e.g. medical team leaders.
        - Ambulance Incident Officer.

Who ?

- The first doctor to arrive at the incident until relieved by a senior clinician who has had appropriate training and/or experience in the role.

Action

- He should don the Medical Incident Officer Tabbard, if available, and report to the senior police officer present (Police Incident Officer).
- Establish the Medical Control Point (this will be with the Ambulance Control Point).
- *Liaise* with:
    - Ambulance Incident Officer.
    - Police Incident Officer.
    - Fire Incident Officer.
    - Designated Hospitals; inform them of:
        - Number of casualties and severity of their injuries.
        - Any special injuries, e.g. burns.
        - Need for a surgical team: for field amputation.
        - Time of dispatch of casualties to the hospital, with as much relevant clinical information as possible (the Ambulance Incident Officer will arrange for the hospitals to be kept advised of incoming casualties; the Medical Incident Officer only has need to pass information or speak to the hospital in relation to those patients with special needs).
- *Assess the problem:*
    - Reconnoitre the scene for:
        - Number and severity of casualties.
        - Trapped casualties.
        - Special injuries:
            - Burns
            - Spinal injuries.
            - Those requiring field surgery.
        - Any toxic risks and ascertain how to treat any contaminated casualties.
    - Agree these findings with the Ambulance Incident Officer.

Management

- Take charge of all Nursing and Medical Rescuers.
- Organise Medical Communications with the Ambulance Service.
- Delegate:
    - A triage doctor:
        - A senior doctor, who should work with the Ambulance Casualty Selection Officer.
    - A senior doctor for the incident scene (Forward Medical Incident Officer):
        - Medical team leader(s) (in a large incident, there may need to be several medical teams).
    - A senior doctor for the Casualty Treatment Area/Casualty Clearing Station.
    - A senior doctor for the Casualty Loading Point:
        - He should work closely with the Ambulance Casualty Loading Officer.
    - A hospital liaison doctor.
- Provide doctors for the confirmation of death, once there are sufficient resources to treat the injured.
- Send in further doctors as requested by Medical team leaders, etc.
- Arrange for the relief of the medical teams after about 4 hours into the incident.
- Consider:
    - The need for surgical teams for field amputations, etc.
    - The need for special medical resources/equipment.
    - The use of paramedics/ambulance technicians (in consultation with the Ambulance Incident Officer).
    - The possible use of St John or Red Cross paramedics, nursing teams or first aiders (in consultation with the Ambulance Incident Officer).
    - The use of nurses to escort patients to hospital.
- Occupational and Environmental Health:
    - Look after the health and safety of members of the other emergency services:
        - Exhaustion
        - Heat exhaustion
        - Hypothermia
        - Feeding
        - Minor injuries, etc.
- Organise a continual medical presence until the whole incident has been closed down.
- Maintain a record of events with times, etc.
- Consider giving a press interview, after consultation with the Police and Ambulance Incident Officers.
- Post incident:
    - Prepare a report for any inquiry, etc.
    - Organise:
        - The medical debriefing.
        - Counselling for:
            - Medical teams.
            - Other members of the emergency services.

Note: - The scene should be disturbed as little as possible so that post-accident forensic investigation into cause of accident/mechanism of injury, etc. can be established.

Gold/silver/bronze system of command and control

- This is a new system of nomenclature for senior officers and Controls involved in the command and control of major incidents, and may be used by all the emergency services.
- In each emergency service, involved in a major incident, there is always only one officer of Gold status, and usually only one of Silver status, but several of Bronze status.

Gold Control

- The major incident desk in control.

Gold Commander

- The overall commander of a service (usually the chief officer, chief executive or director).

Silver Control

- The on scene communications/incident control vehicle/room.

Silver Commander

- The service's Incident Officer at the scene.

Bronze

- The subordinate commanders/officers of a service at an incident.

Hospital organisation

Listed hospitals

- Hospitals listed by the Regional Health Authority as adequately equipped to receive casualties on a 24 hour basis and able to provide, when required, the Medical Incident Officer, the Nursing Incident Officer and/or a mobile Medical and Nursing Team(s).

Receiving hospital(s)

- The hospital(s) selected by the Ambulance Service (from those listed by the Regional Health Authority), to receive casualties in the event of any particular incident.
- These are preferably Major Hospitals and are usually the nearest hospitals to which the first seriously injured casualties will be sent.
- Hospitals to which the overflow of seriously injured casualties, and walking wounded may be sent are also designated Receiving Hospitals.
- The *first* Receiving Hospital *only* may nominate or provide the Medical Incident Officer.

Mobile medical and nursing teams

- All Receiving Hospitals should arrange for a mobile medical and nursing team to be dispatched on request only from the Ambulance Service or Medical Incident Officer. However they should be careful not to deplete staff required from the A&E Department, or elsewhere in the hospital, who will be needed to provide care for gravely injured patients arriving at that hospital. Where appropriate arrangements should include the mobilisation of Immediate Care Schemes.

- *Note:* - In very rural or sparsely populated areas, the local District General Hospital may have to provide both a medical team and the Medical Incident Officer in the first instance. These should be relieved at the earliest opportunity by a medical team and/or Medical Incident Officer from another Listed Hospital or from the nearest Immediate Care Scheme.

Distribution of casualties

- Casualties should if possible be conveyed to the hospital and facilities appropriate to their needs.
- Ideally more than one hospital should always be involved so that there is an even distribution of patients between hospitals from the very start so that one hospital is not overstretched while another is idle.

Action of doctors at a major incident

All doctors

- On arrival at the incident:
  - Park under police supervision and switch off green light (this sequence may be reversed in special circumstances, e.g. at airports).
- Don protective/identifying clothing.
- Log in with police.
- Report to the Medical Incident Officer/Ambulance Control Vehicle.
- Carry out the instructions of senior doctors in a disciplined manner.
- Should *not* give press interviews without prior permission from both the Police and Medical Incident Officers.

The first doctor at the scene

- The first doctor to arrive at the scene should assume the role of Medical Incident Officer, until relieved by a senior doctor who has been specially trained in the role.

Communications for major incidents

- Effective communication is the key to effective management, and is the area where there are most problems in major incident management, especially in the early stages.
- The ambulance service will normally provide all communications for the Medical Incident Officer and medical teams.
- At all times, but especially at major incidents, when air time is at a premium strict radio discipline should be maintained, and all messages kept brief and simple, so as to avoid misunderstandings and confusion.
- The method of communication may vary according to the location, type of incident, and equipment available.
- Callout/en route:
    - Local immediate care scheme frequency
    - Ambulance frequency
    - The Emergency Reserve Channel (ERC).
      (Ideally there may be a national BASICS frequency in the future, so that any BASICS doctor called into any area can communicate with the local scheme.)
- On scene:
    - Between doctors:
        - Runner, VHF/UHF hand held radios.
    - Inter-service:
        - Runner, UHF hand held radios.
    - With hospital via:
        - VHF radio on Ambulance or Immediate Care Scheme frequency.
        - Cellphones, although problems have been encountered due to media overusage blocking the system (see below).
        - British Telecom telephone (landline).

Emergency reserve channel (ERC)

- This is a nation wide ambulance frequency which is usually only used during major incidents or major disasters.
- It enables one ambulance service to communicate with vehicles from any other ambulance services that may be called in to assist it.
- Many Immediate Care doctors also have radios on this frequency, with the permission of their local ambulance service.

ACCOLC (Access overload control)

- This is a filtering sytem used on the Racal-Vodaphone cellular radio system.
- It may be activated (usually by the police) at major incidents, and only allows access for those with prior authorisation.

Priority access

- A similar sytem to ACCOLC, but on the Cellnet cellular radio system.

Triage

Definition: The sorting of casualties into different categories according to the severity of their injuries.

- In the mass casualty situation, the objective must be to do the most good for the greatest number of casualties.
- In many cases the early removal from the scene of the uninjured and walking wounded removes a source of distraction and allows the rescuers to give their undivided attention to the more seriously injured.

Triage Categories						Expected survival %
Red	Priority 1	P1	Critical	Immediate	T1	10%
Yellow	Priority 2	P2	Serious	Urgent	T2	30%
Green	Priority 3	P3	Minor	Delayed	T3	60%
Blue				Expectant	T4	
Black			Dead	Deceased	T0	

Expectant casualties
- Those severely injured casualties who are unlikely to survive even if treated aggressively, but would require a greater than appropriate medical resource in the process, thus depriving potential survivors of treatment.
- Only used in the mass casualty situation.

Uninjured survivors
- It is thought that these should also be included in the categories of casualties, as they too will require special handling and treatment, e.g. counselling.

Triage methods

Self triage
- Walking wounded:
    - These will tend to walk away from the site of the incident and in many civilian incidents may present first at the nearest casualty department or even to casualty departments some considerable way from the incident, as they know that the nearest hospital will be more than busy!
- Crawling wounded:
    - Will try to get away from incident in any way they can.
- Trapped wounded:
    - Those unable to get away from the incident either because they are physically trapped, or as a result of their injuries.

Note: - Some seriously injured patients may collapse some distance from the scene of the incident.

Medical triage
- Categorisation according to the medical condition/injuries/Triage Revised Trauma Score of the injured.

Triage labelling

- A system of casualty labelling according to the patient's triage category.

Triage labelling requirements
- Any labelling system should be:
    - Highly visible:
        - Colours are often difficult to distinguish in poor visibility; the category description should also be clearly shown.
    - Robust and waterproof.
    - Easy to attach and difficult to remove.
    - It should be easy to change the casualties triage category in either direction.
    - It should be easy to fill in casualty details rapidly.
    - Should have space for serial observations.
    - Should allow trauma scoring, if circumstances permit.
    - Uniform amongst all those involved at any incident.

Dynamic/continuous triage

- Triaging should take place continuously especially at the:
    - Incident scene:
        - Initial triage.
        - If trapped, during entrapment and prior to release.
    - Casualty Clearing Station/Casualty Treatment Area.
    - Casualty Loading point.
    - A & E Department.
    - At any other time as indicated by a change in the patient's condition.

The dead

- Should be confirmed dead in the presence of a police officer, and the relevant details recorded on the patient's triage label.
- The body should if possible be left in situ for later photography by the police, for forensic purposes, and eventual removal to the temporary mortuary facilities.

CASUALTY NUMBER
GMAS 000000

CASUALTY ASSESSMENT MODULE

PRIMARY SURVEY   Time   :

Airway   ☐ Clear   ☐ Obstructed

C. Spine   ☐ Normal   ☐ Possible injury

Breathing   ☐ Spontaneous   ☐ Problem

Circulation/ ☐ External   ☐ Possible Internal
Haemorrhage   ☐ None/slight   ☐ Moderate ☐ Severe

Disability: ☐ Alert   Responds to ☐ Visual stimuli
                                            ☐ Pain
                                            ☐ Unresponsive

Exposure/Injuries

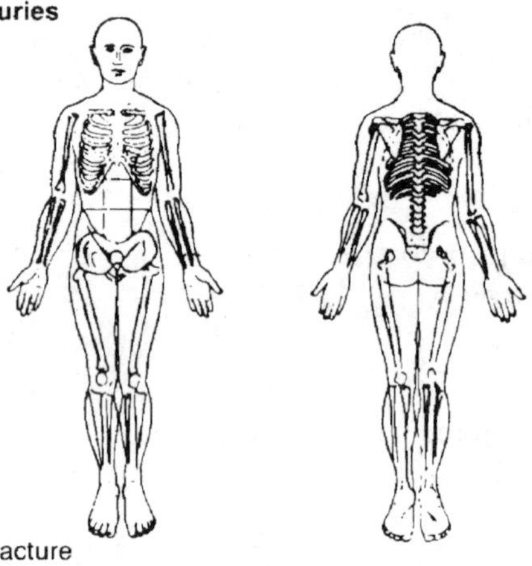

C# Closed Fracture
O# Open Fracture   L Laceration
B Burn (shade area) A Abrasion
F Foreign body   E Eccymosis (bruising)

PRIMARY MANAGEMENT

Airway   ☐ Oropharyngeal ☐ Nasal   ☐ ET Tube
              ☐ C/Thyrotomy   ☐ Oxygen   ☐ Suction
C. Spine   ☐ C. Collar   ☐ Hines

Breathing: ☐ Ventilated   ☐ Chest drain

Circulation Cannula size: Rt............ Lt............
                 IV Fluids   Volume   Time
              ☐ H'mans/N.Saline _____ _____
              ☐ H'maccel/G'fusine _____ _____

SECONDARY MANAGEMENT

Analgesia ☐ Entonox   Dose   Time
Drugs   ☐ _____ _____ _____
(specify) ☐ _____ _____ _____

Splinting ☐ Frac Straps ☐ KED   ☐ Traction
              ☐ Box   ☐ Other (specify)_____

OBSERVATIONS   Time   1)   :

Respiratory Rate —

Oxygen Saturation: Sa O₂% —

Blood Pressure —   - - - - - - -

Pulse Rate —

SECONDARY SURVEY

Eye Opening	Spontaneous	4 ☐
	To voice	3 ☐
	To pain	2 ☐
	None	1 ☐

Best Verbal Response	Oriented	5 ☐
	Confused	4 ☐
	Inappropriate	3 ☐
	Incomprehensible	2 ☐
	None	1 ☐

Motor Response	Obeys command	6 ☐
	Localises pain	5 ☐
	Withdrawal (pain)	4 ☐
	Flexion (pain)	3 ☐
	Extension (pain)	2 ☐
	None	1 ☐

Pupils React R ☐
            (✓ or X) L ☐
1 o Constricted   Size R [   ]
2 O Normal
3 O Dilated   Size L [   ]

Trauma Score: Time   1)   :

COMMENTS:

Signed Crew   **Dr.**

Figure 29-1 Triage card: Casualty assessment

DECEASED

Death Pronounced:

Time: Date:

Name of Doctor:

Signature

Witnessed by PC:

Number:

Name:

Figure 29-2 Triage card: The dead

The press

- Interviews are best avoided.
- Statements to the press should only be given by the Medical Incident Officer, but only after first agreeing the contents with the Police Press Officer, other Incident Officers, and the site owners, where appropriate, so that there is no contradiction or conflict to be exploited.
- Any statement should be brief and factual.
- Avoid giving opinions.
- Do not give details of individual casualties.

30

Aeromedical evacuation

Aeromedical evacuation

Introduction

- All personnel involved in Immediate Care require some understanding of aeromedical problems as there is an increasing tendency to use aircraft, especially helicopters in primary evacuation.
- Once involved with Immediate Care they may also find that their experience and expertise makes them sought after to assist with the secondary evacuation of the seriously injured or ill from abroad. It is essential that they have some grounding in the problems associated with this before they undertake such work.

Rotary wing aircraft: helicopters

Uses

- There is increasingly use of helicopters for *primary evacuation* of casualties especially in:
    - Major disasters.
    - Patients with very severe or multiple injuries.
    - Remote places:
        - Scarce ambulance resources.
        - Long travelling distances.
        - Rough terrain.
- They may also be used for *secondary evacuation*:
    - Hospital to hospital direct short haul transfer:
        - Often used for:
            - Spinal injuries
            - Severe burns.

Helicopter types

- They may be:
    - Civilian:
        - Usually a small helicopter with some provision for transporting casualties.
    - Police:
        - A small helicopter, which may be owned or chartered by the police.
        - Its prime role is traffic control/surveillance, with some provision for carrying casualties.
    - Ambulance service:
        - Small helicopter. Often chartered and specially adapted for ambulance use.
    - Military:
        - Usually Royal Navy or Royal Air Force.
        - This is usually a large helicopter, whose primary role is Search and Rescue, or troop or cargo transportation.
        - They have provision for transporting casualties, but there is little sound insulation so they tend to be particularly noisy.

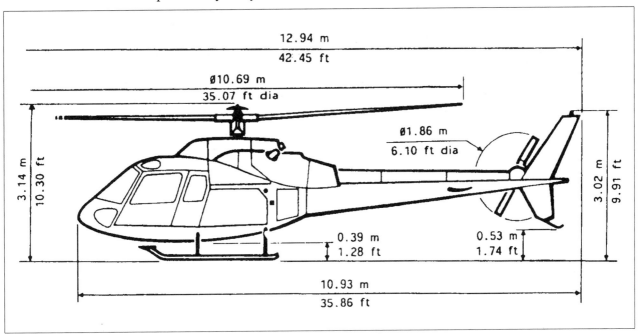

Figure 30-1 The main dimensions of the AS 355 helicopter

Advantages

Access
- Helicopters do not require an airfield or landing strip on which to land.

Speed
- Helicopters are relatively fast compared to road transport.
- Can travel in a straight line.

Range
- Their range is:
    - Wessex/MBB 105: 300 miles.
    - Sea King/Dauphin 2: 600 miles.

Access
- They have:
    - The ability to land in relatively small spaces.
    - The ability to land on rough ground if equipped with skids (on soft ground, the rotors may have to be kept going to provide enough lift to prevent the helicopter from sinking in).
  - A winching facility (military and coastguard helicopters only):
      - A winch can lift up a stretcher from places only accessible from the air:
        - Very rough terrain.
        - Cliffs.

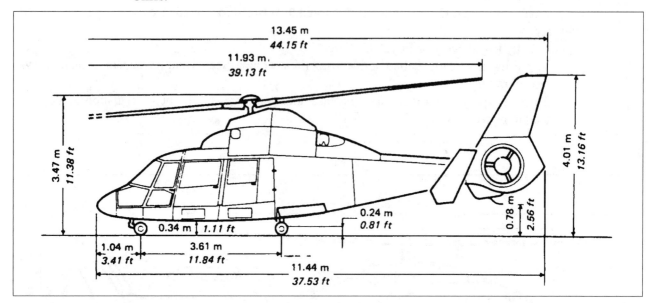

Figure 30-2 The main dimensions of the SA 365 Dauphin helicopter

Disadvantages

Cost
- Helicopters are very expensive to operate.

Range
- Have a relatively short range of action compared to fixed wing aircraft.

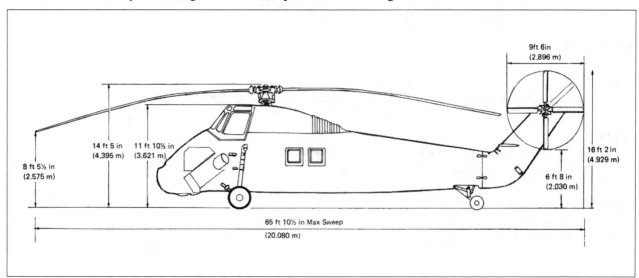

Figure 30-3 The main dimensions of the Wessex helicopter

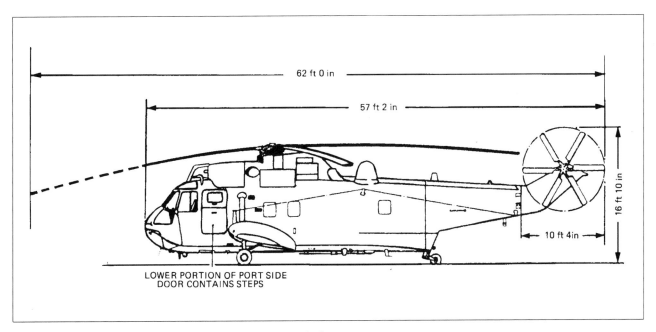

Figure 30-4 The main dimensions of the Sea King helicopter

Static
- The static generated by the aircraft may have to be earthed, and this may cause problems, especially during winching.
- This is size dependent and occurs with the Sea King, but not the Wessex.

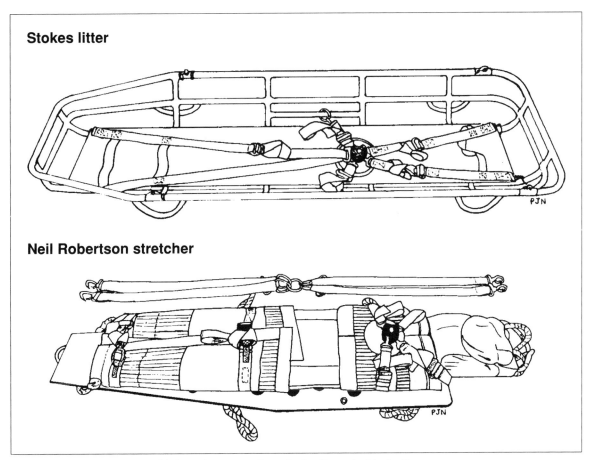

Figure 30-5 Devices in which patients can be winched/carried in helicopters

Rotor blades
- These can be very dangerous for those on the ground, especially if it is sloping.
- All those approaching a helicopter should do so cautiously and under the direct control and guidance of the pilot.
- May generate considerable downdraught, which can be unpleasant for those on the ground. All loose items should be secured.

PRACTICAL POINT: - If the blades are rotating, always approach a helicopter in a crouched position.
- Never go near a rotating tail rotor.

The high levels of noise
- Cabin levels 80-115 dBA (pain >140 dBA):
- This may be uncomfortable, and can necessitate the use of ear defenders for all (this includes the patient, even if he is unconscious).
- Causes difficulty with communication:
    - Necessitates the use of hand signs/headphones.

Vibration
- This may be quite unpleasant.

Flicker
- May cause vertigo, which may be uncomfortable.
- Rarely can induce epileptiform fits.

Wind chill/cold
- This may precipitate hypothermia and aggravate shock:
    - Consider using an insulating (space) blanket.

Other problems
- There also may be problems with:
    - Compatibility of equipment:
        - Different voltage, etc.
    - Interference with the aircraft's avionics:
        - LEDs.
        - Defibrillator discharge (in practice, this does not appear to be the problem that it might seem to be in theory).
    - Lack of space.

Helicopter landing site

Site selection

- The site should be clear of all tall obstacles (25 metres or over):
    - Trees, buildings, pylons.
- The actual landing spot should be firm and at least 15 metres in diameter.
- The maximum slope should be no more than 12%.

Helicopter landing site preparation

- Clear an area 100 metres in diameter.
- Remove or secure all loose material which may be either blown about causing injury or sucked into the engine air intake:
    - Paper debris
    - Stones
    - Medical equipment
    - Leaves and loose branches.
- Keep the area clear of any crowds and animals.
- Indicate the wind direction using smoke if possible.

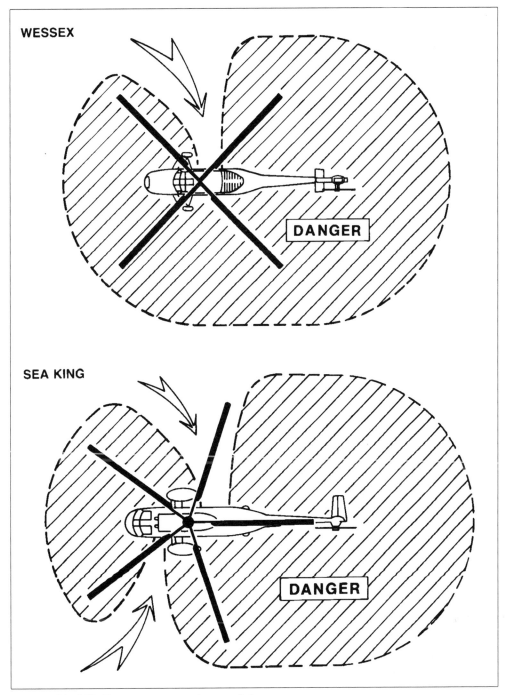

Figure 30-6 Helicopter entry points and danger zones

Landing helicopters

- Most helicopter pilots are skilled and practised in unaided landings, and do not usually require any assistance.
- If the selected site is particularly difficult for any reason guidance may helpful:
    - Guide the helicopter in by standing or kneeling well beyond the edge of the 15 metre landing spot, with your back to the wind and with both arms raised.

Fixed wing aircraft

Uses

- Fixed wing aircraft are usually only used for the secondary transfer or evacuation of patients over relatively long distances.

Types

- The aircraft may be:
    - Piston or jet engined.
    - Pressurised or unpressurised.
- The flights may be:
    - Long, medium or short haul.
    - By air ambulance or scheduled flight.

Advantages

- May be extremely rapid, and the only practical method of long distance patient transport.

Selection of type of aircraft ?

- This depends on:
    - What is available.
    - The finance/insurance that is available.
    - The airport facilities:
        - The length of the runway.
        - The time that the airport is open.
    - The time to be spent in transit:
        - The risk to the patient is directly proportional to the length of time spent travelling.
    - Any compromise between range versus speed, and altitude, e.g. cabin pressurisation for open skull fractures, pneumothorax and diving dysbarism.
    - Whether a stop-over is necessary:
    - Consider the risk of unnecessary exposure of the aircraft crew and other passengers to any endemic health problems in the pick up country.
    - Limits on the crew's flying time.
    - Whether pressurisation is necessary:
        - This depends on the aircraft's altitude.

- Whether there is a problem with:
    - Hypoxia:
        - This is exacerbated by increasing height.
        - ? Therapeutic oxygen supply needed/available, e.g. for patient with:
            - Cardiac failure
            - Myocardial ischaemia
            - Severe anaemia
            - Respiratory disease
            - Cerebral artery insufficiency.
- The reduced ambient temperature.
- Decompression/high flying (low pressure):
    - This should be avoided:
        - In patients with abnormal gas containing cavities whether traumatic, therapeutic/ investigative.
        - Following recent diving:
            - Within 12 hours of "no-stop" diving (<10 metres).
            - Within 24 hours of "stop" diving (>10 metres).
        - In patients suffering from any diving related disease of recent onset.
- Dehydration:
    - This is worse on long flights, due to the low humidity of the aircraft's air conditioned cabin air.
- The risk of "Jet lag":
    - This is the disturbance of circadian rhythms, which is caused by transmeridian flight, i.e. crossing time zones. This is far worse after eastward flights compared with westward flights.
    - It does not occur when travelling along time, i.e. from North to South or vice versa.
- Poor lighting and lack of adequate space in all types of aircraft.
- Drug schedules:
    - There may be problems due to changes in time.
    - It is probably best to maintain these on the departure zone time until arrival at the final destination.
- The different voltage used in the aircraft (28 volt DC).
    - This may cause problems (non functioning) of some essential medical equipment:
        - Monitors
        - Infusion pumps, etc.
- There are special regulations regarding the importation and carriage of "Dangerous cargo":
    - Relevant items are oxygen, mercury, aerosols and flammable materials.
- There is a legal requirement to have a Home Office Licence for the importation and reimportation of "Controlled Drugs".

Planning

- Road ambulance liaison:
    - The collection of the patient from the point of arrival.
- Medico-legal:
    - Obtain permission from the treating doctor abroad for the transfer.
- Make certain that the UK destination is adequate for the patient's needs, and that there will not be any need for a further transfer within the UK.
- If repatriation is for the insurer's economic reasons, make sure that:
    - The patient gives their consent.
    - There is no increased medical risk to the patient in the transfer.
    - The medical care in the UK is as good, if not better, than that abroad.

Problems

- Getting enough accurate information about the patient:
    - Language/translation:
        - From medical foreign language into foreign language into English into medical English.
        - The doctors/officials in the foreign country may be economical with the truth in order to expedite transfer of the patient.

Information required

- Ideally all this information should be obtained before setting off to collect the patient, although invariably not all of it is.
- The name, age, sex, religion and home address of the patient.
- The name, address and telephone number of the patient's general practitioner, and hospital consultant.
- The patient's destination:
    - Hospital, nursing home, etc.
    - It is always advisable to check that there is actually a bed available for the patient.
- The patient's height, size, weight:
    - Can he/she fit in the aircraft?
- The diagnosis, treatment carried out, and the time intervals involved.
- Details of any special requirements both medical and nursing care:
    - Diet
    - Suctioning
    - Intravenous fluids, etc.
    - Monitoring
    - Splinting.
- The available facilities in the hospitals involved in the patient's care, both in the foreign country and the UK (if appropriate).
- The experience and expertise of the hospital staff in the foreign country, and accompanying the patient to and in the aircraft.
- The drugs used and to be used:
    - Names
    - Doses
    - Times given.

In the aircraft

- Patients must have a secure harness fastening them to the stretcher.
- All medical equipment must be made secure:
    - Fixation of the endotracheal tube.
    - Intravenous lines.
- Make sure that you are prepared for all likely medical emergencies:
    - Make sure that there is enough room around the patient.
    - Prepare and place equipment ready to use.
    - Establish intravenous access.
- Prepare yourself for a possible emergency evacuation of the aircraft.

31

Radio communications

Radio communications

Introduction

- Effective communication is the key to the command and control of resources, and an understanding of their use is very important if the delivery of Immediate Care is to be efficient.
- The efficiency of radio communication is dependent on correct procedures being followed and accurate information being given to Control, which will enable the correct decisions to be made about the provision of resources at its disposal and to control them effectively.

Organisation

Control

- This is the central radio, usually in a fixed place, which controls the radio network.
- There is usually a control console which is connected to the transmitter and receiver by a landline.
- The transmitter and receiver are situated adjacent to the radio mast near the top of which is the aerial to which they are connected, and which receives and transmits the radio signals.

Mobile radios

- These are small radio sets which incorporate both a transmitter and a receiver, connected to an aerial.
- They may be:
    - Vehicle mounted: usually permanently fixed in the vehicle, possibily with hands-free operation.
    - Transportable: portable, with good range, but rather heavy and bulky, and may be used in-vehicle.
    - Hand held (portable): usually lightweight with a limited range.

Radio frequencies

Bands

- There are three radio frequency bands used in the United Kingdom by the statutory ambulance services, Immediate Care schemes, voluntary aid societies and motor sport organisations:
    - Low band AM: 77-88 MHz (voluntary aid societies, motor sport organisations).
    - High band FM: 166-176 MHz (statutory ambulance services, Immediate Care schemes, motor sport organisations).
    - UHF: various (statutory ambulance services for short range communications).

Modulation

- Radio waves may be modulated in two ways:
  - FM: frequency modulation
  - AM: amplitude modulation.
- A radio using one kind of modulation cannot usually communicate satisfactorily with a radio using the other kind of modulation.

Radio reception

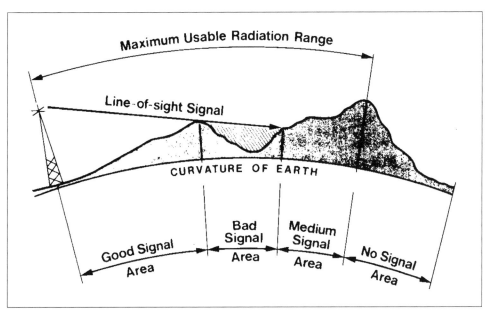

Figure 31-1 Radio reception

Transmitter range

- Radio has a limited range.
- Communication is always best from a high unobstructed location.
- If a mobile cannot hear Control (which usually has a higher powered transmitter and better aerial siting than mobiles), then it is unlikely that Control will be able to receive the mobile.
- If radio reception is poor, e.g. at the limit of the range, or in a radio black spot, move to a more favourable location (usually higher up, or on the opposite side of a hill), before attempting to transmit.

Interference

- Transmission and reception can be upset by weather: thunderstorms, heavy rain, etc.

Radio black-spots/shadows (areas of poor radio reception)

- Can be caused either by the terrain, tall buildings, steel cladding, etc.

Methods of transmission

Single frequency simplex

- This is where both the base station and the mobiles transmit and receive on the same frequency.
- This means that all the radios in a system can hear transmissions from all the other radios.
- Used by the voluntary aid societies, in motorsport, and by ambulance services UHF (short range communications) .

Advantages

- Useful when mobiles need to be able to communicate directly with each other.

Disadvantages

- If two mobiles transmit at once, they will cause mutual interference "heterodyne".
- Two mobiles can engage the whole system and make it difficult for Control to exercise control.

CONCLUSION

- Suitable for systems covering a relatively small area, when mobiles are involved in the same incident or event and need to be able to communicate directly with each other, but radio discipline needs to be strictly enforced. May also be useful in schemes with very few mobiles covering large areas, which are unlikely to interfere with each other.

Two frequency simplex

- In this system the base station transmits on one frequency, and the mobiles transmit on another adjacent frequency.
- This means that all mobiles can receive the base station, but only the base station can receive transmissions from the mobiles (which cannot usually receive transmissions from each other):
    - Base: transmits on frequency A and receives on frequency B.
    - Mobiles: transmit on frequency B and receive on frequency A.
- Used by ambulance services and Immediate Care schemes.

Advantages

- Easier for Control to exercise control.
- Useful when a base station controls a large number of mobiles, and there is usually no need for mobiles to be able to transmit to and receive each other.

Disadvantages

- Occupys two channels.

CONCLUSION

- The system of choice for large systems covering large geographical areas.

Duplex

- The use of a two frequency system, in which both the transmitter and receiver can both operate simultaneously (like a telephone).
- Electronically complicated.
- Used in Cellular radio.

Facilities

Talkthrough

- This is a facility used in two frequency simplex, which enables the base station to retransmit everything that it receives.
- This enables mobiles to hear all transmissions, and for one mobile to communicate with another.
- It is switchable from the base station console and may also be switchable by mobiles using a tone control system (see below).

Encoders/decoders

- These encode or decode a series of audio tones (usually three or five), which can be used to selectively "page" (the radio will emit a bleep similar to a pager) and "open up" a radio from a stand-by (dormant) state (when they are switched on, but their loud speaker is muted).
- The sequence of tones may also be used to activate a pager on the same radio system, so that when a mobile is paged, not only will the radio open up, but the pager will go off at the same time.
- Useful:
    - When a channel or frequency has to be shared with other users, and mobiles do not want to have to listen to irrelevant transmissions.
    - When used in conjunction with a pager, for alerting a radio operator who may not be close to the radio.

Sub-audio tone

- This is an inaudible tone (unique to a particular system), which is transmitted simultaneously with any speech. The receiving radio will only "open up" and switch on its speaker, when it receives this tone. The radio will revert to a "closed down" state with its speaker muted as soon as it ceases to receive the sub-audio tone.
- Its purpose is to only open up radios when there is a transmission on their radio system and is useful when a channel or frequency has to be shared with other users, and mobiles do not want to have to listen to irrelevant transmissions.

Squelch

- This is a control found on older sets, which reduces the amount of receiver interference, but at the same times increases the threshold/strength of signal required for the radio to receive a transmission.

Callsigns

Fixed stations

- Fixed stations are usually called "Control" or "Base", with a prefix indicating the name of the service, e.g. Essam Control (Essex Ambulance Control), SWAG Base (Saffron Walden Accident Group Base).

Mobiles and portables

- Mobiles and portables are usually given letter names of the the NATO phonetic alphabet or numbers of the NATO figure pronunciation (see below). This may be:
    - Preceded by a prefix indicating the name of the service, e.g. Essam 181 (Essex Ambulance Service mobile 181).
    - Preceded or followed by an indication of the status of the mobile, e.g. Medic SWAG 01 (Doctor 01 from the Saffron Walden Accident Group), Essam 181 Papa (Essex Ambulance Service mobile 181 with a paramedic on board).
    - Callsigns usually belong to an emergency vehicle, rather than to members of its crew.
    - Doctors and officers in the emergency services usually have their own individual callsigns.

Note:- Always use *full* callsigns, when starting and closing any exchange of messages.

Radio procedure

Introduction

- Correct Control, vehicle and individual "callsigns" must be used at all times and *never* the names of control operators, vehicle crews or doctors.
- Messages should be spoken in a way that will ensure the receiver has full understanding of them.
- The three characteristics of a good radio message are:
    - Clarity:
        - Pronounce words distinctly and slowly.
    - Accuracy:
        - In the situation where communcations are difficult, or the pronunciation of words, names or numbers is difficult and liable to cause uncertainty in the mind of the receiver, the word or name should be spelt out using the N.A.T.O. phonetic alphabet or in the case of numbers use the N.A.T.O. figure pronunciation (see below).
    - Brevity:
        - Messages must be as brief as possible, using well recognised abbreviations and codes.
- The following factors are therefore important:
    - Rhythm
    - Rate:
        - Normal speed of talking is 40-60 words per minute.
    - Volume:
        - keep your mouth close to the microphone and speak across it (do not shout or whisper).
    - Pitch
- Never use obscene language or swear words over the air. This is an offence under the Radiotelephone Licensing Regulations, and offenders may be prosecuted.

Proper use of radio

- Radios should be switched on the moment the vehicle becomes mobile.
- Remember, only one mobile or radio user can use the radio frequency or channel at one time and that messages of a non-urgent nature could be blocking another mobile's urgent call for assistance.

Preliminary call

- This is a transmission to ensure that communications are possible before air space is wasted in passing a message which cannot for one reason or another be received.
- It is essential to stop and think before commencing a radio message - plan it, and until you get enough experience write it down on paper to prevent confusion (if circumstances permit).
- Before transmission, make sure that the channel is clear:
    - Always listen before transmitting. If you are not certain if the channel is in use, ask briefly.
    - Operators should *never* attempt to call Control when another transmission is in progress, except in life threatening emergencies, when the call should be prefixed "Safety", Priority" or "Priority Urgent" (in motorsport).
- Then call once only using the full call signs, and always giving your own call sign after that of the station you are calling.
- When a doctor or vehicle initiates a call to control the following procedure should be used:
    - Control "call sign" (this is usually repeated once), followed by the doctor's or vehicle's "call sign".

Example
"Essam Control, Essam Control, Medic 01, over".
"Medic 01, Essam Control, go ahead, over."

Messages
- Each message should end with "over".

Acknowledgements

- Every message must be acknowledged, otherwise the calling station may think the exchange is incomplete and may continue to keep the channel clear of other users.

Closing

- At the end of a message or series of messages, stations may end with either the words:
    - "Standing by" indicating that they will continue to monitor that radio frequency *or*
    - "Over and out" indicating that they do not expect any further communications.

Locations

- When giving a location, reference should be made to distances, cross roads, road junction numbers, and well known buildings along with the area location.

N.A.T.O. phonetic alphabet

A	ALPHA	N	NOVEMBER
B	BRAVO	O	OSCAR
C	CHARLIE	P	PAPA
D	DELTA	Q	QUEBEC
E	ECHO	R	ROMEO
F	FOXTROT	S	SIERRA
G	GOLF	T	TANGO
H	HOTEL	U	UNIFORM
I	INDIA	V	VICTOR
J	JULIET	W	WHISKEY
K	KILO	X	X-RAY
L	LIMA	Y	YANKEE
M	MIKE	Z	ZULU

Numeral pronounciation

1	WUN	6	SIX
2	TOO	7	SEV-EN
3	THUREE	8	ATE
4	FOUR	9	NINER
5	FIYIV	0	ZERO

Signal strength

- This is used when checking signal strength and radio reception with another radio.

    1 Unreadable
    2 Very noisy and barely readable
    3 Noisy but readable
    4 Good, but slightly noisy
    5 Loud and clear (OK)

Kilo code

- This is a code system which is used by some ambulance services, but there is little uniformity between different services.
- It is used to save air time and prevent confidential information being understood.

    Kilo 1   Death unconfirmed by a doctor
          2   Death confirmed by a doctor
          3   Overdose not seen by a doctor
          4   Overdose seen by a doctor
          5   Myocardial infarction
          6   Unconscious patient
          7   Abortion
          8   Psychiatric patient
          9   AIDS patient
          10 Terminally ill patient

Common abbreviations/expressions used in radio communications

ETA   Estimated time of arrival

ETD   Estimated time of departure

RTB   Return to base

Say again   Repeat your message

Roger   Message understood

Over   Used at the end of each message, apart from the final one.

Standing by Used at the completion of an exchange of messages, indicating that the radio is expecting further transmissions and will remain "opened up".

Wait   Indicates that you are unable to reply immediately. It is normally followed by an indication of time, e.g. wait one (minute).

Go ahead   Usually used after a "wait" period.

Notes

32

Counselling disaster and accident victims

Counselling disaster and accident victims

Introduction

- Those involved with Immediate Care should be aware of the need for counselling for all those involved in incidents resulting in serious physical or emotional trauma, because they may be involved both as a sufferer and in the treatment of sufferers.
- It is now well recognised that the best counsellors are not only those trained in counselling, but also those who were themselves involved in the actual or similar events, and as such, those involved in Immediate Care who are not affected, may have a unique and very special role.
- Counselling, however, should not be thrust unthinkingly on all those involved in horrific events, but there should be an understanding that they may require help and if so should not feel embarrassed or awkward about asking for it.
- Many of those involved in Immediate Care may in fact give themselves and their colleagues a kind of counselling, by discussing the event with their colleagues or others involved in it, or even by holding informal or formal debriefing sessions, at which feelings can be vented in a non threatening and non judgemental environment.
- It should be remembered that even the experts may be upset by "the Big One".

Post-traumatic stress disorder (PTSD)

Incidence

- 40-70% of all those directly involved in a disaster, experience symptoms during the following month.
- 20% may experience chronic levels of anxiety for more than 2 years.
- Long term effects (lasting up to 5 years) are possibly most common in those involved in fires or explosion at sea.
- Up to 70% of rescuers may be affected.
- Associated with an increase in physical and psychiatric illness and accidental and non-accidental death.

Aetiology

- The causative event does not have to be a major disaster, but may also be a particularly traumatic event which can include:
    - Serious injury accidents
    - Torture
    - Rape
    - Assault

- Those at risk may also include:
  - Battle shocked soldiers
  - Highjack victims
  - Concentration camp survivors
  - Hostages
- Disasters which expose their victims to a prolonged risk of death or mutilation are more likely to produce severe and prolonged effects.
- It is not only the victims themselves that may suffer from this condition, but also their friends, relatives, and emergency services personnel and rescue workers.
- Community workers and members of the voluntary agency members involved in the care of the survivors of a disaster may also be at risk.
- Emergency services personnel are more likely to suffer from PTSD if:
  - They are unable to do anything active to help the survivors.
  - There are gruesome tasks involving multiple deaths, mutilated bodies or the deaths of young children.
  - There is poor organisation and management of the disaster with a lack of command and control, and explanation of their tasks, leading to frustration over lives than cannot be saved, equipment failure, delays and overwhelming demands being made on them.
- Those involved in a near miss situation (i.e. those who but for some accident of fate would have been a victim) may also be affected.

Pathopsychology

- The traumatic event is by definition, one which is distressing for all those involved with it, and in particular gives them feelings of acute fear, terror, and usually a sense of helplessness, and impotence.
- Characteristics of the distaster, the rescue operation and the sufferer may all affect the degree of stress experienced.
- PTSD can affect normal individuals; it is the event which is abnormal.
- Those with a predisposition for pre-morbid depressive or neurotic traits are more likely to be affected and probably also more severely affected than those without such personality traits.
- Psychopathic personalities may to a certain extent be protected.
- Head injury with retrograde amnesia seems to protect patients from the condition.
- Some of the effects may be worse in those who are uninjured and in those involved in the near miss situation, who may have feelings of guilt about having survived.
- Those most at risk include:
  - The unemployed
  - Those from lower socioeconomic class
  - Those from large families
  - The divorced and those with littlle support
  - Females
  - The young, especially children (including those born from victims shortly after the disaster)
  - The elderly (because of their reluctance to ask for help).

Prognosis

- The overall prognosis is:
  - Good if treatment is early and specific.
  - Bad if symptoms and treatment are each delayed more than 6 months.

Symptoms

- The onset of symptoms may be delayed by up to 6 months after the event (many patients will avoid seeking medical help in an effort to avoid anything to do with their experience).
- Symptoms must have been present for at least 1 month before the diagnosis can be made.

Presenting symptoms

- May include:
    - *History of:*
        - Anxiety
        - Depression
        - Exhaustion
        - Poor concentration
        - Marital problems
        - Palpitations
        - Irritability
        - Sudden outbursts of anger
        - Alcohol abuse.
    - *Appears:*
        - Apathetic
        - Withdrawn.

Diagnosis

- Five groups of symptoms have been identified, although in the USA only three are recognised:
    - The traumatic event is repeatedly and persistently relived, with recurrent intrusive thoughts or images (flashbacks) of the event including vivid dreams and/or nightmares (Repetition syndrome).
    - Intense psychological distress at any exposure to events associated with or connected to the trauma.
    - Increased arousal or symptoms of anxiety, with disturbed sleep and difficulties with concentration, and an exaggerated startle reflex (excitability).
    - The patient's distress can only be reduced, and even so only temporarily, by attempting to block out thoughts about the experience or exposure to situations connected with the disaster (avoidance).
    - Loss of pleasure and enjoyment in usual activities including personal relationships, depressive symptomatology, suicidal thoughts, and a sense of estrangement from others who have not experienced the same trauma.

Management

- The treatment of PTSD is based on two principles:
    - The provision of support, preferably in groups, helps the patient to understand that he is not alone (the key is talking about and sharing the experience).
    - The prevention of avoidance behaviour, and encouragement and support for patients to face any situations about which they have become phobic.

Primary intervention

- Immediately following a disaster, victims may experience:
    - Confusion
    - Fear
    - Shock
    - Disorientation
    - Feelings of being overwhelmed
    - Anger.
- They have a basic need for:
    - Comfort
    - Reassurance:
        - Good communication conveying rapid accurate information about:
            - What has happened to their fellows
            - What has happened to them
            - What is still happening/going to happen, e.g. operations, discharge from hospital.
    - Protection
    - Security
        - Reuniting them with their natural group:
            - Friends, relatives, co-workers
- Early psychological intervention may have several advantages:
    - Personal experience of the disaster and its immediate aftermath may increase credibility (as may experience of similar disasters).
    - Allows the professional to be seen and regarded as part of the medical team, rather than as a distant and possibly threatening figure to whom the victim is referred later.
    - Assist in the forming of a special relationship (bonding) between victim and helper.
    - May facilitate psychological triage:
        - Identify those most at risk of developing problems later.

Secondary intervention

- This should be started once the basic threat to survival has ended and basic needs met.
- Should generally only be in response to symptoms.

Specific techniques

Individual or group counselling (possibly best):
- Eases the expression of feelings
- Helps in the understanding of reactions and methods of coping
- Informs the victims what they may expect of themselves
- Identifies specific problems and suggests realistic solutions
- Inspires hope for the future
- Allows identification of positive achievements and progress
- Must help the patient to take a realistic and unbiased view of what has happened to him and prevent him from seeing himself as a "permanent victim" for the rest of his life.

Desensitisation

Learning relaxation techniques

Psychotherapy

Tricyclic antidepressants (may also improve sleep quality and prevent nightmares)

Debriefing of rescuers/emergency services personnel

- The aim should be to:
    - Review the helper's role
    - Ease the expression of feelings
    - Explore particular problems and their solutions
    - Identify positive gains
    - Explore the consequences of disengagement
    - Identify those at risk.

Method
- Begin by reporting factual information.
- Then lead on to more delicate issues such as their psychological and emotional reactions following the incident.
- Debriefing should be conducted in a thoroughly professional manner, and should be considered a natural extension of the normal procedure following a disaster.
- Discussion should be encouraged to be as honest and open as possible, which will require a constructive and non judgemental attitude on the part of the group leader and other senior personnel.
- Debriefing will be most effective if sessions are organised in naturally occurring groups, which encourages comaraderie, rather than a group of individuals who have little in common.

Note:- Successful debriefing makes demands on the group leader; he/she should have:
    - Some personal knowledge of the specific disaster and its effects.
    - A knowledge of the psychological reaction to trauma and of group dynamics.

33

Organisation of immediate medical care

Organisation of immediate medical care

Liaison

- For any Immediate Care scheme to be effective, there must be good liaison with:
  - Ambulance Service
  - Police
  - Fire Service
  - Local A & E Departments
  - Other local immediate care schemes

Equipment

- The equipment used in or by a scheme depends on:
  - The funds available:
    - In general, equipment must give value for money, and when setting up a scheme it is best to provide relatively basic equipment initially, and then slowly add to it as the doctor's experience grows.
  - The equipment carried by the local Ambulance Service. It may be either:
    - Additional
    - Complementary
    - Should always be compatible.
  - The experience and training of the doctors involved.
  - The physical size of the doctor's car.
    - It should be realised that there is a limit as to how much can be squeezed into the average car boot, and some items which are bulky and be used only on rare occasions are probably best issued to the busier and more experienced doctors.
  - Although given to an individual doctor for his personal use, the equipment should continue to be the property of the scheme.
  - The actual choice of equipment is discussed in another section (see below).

Green beacons

The Law

- The relevant regulations are contained in "The Road Vehicles Lighting Regulations 1984, Statutory Instrument number 812", which state that:
    - Any vehicle being used by a Registered Medical Practitioner for the purposes of an emergency, may display one or more green lamps. Doctors who are not fully registered are excluded.
    - Each green lamp or warning beacon is a device capable of emitting a flashing or rotating beam of light throughout 360 degrees in the horizontal plane.
    - Only those people entitled to use a green beacon may in fact have one fitted to their vehicle, whether or not it is in working order.
    - Each beacon must be visible at a reasonable distance from the vehicle, be mounted not less than 1200 mm above the ground and must flash at a rate between 60 and 240 equal times per minute.
    - Although not specified in this legislation, no vehicle may use bulbs in their headlights or beacons exceeding 55 watts.

Twin tone horns/sirens

- At present there is no facility in law for doctors to use either twin tone horns or sirens, or for anybody to legally give them permission.
- Many doctors, however, use these devices with the unwritten "permission" of their local Chief Constable, on the understanding that if the privilege is ever abused, it would result in action being taken against them.

Identity cards

- It is advisable for all doctors to carry identity cards (obtainable from BASICS headquarters).
- The reasons for this are as follows:
    - The card identifies the holder as being a BASICS doctor. Especially at major incidents, there may be large numbers of doctors volunteering their services. These may include imposters and doctors inexperienced and untrained in Immediate Care. The police and ambulance services need to identify the genuine doctors who are going to be useful to them.
    - In addition, if there is any element of security risk, the police will only allow doctors who are either known to them or who have identification into the scene.
    - Ideally there will at some time in the near future be a register of all BASICS ID card holders, held at a central point which is contactable on a 24 hour basis for verification purposes.

Training

Introduction

- The value of proper training in Immediate Care should not be underestimated. Although it shares a lot of common ground with several other disciplines, especially anaesthetics, accident and emergency medicine, and orthopaedics, it really is a discipline in its own right and has some subject matter that is unique.
- Because it is such a practical subject, like many other branches of medicine, it is difficult to learn by theory alone. By its very nature, and unlike many other disciplines, there is usually little time for much thought and so those involved in Immediate Care have to learn to get it right automatically. Such automatism can only be developed by constant practice, and working to protocols.

Training on the job

- The best way to train for Immediate Care is to do it. However it is important to remember that every incident is unique, and should be treated as part of the learning process.

Follow up
- If possible every casualty, other than those with minor injuries, should be followed up in hospital to find out what their actual injuries were, and to try to evaluate the benefit of the Immediate Care that was given, and to see if anything else could have been done, or if it was, whether it might not have been done better or differently.

Debriefing
- If possible most incidents should be discussed afterwards in an honest constructive and critical way with the other members of the emergency team present, especially the ambulancemen, as this will help everyone understand each other's roles, and so improve the treatment for the one person who really counts: the patient. This must be tackled delicately initially, as it is very easy for one's motives to be misunderstood before good relationships are established.
- May act as a mutual counselling session following particularly horrific accidents/incidents.

Theoretical training

- The value of theoretical training should not be underestimated, although Immediate Care is such a practical subject. For the experienced doctor it may be particularly useful for describing recent advances in Immediate Care.

Practical training

- Practical training is particularly useful for procedures, such as intubation, intravenous cannulation, cricothyrotomy and insertion of chest drains, which may only be carried out infrequently on live patients, and where a special technique is necessary.
- It is also invaluable for practising Basic and Advanced Life Support including recognition of arrhythmias, defibrillation and administration of cardiac drugs, using mannikins.
- Any doctor who is issued with a defibrillator should be trained and certified in Advanced Cardiac Life Support.
- The value of joint training, especially the ambulance service and possibly the fire service (in extrication) should be not underestimated and will not only improve technical skills and the understanding of each other's roles, but will also help develop a team approach.

Hepatitis B/HIV disease

Introduction

- The prevalence of the HIV is growing rapidly in the UK, whilst that of Hepatitis B is relatively static, averaging about 1000 reported cases per year.
- So far, as is known, no member of the emergency services has been contaminated or infected with either virus in the course of their duties, but the potential for being infected is a very real one.

Pathophysiology

- Both the viruses responsible for Hepatitis B and HIV disease can be found in the body fluids of infected individuals, although so far only blood contamination has resulted in infection.
- Infection usually enters the body through a defect in the dermis, e.g. a scratch or minor laceration, or through the mucous membranes. Such minor injuries are often sustained by emergency services personnel at an incident site, from broken glass, sharp metal, etc.

Hepatitis B immunisation

- It is strongly recommended that all those involved in Immediate Care be vaccinated against Hepatitis B, and their status be checked at regular intervals (every 3-5 years).
- Vaccination is effective in preventing infection in individuals who produce antibodies. Ten to fifteen percent of those over 40 years of age do not respond, with a smaller proportion in younger people.
- The vaccination course consists of the initial dose, followed 1 month later by another, and a third 6 months after the first. The response to immunisation should be checked 2-4 months later, and a booster dose given if the individual has a low response.
- Non-responders should be considered for Hepatitis B immunoglobulin (HBIG) administration, if exposure takes place.

Protection

Prevention of contamination

- All those involved in Immediate Care should wear latex protective gloves, to protect themselves from contamination with infected blood.
- Many doctors, however, prefer not to wear gloves as they feel that it makes delicate manipulation of instruments difficult. In these circumstances it is advisable to wash the hands thoroughly after dealing with the incident, especially if there are any minor lacerations.
- All sharps should be put in a safety bin at the earliest opportunity. Most ambulance services equip their ambulances with these, and Immediate Care doctors are also advised to carry them.

Treatment of contamination

- There is no known treatment for contamination with blood containing the HIV other than washing the exposed areas with copious water and antiseptic solution.
- Those contaminated with blood thought to be contaminated by Hepatitis B should be given anti Hepatitis B immunoglobulin (HBIG), which provides passive immunity, immediately, together with immunisation, if they have not previously been immunised.

Tetanus immunisation

Introduction

- Tetanus is an acute disease, with an appreciable mortality. Tetanus spores are found in the soil and may be introduced into the body during injury, especially puncture wounds; but also through burns and trivial and often unnoticed scratches and abrasions.
- By the very nature of their work, everyone involved in Immediate Care is at risk of being infected.
- The staff of casualty units should be aware of the risk of tetanus contamination in any patients under their care and advise and treat them as necessary.

Guidelines for the administration of tetanus toxoid (TT) and adsorbed tetanus human immunoglobulin (TIG)

Immunisation status	Wound type	Recommendations
Unimmunised or incompletely immunised	Low risk	One dose of TT followed by complete immunisation (Second dose 4 weeks later; third dose at 4-6 months) *Note:* - In order to maintain satisfactory protection a reinforcing dose should be given 10 years after the initial dose and again 10 years later. - Reinforcing doses at less than 10 year intervals are *not recommended*, since they have been shown to be unnecessary and can result in considerable local reactions.
	Tetanus prone: When the wound/burn is neglected for more than 6 hours. If there is a puncture wound, evidence of sepsis, direct contact with soil, or there is a significant amount of devitalised tissue.	One dose of TT plus 250 u TIG (500 u if more than 24 hr since injury or there is a high risk of contamination) followed by a complete course of immunisation. The remaining two injections should be given at *monthly* intervals. *Note:* - Use separate syringes and limbs as sites of injection for TT & TIG.
Full first course + booster within preceding 10 years	Low risk	No vaccine necessary.
	Tetanus prone	If there is a high risk of tetanus, e.g. after contamination with manure: one dose of adsorbed vaccine.
	Neglected more than 24 hours	One dose TT plus 250-500 u TIG administered at a different site.
Last of 3 dose course *or* Booster more than 10 years previously	Low risk	One dose TT.
	Tetanus prone	One dose TT plus 250-500 u TIG administered at a different site.

Note:- In patients under 6 years of age, substitute DPT for TT.
- Patients with an impaired immunity may not respond to the vaccine and may require additional TIG.

Callout policy

Selective callout

- Doctors are only called out to incidents which have either been assessed by an ambulance crew at the scene, or when persons are known either to be trapped or seriously injured.

Advantages:
- Doctors are only called out when they are known to be needed.
- Extended trained ambulance persons/paramedics may be able to cope adequately on many occasions.

Disadvantages:
- In rural areas, it may take the ambulance a considerable time to get to the incident. Even if there are seriously injured patients, who need Immediate Care, it may not make sense for the ambulance to wait for a doctor, who may have to travel a similar distance to the ambulance, especially if the hospital is not that far away.
- There will nearly always be a delay before the doctor reaches the scene. It is now accepted that the earlier Immediate Care begins, the more effective it will be.
- Doctors may only be called out rarely, and gain little experience. "We are all only good at doing what we do often; and there is no substitute for repeated experience". A small number of callouts tends to lead to poor doctor morale and loss of enthusiasm, poor working relationships and poor discipline.

CONCLUSION: - The method of choice for urban areas, where both the ambulances, doctors and hospitals are near the incident, and little time is spent in transit.

Non-selective callout

- Doctors are routinely called to every incident regardless of the initial assessment, except for obvious trivia.

Advantages:
- Doctors reach the scene early, so that immediate treatment begins early.
- Doctors attend many incidents, and even if their presence may not be strictly necessary in a considerable percentage of calls, they gain considerable experience and expertise in Immediate Care.
- On some occasions doctors may save ambulance time by either deciding that a patient does not require treatment or in the case of casualties with minor injuries only, divert the ambulance to their surgery or local cottage hospital for treatment.
- Doctors also develop a close working relationship with the ambulance crews, so that when there is a major incident, they all work together as a team.
- A large number of sucessful callouts leads to good doctor morale and good discipline.
- Doctor callout becomes a routine for ambulance control, so time is not wasted deciding whether or not a doctor is required.

Disadvantages:
- On some occasions, the callout may be a waste of doctor time, although, even if their attendance is not strictly necessary, it is very seldom ever a complete waste of time.
- Doctor callout may take up ambulance control time, which can be at a premium.

CONCLUSION: - The callout method of choice for rural areas.

Limited selective callout

- This is when the control officer has a list of priorities and decides from the incoming information from the public, whether or not a doctor is required.
- It is really a variation of selective callout and suffers from the same disadvantages, as well as the fact that the initial information from the public is often innaccurate.
- It could however be developed using flow diagrams and carefully applied criteria to a very satisfactory callout system, especially for medical emergencies.

Commitment of doctors

Introduction

- Whether an Immediate Care Scheme uses an on call rota, a continuous on call commitment, or a mixture of the two, it will depend on the personal preferences of the participating doctors.

Rota
- The on call commitment is shared between several doctors, usually partners in the same practice.

Advantage:
- There is nearly always a doctor available in each area.

Disadvantages:
- No one doctor really gets enough experience to be good at Immediate Care, and it is rare to find that all doctors in a partnership are equally enthusiastic about practising Immediate Care.
- It is usually too expensive to equip all the doctors in one area to a high standard.

Continuous
- Every doctor is on call continuously, except when he is either out of the area, or not available for personal reasons.

Advantage:
- In each area there are one or two doctors who get a lot of experience, have high morale and discipline and can be equipped to a high standard.

Disadvantage:
- It can be a very considerable commitment for a doctor to be on call continuously, and can put a strain on personal and professional relationships.

CONCLUSION: - If possible a small number of highly committed and highly professional doctors who attend a relatively large number of incidents, is desirable to provide a professional service, but may be an unrealistic ideal in some areas.

Medico-legal aspects of immediate care

- At present the practice of Immediate Care is considered a normal part of hospital and general practice, and there have been no cases of doctors being sued for medical negligence. However, with an increasingly litigation minded population, the time may come when doctors are at risk of being sued.
- A registered medical practitioner is expected to provide "appropriate and prompt action upon evidence suggesting the existance of a condition requiring urgent medical intervention".
- GPs are expected as part of their terms of service to provide emergency treatment to any person who requires it within their practice area. A practitioner with special skills in resuscitation, who offers assistance, takes on a duty of care, and must exercise it within the constraints imposed by the prevailing circumstances.
- Having taken on the duty of care to a patient, a doctor is expected to provide a reasonable standard of treatment. "A doctor is not negligent, if he is acting in accordance with a practice accepted as proper by a responsible body of medical men skilled in that particular art, merely because there is a body of such opinion, that takes a contrary view".
- It is advisable for all doctors actively involved in Immediate Care to make sure that they are trained and competent in its practice. Training should include proper instruction, supervised practice and self audit.
- Records should be made and retained, as they would be for any other branch of medicine.
- It should be remembered that once he has seen a patient, that doctor becomes legally responsible for the medical management of that patient, until the patient is handed over into the care of another doctor. He may also be considered legally responsible for the actions of any ambulance persons present, who may be considered to be working under his direction as far as the actual medical management of the patient is concerned.

Notes

34

Immediate medical care equipment

Immediate medical care equipment

Introduction

- This is a very brief and basic list of the various types of equipment used in Immediate Care, together with some of the manufacturers. It is by no means exhaustive, and the omission of a product does not mean that it is not recommended.
- There may be positive advantages in using equipment from a common manufacturer, which may facilitate interchange of equipment or parts of equipment, e.g. ECG chest leads.
- It is easy to get carried away by new and increasingly complex equipment. The value of any new item of equipment is unproven, and there needs to be careful pre-hospital and hospital evaluation of its role in Immediate Care before purchase.
- If new equipment is introduced, then to be used effectively, there needs to be instruction in its use not only for the ambulance service, but also for Immediate Care doctors and possibly even the fire service, so that all the members of the team are familiar with its use and applications.

Key: * - Basic Equipment: suitable for most doctors.
       ** - More Advanced Equipment: more expensive and probably best reserved for doctors who are called out a lot and are more experienced.
        + - Not recommended.

Radio equipment

- Radiopagers:
    - Commercial:
        - Cellular
    - VHF
- Hand portables:
    - UHF:
        - Short range, only used for on-site communication
    - VHF:
        - Long range, but there may be problems with "shadowing"
    - Cellular.
- Car radios:
    - UHF:
        - usually only used as a relay
    - VHF with selective calling, status reporting, etc.
    - Cellular

Vehicle equipment

Green beacons

- Light source may be either:
    - Quartz Halogen bulb with:
        - Rotating reflector
        - Stroboscopic tube
        - * Single light:
        - ** Multiple lights
        - ** Bar light
- Mounting:
    - * Magnetic:
        - May fall off due to buffeting at high speeds
    - ** Permanent:
        - Bolt on.
        - Gutter mounting

Audible warning devices/sirens

- * Air operated (pneumatic):
    - Cheap, need maintaining
    - Not so loud
- ** Electronic:
    - Expensive, but very audible

Protective identifying clothing

- * Jackets which meet the BSI standard
- * Tabards
- ** Over trousers
- Boots
- Gloves:
    - * Latex
    - ** Rubber: debris gloves
- ** Goggles
- ** Fire-resistant suits (usually a "Proban" coated overall)
- ** Chemical-resistant suits (Germa Clothing Range)

Rescue equipment

- * Shears/scissors
- * SOS Rescue Device
- ** Seat belt cutter

Patient management equipment

Airway management devices

- * Oropharyngeal Airways:
    - Guedel
- Nasopharyngeal airways:
    - * Latex.
    - ** Linder balloon
- Oropharyngeal/Nasal airway: Dual Aid
- + Ventilation airways:
    - SALAD/Safar
    - Brook airway (basic and professional)
    - Vent Easy
    - Lifeway (Sussex)
- + Oesophageal airways:
    - Oesophageal Obturator airway
    - Oesophageal Gastric Tube airway
- ** Modified Oesophageal Airways:
    - Pharyngeal Tracheal Lumen Airway
    - Combi tube
    - Laryngeal Mask Airway
- Cricothyrotomy devices:
    - * Large intravenous cannula: 12-16 G
    - ** Minitrach II
    - ** Quicktrach
- **Small tracheostomy tube: 5
- * Endotracheal introducers:
    - Gum elastic bougie (facilitates intubation)
    - Malleable plastic introducer
- Suction:
    - * Hand operated
    - * Foot operated
    - ** Oxygen driven from ventilator
    - ** Electric/battery operated

Ventilation management devices

- * Mask: Pocket mask with oxygen inlet and valve
- * Bag and mask (preferably with an oxygen reservoir and additional paediatric mask)
- * Oxygen cylinder with multiflow ability and high concentration mask, plus recharging device
- ** Ventilators
- ** Chest drainage kits
- * Laryngoscopes:
    - Welch Allen Disposable
    - Penlon (plastic)
    - Plastic with interchangeable blades
    - Metal with adult and paediatric blades (may have bulb or fibre optic illumination)

Circulation care devices

- * Wide bore cannulae: 12, 14, 16 G
- ** With dilator for very rapid infusion
- ** Intraosseous needles
- * Giving sets
- ** IV Push - Pressure Infusor
- * Elbow splint: Armlok
- ** Wrist splint
- Tourniquet:
  - * For phlebotomy
  - ** For haemorrhage control
- * Fluid warmers:
  - Reusable hot pack
  - Infupack
- ** Pneumatic Anti Shock Garment: Gladiator
- * Hooks for drips:
  - Butchers
  - Magnetic

Splints for the management of fractures

- * Cervical spine:
  - Stifneck
  - Philadelphia
  - Necloc
  - Hines
  -+ Loxley
- * Femur: Traction splints:
  - Pneumatic (bicycle pump):
    - Donway splint
  - Spring tension:
    - Sager
  - Locked winder:
    - Conway Trac 3
  - Winder and ratchet:
    - Hare (latest versions as Conway)
- * Lower leg:
  - Box: adult and paediatric
  - Frac straps

Extrication devices **

- KED
- RED
- Fallon
- ED 2000
- XP1

Monitoring equipment

- - * Stethoscope
- - * Torch
- - * Sphygmomanometers:
  - - Aneroid
  - - Audio
- - ** Pulse oximeter
- - ** Multi measurement devices:
  - - Non invasive BP
  - - ECG
  - - Oximetry
  - - Temperature

Equipment for medical emergencies

- - ** Defibrillators
- - * Nebulisers
- - * Blood glucometers:
- - * Peak flow meter: Mini Wright

Equipment containers

- - Preferably lightweight.

Recording information/reporting

- - * BASICS report forms
- - * BASICS triage labels
- - ** Cameras: still, instant, polaroid

Miscellaneous equipment

- - Lights:
  - - * Flood/spotlight:
    - - Hand held:
    - - Magnetic
  - - ** Head light.
- - Space blankets:
  - - * Single use
  - - ** Heavy duty
- - Labels for equipment cases
- - Book: Dangerous Chemicals: a First Aid Guide

Drugs for immediate care

Cardiovascular system

Diuretics

- Frusemide: 10 mg/ml 2/5 ml amp.

Antiarrhythmic drugs

- Lignocaine: 100 mg/5 ml.
- Atropine: 1 mg/10 ml.
- Calcium chloride: 10 ml 10%.

Nitrates

- Glyceryl trinitrate spray.

Sympathomimetics

- Adrenaline: 10 ml 1:10,000.

Anti-coagulants

- Hepsal (should be stored in a refrigerator).

Antiplatelet drugs

- Aspirin 75, 300 mg.

Thrombolytics

- Anistreplase (should be stored in a refrigerator).

Intravenous infusion fluids

- Crystalloid:
    - Hartmann's solution
    - N-Saline
- Colloids:
    - Haemaccel
    - Gelofusine.
- Buffering solution:
    - Sodium bicarbonate: 50 ml 8.4%.

Respiratory system

Bronchodilators

- β_2 adrenergic agonists:
    - Salbutamol:
        - Nebules: 2.5/5 mg.
- Adrenoceptor stimulants:
    - Adrenaline: 1 ml 1:1000.
- Anticholinergic:
    - Ipratropium bromide:
        - Nebuliser solution: 0.25 %.
- Methylxanthene:
    - Aminophylline: 250 mg/10 ml.

Steroids

- Hydrocortisone: 100 mg.
- Prenisolone: tabs 5 mg.

Antihistamines

- Chlorpheniramine: injection 10 mg/ml.

Central nervous system

Analgesics

- Opiates:
    - Diamorphine (should be administered with an anti-emetic, e.g. metoclopramide)
    - Cyclimorph 15
    - Nalbuphine.
- Opiate antagonist: naloxone.
- Gases: nitrous oxide/oxygen.
- Non steroidal anti-inflammatory: diclofenac.

Anaesthetics/sedating agents

- Diazepam:
    - Intravenous injection: 5 mg/ml 2ml.
    - Rectal tubes: Stesolid: 2 mg, 4 mg/ml 2.5 ml.
- Midazolam: 10 mg/2 ml/5ml.
- Ketamine.

Infections

Penicillin
- Procaine penicillin injection.

Chloramphenicol

Endocrine system

- Diabetes, treatment of hypoglycaemia:
    - Glucose: 50 ml 50%.
    - Glucagon: 1 mg.

Obstetrics/gynaecology

Oxytocic

- Ergometrine: 500 µg/ml.

Skin disinfectant/cleanser

- Povidone iodine dry spray (Betadine)

Notes

Bibliography

Books: Title	Author	Publisher	Date
ABC of Antenatal Care	Chamberlain	British Medical Journal	1992
ABC of Diabetes: *Second Edition*	Watkins	British Medical Journal	1988
ABC of Major Trauma	Edited: Skinner	British Medical Journal	1991
ABC of Poisoning	Henry & Volans	British Medical Journal	1985
ABC of Resuscitation: *Second Edition*	Edited: Evans	British Medical Journal	1990
ABC of Spinal Cord Injury: *Second Edition*	Edited:Grundy et al	British Medical Journal	1993
Accidents and Emergencies in Children	Morton and Phillips	Oxford University Press	1992
Accident & Emergency Diagnosis & Management	Brown	Heinemann	1987
Accident & Emergency Medicine: *Second Edition*	Rutherford et al	Churchill Livingstone	1989
Accidents & Emergencies	Kirby	Castle House	1988
ACLS Manual		American Heart Assoc	1989
Advanced Life Support Manual	Edited: Handley	Resuscitation (UK)	1993
Advanced Trauma Life Support Course		American Coll of Surg	1988
Basic Rescue and Emergency Care		American Academy of Orthopaedic Surgeons	1990
Burns: The First Five Days	Settle	Smith & Nephew	1986
British National Formulary *Number 25 (March 1993)*		British Medical Assoc & Pharmaceutical Soc of GB	1992
Cardiopulmonary Cerebral Resuscitation	Safar & Bircher	Saunders	1988
Cardiopulmonary Resuscitation	Skinner & Vincent	Oxford University Press	1993
Care of the Acutely Ill & Injured	Edited: Wilson & Marsden	John Wiley	1989
Clinical Forensic Medicine	Edited: McLay	Pinter	1990
Common Obstetric Emergencies	Gibb	Butterworth Heineman	1991
Current Emergency Diagnosis & Treatment	Edited: Ho and Saunders	Appleton & Lange	1990
Dangerous Chemicals: A First Aid Guide: *Second Edition*	Edited: Houston	Wolters Samson	1986
Disasters	Walsh	Edward Arnold	1989
The ECG Made Easy: *Second Edition*	Hampton	Churchill Livingstone	1992
The ECG in Practice: *Second Edition*	Hampton	Churchill Livingstone	1992
Emergency Care and Transportation of the Sick and Injured: *Fifth Edition*	Edited: Heckman	American Academy of Orthopaedic Surgeons	1992
Emergencies in General Practice	Moulds, Martin & Bouchier Hayes	MTP Press	1985
Emergencies in the Home	Various	British Medical Journal	1990
Emergency Care in the Streets: *Fourth Edition*	Caroline	Little Brown & Co	1991
Guide to Major Incident Planning	Edited: Hines & Robertson	BASICS	1986

Guide to the Misuse of Drugs Act 1971 and the Misuse of Drugs Regulations		Department of Health	1989
Haemaccel Lecture Series: Vols 1 & 2	Various	Hoechst	1987
Immediate Care	Zorab & Baskett	Saunders	1978
Immunisation against Infectious Diseases *1992 Edition*	Dept of Health	HMSO	1992
Lecture Notes on Accident & Emergency Medicine	Yates & Redmond	Blackwell	1985
The Management of Acute Pain	Park and Fulton	Oxford University Press	1992
The Management of Major Trauma	Robertson & Redmond	Oxford University Press	1991
The Management of Wounds and Burns	Wardrope & Smith	Oxford University Press	1992
Medical Aid at Accidents	Snook	Update	1977
Medicine for Disasters	Edited: Baskett & Weller	John Wright	1988
Obstetric Emergencies	Edited: Benrubi	Churchill Livingstone	1990
Pre-Hospital Trauma Life Support: *Second Edition*	Prehospital TLS	Committee of the National Association of EMTs	1990
Rescue Emergency Care	Edited: Easton	Heinemann	1977
Resuscitation Handbook: *Second Edition*	Baskett	Lippincott/Gower	1993
Resuscitation of the Newborn pts 1&2	Royal Colleges		1989
Royal Free Coronary Care Protocol Book		Sponsored by Hoechst	1989
RTA: Persons Trapped	Watson	Greenwade	1991
Simpsons Forensic Medicine: *Tenth Edition*	Knight	Edward Arnold	1991
Trauma: Pathogenesis & Treatment	Edited: Westaby	Heinemann	1989
Yearbooks of Emergency Medicine	Wagner	Year Book Medical Pub.	1990/91/92

Journals

Archives of Accident & Emergency Medicine
The British Journal of Accident and Emergency Surgery
The British Medical Journal
Care of the Critically Ill
Injury: The British Journal of Accident Surgery
Journal of the British Association for Immediate Care
Resuscitation: Journal of the European Resuscitation Council

Monographs

Monographs of the British Association for Immediate Care:
    1 Chest Injuries *Second Edition*
    2 Pain Relief
    3 Rescue From Remote Places I
    4 Rescue From Remote Places II *Second Edition*
    5 Entrapment in Road Traffic Accidents
    6 Head Injury

The above list is is by no means exhaustive, but reading most of the above should give the reader a very good grounding in the ever developing art and science of Immediate Care.

Index

Notes